Fostering
Emotional Well-Being
in the Classroom

# Fostering
# Emotional Well-Being
# in the Classroom
### Third Edition

Randy M. Page     Tana S. Page
*Brigham Young University*

**JONES AND BARTLETT PUBLISHERS**
*Sudbury, Massachusetts*
BOSTON     TORONTO     LONDON     SINGAPORE

*World Headquarters*
Jones and Bartlett Publishers
40 Tall Pine Drive
Sudbury, MA 01776
978-443-5000
info@jbpub.com
http://health.jbpub.com

Jones and Bartlett Publishers Canada
2406 Nikanna Road
Mississauga, ON L5C 2W6
CANADA

Jones and Bartlett Publishers International
Barb House, Barb Mews
London W6 7PA
UK

**Production Credits**
Acquisitions Editor: Kristin L. Ellis
Production Editor: Julie C. Bolduc
Editorial Assistant: Nicole Quinn
Senior Marketing Manager: Nathan Schultz
Assistant Marketing Manager: Ed McKenna
Manufacturing Buyer: Therese Bräuer
Cover Design: Philip Regan
Printing and Binding: Malloy Lithographing, Inc.
Cover Printing: Malloy Lithographing, Inc.

Cover photos:
    (l) © Eyewire; (c) © Digital Vision; (r) © Eyewire

Chapter-opening drawings by the following students:
    Chapter 1, Lindsay Mayburry
    Chapter 2, Jennifer Peterson
    Chapter 3, Ashleigh Hebert
    Chapter 4, Casey Taylor
    Chapter 5, Beau Mosman
    Chapter 6, Nathaniel Page
    Chapter 7, Beau Mosman
    Chapter 8, Jamie Patten
    Chapter 9, Andrea Reese

Interior photos:
    p. 20, Michael Newman/PhotoEdit; p. 22, Mary Kate Denny/PhotoEdit; p. 117, Richard Hutchings/PhotoEdit; p. 165, David Young-Wolff/PhotoEdit; p. 179, Geostock/Getty; p. 319, SW Productions/Getty; p. 338, Cleo Freelance Photo, The Picture Cube

**Library of Congress Cataloging-in-Publication Data**
Page, Randy M.
    Fostering emotional well-being in the classroom / Randy M. Page, Tana S. Page.
      p. cm.
Includes bibliographical references and index.
    ISBN 0-7637-0055-X (alk. paper)
1. Students—Mental health. 2. Mental health promotion. 3. Self-esteem in children.
4. Self-esteem in adolescence. 5. Classroom environment. I. Page, Tana S. II. Title.
    LB3430 .P34 2002
    371.4′04—dc21
                                                    2002151294

Printed in the United States of America
06 05 04 03 02   10 9 8 7 6 5 4 3 2 1

# Contents

# Preface

This third edition of *Fostering Emotional Well-Being in the Classroom* is designed to help you as prospective teachers, current teachers, and parents to make a positive impact on the lives of young people. This edition specifically provides up-to-date and comprehensive coverage of the critical issues affecting the well-being of today's youth. It is a valuable resource for parents and for teachers of all disciplines at both the elementary and secondary level. It is an excellent text for courses in school health, health education methods, child and adolescent health, emotional health and development, child and family development, youth at risk, and classroom management and discipline.

The chapters in this edition have been rearranged so that Chapter 1 outlines the underlying principles that form the basis of an emotionally healthy classroom. These principles are often overlooked in teacher education courses. This chapter stresses that emotional climate is critical to optimal student learning and growth. Chapter 1 puts first things first by giving you specific guidance in how to create an emotionally healthy climate in your classroom, school, and home.

Chapter 2 presents the skills that help young people live happy and productive lives. These skills help young people avoid many situations that place them at risk of injury or poor health status. It is essential that curricula addressing stress, nutrition, sex, drugs, violence, and suicide help young people develop these skills. We have placed these skills in the front of the book so that you are familiar with them as you study the content chapters that follow. Chapter 2 also contains many activities that will help you teach these critical skills to students. These activities can be adapted to fit into lesson plans addressing many different health and well-being topics. For example, you can use many of the self-esteem and self-worth activities in teaching topics such as stress, nutrition, sex education, drug abuse prevention, or violence prevention.

Media literacy information in this third edition has been updated and expanded. Chapter 2 now contains sections on media exposure, limiting media exposure, evaluating media messages, the world of advertising, targeting kids, school-based advertising and marketing, online kids, and online safety tips. We have also added new sections on media in Chapters 3 through 7.

Chapters 3 through 9 have been updated, and this edition addresses several new issues and topics, including new information on working with children with special needs and chronic health conditions; controversies regarding attention deficit hyperactivity disorder; asset development; relationship building; decision making; community and world stressors; sleep deprivation; overscheduling; teacher burnout; the epidemic of obesity; type 2 diabetes; junk food in schools; new dietary guidelines; the *Surgeon General's Call to Action to Promote Sexual Health and Responsible Sexual Behavior*; teaching activities for sex education; emotional consequences of promiscuity; substance abuse trends and prevention programs that work; Al-Anon and Alateen; the surgeon general's report on youth violence; bullying in schools; Megan's Law; depressive disorders; assisting depressed youth; and self-injury.

This text exposes you to a myriad of potential problems and issues facing today's school-age youth. Examining these problems can leave one feeling overwhelmed at the prospect of meeting so many needs. As this text addresses these problems and issues, we hope it empowers and inspires you by giving you the specific tools and skills that help you make a difference in the lives of young people.

# Acknowledgments

We are very grateful for all of those who helped bring about this third edition of *Fostering Emotional Well-Being in the Classroom*. Kris Ellis at Jones and Bartlett was a great source of support and guidance. Julie Bolduc, our Production Editor, was meticulous in her care of the manuscript. We recognize that the talents and efforts of Kris and Julie greatly enhanced the quality of this book. Two budding artists, Beau Mosman and Jamie Patten, provided new artwork for Chapters 5, 7, and 8. The comments and suggestions of students and reviewers, past and present, helped facilitate many changes in this edition.

Diane Davis
   Bowie State University
Brian Geiger
   University of Alabama—Birmingham
Steven Godin
   East Stroudsburg University
Marsha Greer
   California State University—San Bernardino
Melissa Hedstrom
   Western Oregon University
Linda L. Hendrixson
   East Stroudsburg University
Tammy James
   West Chester University
Jeanette Tedesco
   Western Connecticut State University
Karen Vail-Smith
   East Carolina University
David M. White
   East Carolina University

Once again, we thank our terrific children—Michaelene, Nate, Emily, and Chris—who inspire us, teach us, and help make each day a joy. Thanks for your patience, support, and willingness to spend countless hours discussing with us the content in this book.

# CREATING AN EMOTIONALLY HEALTHY CLASSROOM

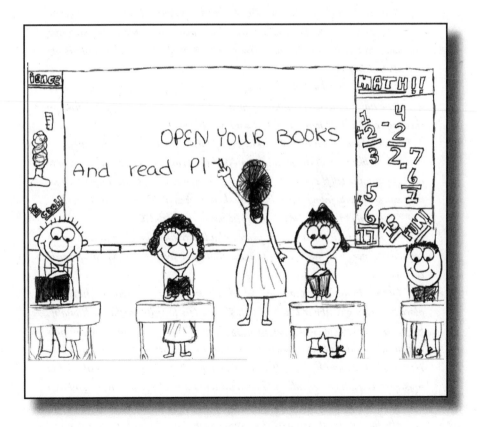

# *Cipher in the Snow*

*It started with tragedy on a biting cold February morning. I was driving behind the Milford Corners Bus as I did most snowy mornings on my way to school. It veered and stopped short at the hotel, which it had no business doing, and I was annoyed as I had to come to an unexpected stop. A boy lurched out of the bus, reeled, stumbled, and collapsed on the snowbank at the curb. The bus driver and I reached him at the same moment. His thin, hollow face was white, even against the snow.*

*"He's dead," the driver whispered.*

*It didn't register for a minute. I glanced quickly at the scared young faces staring down at us from the school bus. "A doctor! Quick! I'll phone from the hotel..."*

*"No use. I tell you he's dead." The driver looked down at the boy's still form. "He never even said he felt bad," he muttered, "just tapped me on the shoulder and said, real quiet, 'I'm sorry, I have to get off at the hotel.' That's all. Polite and apologizing like."*

*At school, the giggling, shuffling morning noise quieted as the news went down the halls. I passed a huddle of girls. "Who was it? Who dropped dead on the way to school?" I heard one of them half-whisper.*

*"Don't know his name; some kid from Milford Corners," was the reply.*

*It was like that in the faculty room and the principal's office. "I'd appreciate your going out to tell the parents," the principal told me. "They haven't a phone and, anyway, somebody from school should go there in person. I'll cover your classes."*

*"Why me?" I asked. "Wouldn't it be better if you did it?"*

*"I didn't know the boy," the principal admitted levelly. "And in last year's sophomore personalities column I note that you were listed as his favorite teacher."*

*I drove through the snow and cold down the bad canyon road to the Evans place and thought about the boy, Cliff Evans. His <u>favorite teacher!</u> I thought. <u>He hasn't spoken two words to me in two years!</u> I could see him in my mind's eye all right, sitting back there in the last seat in my afternoon literature class. He came in the room by himself and left by himself. "Cliff Evans," I muttered to myself, "a boy who never talked." I thought a minute. "A boy who never smiled. I never saw him smile once."*

*The big ranch kitchen was clean and warm. I blurted out my news somehow. Mrs. Evans reached blindly toward a chair. "He never said anything about bein' ailin'."*

His step-father snorted. "He ain't said nothin' about anything since I moved in here."

Mrs. Evans pushed a pan to the back of the stove and began to untie her apron. "Now hold on," her husband snapped. "I got to have breakfast before I go to town. Nothin' we can do now anyway. If Cliff hadn't been so dumb he'd have told us he didn't feel good."

After school I sat in the office and stared bleakly at the records spread out before me. I was to close the file and write the obituary for the school paper. The almost bare sheets mocked the effort. Cliff Evans, white, never legally adopted by step-father, five young half-brothers and sisters. These meager strands of information and the list of D grades were all the records had to offer.

Cliff Evans had silently come in the school door in the mornings and gone out the school door in the evenings, and that was all. He had never belonged to a club. He had never played on a team. He had never held an office. As far as I could tell he had never done one happy, noisy kid thing. He had never been anybody at all.

How do you go about making a boy into a zero? The grade school records showed me. The first- and second-grade teachers' annotations read "sweet, shy child", "timid but eager." Then the third-grade note had opened the attack. Some teacher had written in a good, firm hand, "Cliff won't talk. Uncooperative. Slow learner." The other academic sheep had followed with "dull"; "slow-witted"; "low I.Q." They became correct. The boy's I.Q. score in the ninth grade was listed at 83. But his I.Q. in the third grade had been 106. The score didn't go under 100 until the seventh grade. Even shy, timid, sweet children have resilience. It takes time to break them.

I stomped to the typewriter and wrote a savage report pointing out what education had done to Cliff Evans. I slapped a copy on the principal's desk and another in the sad, dog-eared file. I banged the typewriter and slammed the file and crashed the door shut, but I didn't feel much better. A little boy kept walking after me, a little boy with a peaked, pale face; a skinny body in faded jeans; and big eyes that had looked and searched for a long time and then had become veiled.

I could guess how many times he'd been chosen last to play sides in a game, how many whispered child conversations had excluded him, how many times he hadn't been asked. I could see and hear the faces and voices that said over and over, "You're dumb. You're a nothing, Cliff Evans."

A child is a believing creature. Cliff undoubtedly believed them. Suddenly it seemed clear to me: When finally there was nothing left at all for Cliff Evans, he collapsed on a snowbank and went away. The doctor might list "heart failure" as the cause of death, but that wouldn't change my mind.

*We couldn't find ten students in the school who had known Cliff well enough to attend the funeral as his friends. So the student body officers and a committee from the junior class went as a group to the church, being politely sad. I attended the services with them, and sat through it with a lump of cold lead in my chest and a big resolve growing through me.*

*I've never forgotten Cliff Evans nor that resolve. He has been my challenge year after year, class after class. I look up and down the rows carefully each September at the unfamiliar faces. I look for veiled eyes or bodies scrounged into a seat in an alien world. "Look, kids," I say silently. "I may not do anything else for you this year, but not one of you is going to come out of here a nobody. I'll work or fight to the bitter end doing battle with society and the school board, but I won't have one of you coming out of here thinking himself into a zero."*

*Most of the time—not always, but most of the time—I've succeeded.*

Source: Written by J. E. Mizer, "Cipher in the Snow," *NEA Journal*, 50: 8–10, 1964. Reprinted with permission. A movie of this story also exists and has the same title.

Consider the fact that between the ages of 6 and 17, children spend more time with their teachers than with their parents. The potential for having a positive influence upon students is great, as is the need. Although it is an unrealistic expectation to succeed in helping every "Cliff Evans" (see "Cipher in the Snow") feel better about himself or herself, there are countless young people who have been, and are yet to be, touched by a special teacher who makes a big difference in their lives. The purpose of this chapter is to give you information and insights into how to create an emotionally healthy climate in your classroom—how to become a teacher who makes a difference.

## Circle of Influence

Have you ever stopped to think about your circle of influence? To better understand the concept, do the following activity. Use a sheet of paper and draw a large circle on it (or, if you want, create a circle in your imagination). Label the circle as **circle of concern.** Inside the circle write everything you are concerned about—from world peace to what you are going to eat for your next meal. Your circle might contain items such as these: kids living in dysfunctional situations, teen pregnancy, hatred, violence, bigotry, drug abuse, poverty, apathy, conflicts with roommates or family members, car problems, money for next semester, lack of parking on campus, an egotistical professor, a family member's health, obtaining a meaningful position within your career, paying bills, meeting deadlines, lack of time, or finding a soul mate. You will find that you can probably easily fill the entire circle with your specific concerns.

Next, draw a smaller circle within this large circle. Label this as your **circle of influence.** This smaller circle represents what you have control over—what you can influence. Now, think about the items within your circle of influence and ask yourself the following questions: Which of these concerns can you personally influence? Which items belong in the circle of influence and which belong in the outer circle of concern? Finally, and most importantly, ask yourself, "Where do I put *most* of my efforts, thoughts, and actions? Are they within my circle of influence or within my circle of concern?"

**Proactive people** (see Chapter 2) focus their thoughts and activities inside their circle of influence. They spend their time and energy on things they can do something about, and as a result their circle of influence grows over time. **Reactive people,** on the other hand, spend most of their time in their circle of concern. They focus on the weakness of other people, problems in their environment, and circumstances over which they have no control. Their focus creates blaming and accusing attitudes as well as feelings of victimization. Focusing on one's circle of concern causes one's circle of influence to shrink for lack of attention.[1]

Teachers often deeply feel the effects of social problems on a very personal level. Within their own classrooms they witness the devastating effects of dysfunctional homes, poverty, drugs, violence, teen pregnancy, and other problems affecting our communities and society. Because teachers care about people, they are prone to have very large circles of concern. However, focusing more on one's circle of concern rather than on the inner circle of influence can create feelings of being overwhelmed, disempowered, and "burned out." Novice teachers are especially susceptible to becoming fixated upon their circle of concern as they begin dealing with students and their problems.

Spanish Harlem (New York City) junior high teacher Bill Hall provides an excellent example of how one teacher made a positive difference in the lives of his students by being circle-of-influence focused.[2] It would have been easy for Bill to fall into the trap of being circle-of-concern focused. He taught in a neighborhood where infant mortality rates were high, the average male life expectancy was even less than in Bangladesh, and where language and a few walls separated the stark contrast of poverty and affluence. Rather than focusing on these conditions, Bill placed his energy on what he could do, his circle of influence. Bill organized an after-school chess club to help students better learn English. Many of his students had recently arrived from Central and South America, Pakistan, and Hong Kong and could speak only minimal English. This chess club became know as the Royal Knights of Harlem.

The members of the club not only learned English, but grew in confidence as they came to see themselves through Bill's eyes. Their schoolwork improved as they become more proficient at chess. In its first year the club finished third at the state finals in Syracuse, becoming eligible for the junior high school finals in California. Bill raised funds to fly the team to California, where they finished seventeenth out of 109 teams in the national competition. Then his team met a girl from the Soviet Union who was the Women's World Champion. The team reasoned that if this girl could come all the way from Russia, why couldn't they go there? The team traveled to Russia with the corporate help of sponsors, particularly Pepsi-Cola. There the Royal Knights of Harlem won about half of their matches and uncovered a homegrown advantage in the special event of speed chess. Remember, these were not chess protégés, but rather students who were selected for their need to learn English.

Bill never dreamed that all of this would happen within a few short years of starting the chess club. Nor did he foresee the day that his junior high auditorium would be chosen by a Soviet dance troupe as the site of a New York performance because of his chess club's tour in Russia. But, all of this did happen because Bill chose to be circle-of-influence focused. As time passed, his circle of influence naturally grew. When the Royal Knights were asked by one interviewer what they were doing before Bill Hall and chess playing had come into their lives, one boy said, "Hanging out in the street and feeling like shit." "Taking lunch money from younger kids and a few drugs now and then," admitted another. "Just laying on my bed, reading comics, and getting yelled at by my father for being lazy," said a third. When asked if there was anything in their schoolbooks that made a difference, one explained to the agreement of all, "Not until Mr. Hall thought we were smart and then we were" (pg. 139).[2]

They *were* smart and Bill Hall helped them discover their potential. Others too came to realize it. Just before graduating from junior high, these Royal Knight members received numerous offers from high schools to join their "gifted" student programs. One private school from California even provided a full-ride scholarship. At the time of junior high graduation, club members were convinced they could do anything and had career aspirations of law, accounting, teaching, and computer science.

It is common for we educators to wish that we could take our students out of less than ideal circumstances. But this is rarely possible. Bill Hall made a difference by working within his circle of influence—by showing his students that they had the power within them to rise above their circumstances. We can all expand our ability to influence, and thus make a difference, by focusing on what we can do—not on what others should be doing.

Education is all about influencing others. Figure 1-1 depicts our **pyramid of influence** as teachers. It is interesting to note that even though most of our course work in preparation for entering the teaching profession centers on the tip of the pyramid, it is the least influential area. We spend a great deal of energy learning how to write effective objectives and lesson plans, prepare materials, present information, and evaluate student learning. These are vitally important skills for educators. More vital and

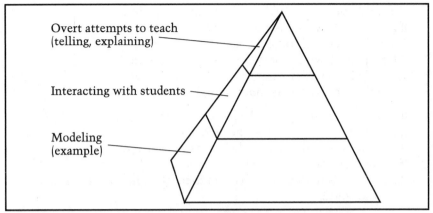

Overt attempts to teach
(telling, explaining)

Interacting with students

Modeling
(example)

Source: Adapted from S. R. Covey, *Principle Centered Leadership*. New York: Fireside, 1990, pg. 120.

**FIGURE 1-1    A teacher's pyramid of influence**

perhaps overlooked are the larger two areas of the pyramid. The foundation for influencing others is modeling, that is, being an example of what we are trying to teach. This includes the obvious, such as a teacher reading while having students do silent sustained reading or being a nonsmoker while discussing the harmful effects of tobacco. It also includes less obvious and, unfortunately, sometimes negative acts such as modeling dislike for things or people. The large midsection of the pyramid of influence deals with interacting with or relating to students. Our ability to influence here is exemplified by the saying "I don't care how much you know until I know how much you care." We will now take a closer look at modeling and interacting.

## Modeling a Healthy Personality

The importance of modeling healthy personality characteristics and emotional health skills cannot be overemphasized. Modeling is a major means by which skills are taught and learned. Observing how others act provides a pattern for youth to follow when in similar circumstances. Next to parents, educators, whose behavior patterns are watched and imitated, are often the most influential adults in a young person's life. Students often learn more from what we do than what we say. The way an educator reacts to frustration or stress can make a lasting impression on a young person. Both displays of positive coping skills as well as negative responses have modeling effects. Therefore, educators must give serious attention to their emotional health and to their own practices and skills. Consider the following poem, adapted from Dorothy Law Nolte.

If a child lives with criticism, he learns to condemn.
If a child lives with hostility, he learns to fight.
If a child lives with ridicule, he learns to be shy.
If a child lives with shame, he learns to feel guilty.
If a child lives with tolerance, he learns to be patient.
If a child lives with encouragement, he learns confidence.

If a child lives with praise, he learns to appreciate.
If a child lives with fairness, he learns justice.
If a child lives with security, he learns to have faith.
If a child lives with approval, he learns to like himself.
If a child lives with acceptance and friendship, he learns to find love
   in the world.

Because school-age children and adolescents spend more time in the classroom than in any place other than the home, it is wise for you as an educator to evaluate your own emotional health and discern what behaviors you are modeling, what you are teaching your students. Do you model the attributes of an emotionally healthy personality? Do you exemplify emotional intelligence, proactivity, problem solving, goal setting, interpersonal relationships, self-worth, and other skills for emotional well-being? Reviewing the characteristics of effective teachers in Box 1-1 and completing the Emotional Health Inventory in Box 1-2 will help you assess the emotional health traits you exemplify in the classroom.

---

IN THE
CLASSROOM

*1–1*

## Characteristics of Effective Teachers

Effective teachers:

◆ Are deeply interested in the students and in the material being taught
◆ Frequently conduct class discussions and do not lecture very much
◆ Relate to students on their level, do not talk down to them, and make students feel comfortable about talking with them
◆ Inject humor, variety, and drama into lessons
◆ Make course work relevant, meaningful, and important to students
◆ Are fair
◆ Are open
◆ Are adaptable to change
◆ Have high behavioral and academic expectations for students

## Emotional Health Inventory

How is your emotional health? Review the following questions to see how you stand and in what ways you can improve.

1. Are you realistic in your view of self and others? Do you feel equal to others as a person, neither superior nor inferior, irrespective of differences in specific abilities, family backgrounds, or attitudes of others toward you? Do you have a sense of security in your life?
2. Can you accept praise without the pretense of false modesty ("Well, anyone could have done it") and compliments without feeling guilty ("Thanks, but I really don't deserve it")?
3. Do you have a good sense of humor? Can you laugh at yourself?
4. Do you have values and principles that you live by and are willing to defend? Do you feel secure enough to modify your beliefs if new experience and evidence suggest that they are in error?
5. Are you concerned with problems outside of yourself? Do you extend yourself to help solve these problems?
6. Are you proactive, taking responsibility for your own life rather than blaming your behavior on circumstances, conditions, or conditioning?
7. Are you able to feel and appropriately express a wide range of emotions (anger, love, resentment, acceptance, sadness, happiness)?
8. Can you receive and give love and affection, recognizing that love is also a verb?
9. Are you able to sense others' feelings? Are you sensitive to the needs of others, to accepting social customs, and to avoiding prejudices?
10. Are you able to control your impulses and delay gratification?
11. Are you able to appropriately calm yourself when feeling anxious, frustrated, or angry?
12. Do you use an assertive communication style as well as good listening skills?
13. Do you set and accomplish goals with a zest for living?
14. Are you able to solve problems as they arise in life? Do you retain confidence in your ability to deal with problems, even in the face of failures and setbacks?

## Interacting with Students

How we interact with students affects the degree of our influence in and out of the classroom. Frank O'Malley, an English professor at Notre Dame for four decades, was a teacher who made a difference in the lives of his students. He taught reading, writing—and caring. At the beginning of each semester he would memorize each student's name and have everyone submit a brief autobiography so that he could understand them better. He focused on the fact that as a teacher he was assisting the growth of unique minds and spirits. He read each paper closely and covered each with red-inked comments of both criticism and praise. He taught his students to exceed their own expectations under his prodding. He gave them a vision of great literature, but also a vision of how they could excel.[3]

We need more Frank O'Malleys in education today, teachers who know and care for each of their students (not just the standouts), teachers who set high behavior and academic standards for all their students and who take the time and energy to help students achieve that higher expectation. As William Glasser said, "When you study great teachers . . . you will learn much more from their caring and hard work than from their style" (pg. 38).[4]

While serving as Secretary of Education, William Bennett took the sound advice of his wife and visited on a weekly basis schools that had been identified as exemplary. These schools were located in all sorts of settings, including many from poorly funded inner cities. Bennett visited these schools for the purpose of finding out why they were successful. Two children at Garrison Elementary School in the South Bronx seemed to sum up Bennett's findings for what makes for a successful school when they told him they went to "America's greatest school" because "there's no messin' around, no foolin' around, and everybody loves you" (pg. 75).[5]

Teachers that make a difference interact with students in ways that create high academic expectations, high behavioral expectations, and a feeling of love, belonging, and community. We will now look at interacting with students in terms of expectations, discipline, dealing with put-downs, and sensitivity to multicultural diversity.

## Expectations

Expectations can lead people to form negative or positive self-fulfilling prophecies. **Self-fulfilling prophecies** are expectations about future behavior and performance that emanate from labels and self-image. Children that are labeled "dumb" are likely to live up to that expectation, just as children labeled "bright" are likely to prove that prophecy correct. Labels and expectations for new students can be formulated by a teacher even before the beginning of an academic year. A label can form in a teacher's mind through discussions with previous teachers, school administrators, students, or parents. The reputations that older siblings establish in school get passed on to younger brothers and sisters. School records of performance and teachers' impressions are also sources of predetermined labels. Cliff Evans, in the story at the beginning of this chapter, is an example of the tragic effect negative labels and expectations can have.

Rosenthal and Jacobson conducted some of the early work relating teacher expectations to student performance and behavior in school.[6] Students in an elementary school were given the "Test for Intellectual Blooming." In each of the classes, an average of 20% of the children were identified as having test scores that suggested they would show unusual academic gains during the school year. The identified children had actually been picked at random from the total population taking the test. Eight months later all the children in the school were retested. Those children whom the teachers expected to show greater intellectual growth had significantly higher scores than other children in the school. This resulted, apparently, from the teachers interacting more positively and favorably with the "brighter" children.

Although Rosenthal's original expectancy research has been criticized for shortcomings in design and methodology, none of the criticisms have denied that teacher expectations have a significant influence on student performance, a fact supported by many subsequent studies. Hamachek cites studies which demonstrate that teachers tend to expect, and therefore get, the same performance from younger siblings that they had come to expect from older brothers and sisters.[7] Hamachek also reviews how children whose IQs have been overestimated by teachers showed higher reading achievement. This was especially true of first-grade teachers who expected the girls to outperform the boys. Teachers who did not have this expectation found no significant difference between the sexes in aptitude for learning to read.

Physical attractiveness also influences teacher expectations and interactions. Teachers are more likely to interact with and respond more positively to attractive children. Some research studies show that even the academic grades assigned to students are influenced by the attractiveness of the students. Dobson describes a study involving a group of adults who were shown photographs of children and asked to select the child most likely to have created a classroom disturbance or act of misconduct.[8] Unattractive children were much more likely to be selected as offenders than attractive children. Likewise, unattractive children were perceived as more dishonest than their attractive classmates. Dobson describes another study which demonstrated that the way adults handle discipline problems often varies in accordance to the attractiveness of the child. Misbehavior was more likely to be treated in a more permissive manner when a "cute" child was involved. Conversely, "ugly" classmates were more likely to receive harsh or severe disciplinary action.

Physical attractiveness also affects how students interact with each other. These interactions, in turn, contribute to the emotional climate of the classroom. Early in life children learn the high value that society places on beauty. Popular children's stories (e.g., *The Ugly Duckling, Sleeping Beauty, Rudolph the Red-Nosed Reindeer, Dumbo the Elephant, Snow White and the Seven Dwarfs,* and *Cinderella*) reinforce this value.

Unattractive children are often mocked and teased by other children. During adolescence—a period of rapid changes in body appearance, form, and size—youth often become fixated on physical appearance. They want to look like the media images of firm, sleek, beautiful bodies displayed everywhere. This is a time when peer perceptions become dominant, when expectations for conformity are intense, and deviations are not easily tolerated.

Teachers must be careful with the nonverbal messages they send to their students concerning the students' competence and lovableness. First, teachers have to be honest with themselves about any negative feelings or expectations they have. Although you would never dream of telling a student he or she is "dumb" or "ugly," these perceptions can be communicated nonverbally without your even knowing it. Communication experts tell us that more than half of what we communicate is conveyed by our body posture and facial expressions, and that the tone of voice is by far the most important part of our verbal message.

As a teacher, you should take a hard look at the expectations you have for your students. Strive to remove negative labels that have been established by previous teachers, experiences, or older siblings, and try to replace negative expectations with positive ones. It is critical to realize that many children in our school systems have rarely or never been viewed in a positive light by a significant adult. The likelihood of positive performance in children increases as they feel warmth from others and believe that they are regarded as capable.

## Discipline

Erroneously, discipline is often thought to be synonymous with punishment. The true purpose of **discipline,** however, is the training of self-control. Feeling in control helps children develop positive self-esteem. Students best learn self-control from people who exemplify it. Therefore, the key to positive and effective discipline lies in the character of the teacher. Disciplinary efforts tend to be unfair and ineffective when teachers display angry or harsh behavior. Teachers with few controls, who do not enforce classroom rules, nurture unpleasant and unruly environments. Successful teachers demonstrate warm, friendly attitudes toward students, have an air of self-assurance that demands respect, and have well-defined behavioral expectations of their students. Such teachers have classroom environments wherein students are comfortable and ready to learn.

*Teacher Behavior*   We usually think of discipline in terms of student conduct. Before addressing student behavior, please carefully review the Ten Commandments of teacher behavior. Following these rules helps teachers create a positive emotional climate in the classroom:

1. Know students' names. Call students by name, become familiar with their interests and talents, and show respect for each student.

2. Ask, "So what?" when preparing lessons. Make learning and the subject matter relevant, challenging and fun to students.

3. Establish and maintain routines for taking attendance, opening class, and so on. Begin class promptly.

4. Use the three Fs for good discipline: be firm, fair, and friendly.

5. Don't expect problems; don't look for them. Expect students to be competent, capable, and eager to learn. It is better to be proven wrong than to have students live up to negative expectations.

6. When problems arise, handle them immediately and consistently before they escalate into larger ones. For example, you can walk toward, stop and look at, or call a misbehaving student by his or her last name. Don't use major "artillery" for minor infractions.

7. Avoid sarcasm, ridicule, and belittling remarks, and help students do likewise.

8. Correct students in private. Avoid all suggestion of criticism, anger, or frustration.

9. Involve students in the setting of individual academic goals.

10. Encourage hydraulic-lift experiences in and out of the classroom (see Figure 1-3).

***Student Behavior*** Now let us address behavioral expectations for students. Clearly defining rules for students at the beginning of the academic year gives them a sense of security and can curtail discipline problems. It has been said that cows in a new pasture will seek out the fences to see how far they can roam. So it is with students. For this reason, it is imperative that teachers clearly define the boundaries (classroom rules) for students. It is inevitable that some students will test the "fences" to see how strong they are (whether the teacher will in fact enforce the established rules). A student contract is often useful in establishing classroom rules. Box 1-3 contains an example of a student behavior contract that has been used in a junior high setting.

Many teachers believe that students are more willing to follow rules that they help to make. It is often helpful to involve students in a discussion about classroom rules on the first day of class. Encouraging their input enhances the children's sense of having some control. Elementary students can take turns writing their rules on a large sheet of paper to hang in a prominent place in the classroom. The process by which rules are developed is perhaps not as important as making sure that they are clearly defined from the beginning and that they are consistently and fairly enforced.

IN THE
CLASSROOM
*1-3*

# Classroom Policy and Procedure

1. Bring pencil/pen and notebook daily.
2. Assignments done in class will not be accepted late. Homework assignments will be accepted late but with points taken off.
3. When you have been absent, it is *your* responsibility to find out what you have missed, turn in assignments, and make up tests.
4. Candy and gum are not permitted in the classroom.
5. Be in class on time, which means in your seats when the bell rings, or have a late excuse.
6. The bell does not dismiss students; I do.
7. Take care of drinks and restroom needs during class changes.
8. Sharpening of pencils is to be done before class, never during a lecture or discussion.
9. Do NOT touch any audiovisual or computer equipment unless I authorize you to do so.
10. If you are failing in your course work or are not turning in assignments, I will notify your parents.
11. No student is prejudged. That is, I do not read student files beforehand to see who and what problems may be coming in. I assume all students are capable of A work. I also assume that no student is a behavioral problem. If there are any such problems those persons will have to show me and the class who they are. Problems, should there be any, will be dealt with accordingly.
12. These behaviors will result in points being subtracted from your grades:
    a. Excessive talking
    b. Disruptive behavior
    c. Chewing gum or candy
    d. Failure to follow instructions
    e. Unexcused tardiness

## Student Contract

I have listened to and read the classroom policy and procedure regarding citizenship, behavior, and course work. I agree to adhere to this contract and understand that each violation will result in losing 5 points. This will be reflected in my final grade.

Signed: _____    Date: _____

## Dealing with Put-Downs

Put-down or harassment-type comments and behaviors can destroy the positive emotional climate of a school faster than almost anything else. The next time you are in the classroom, on the playground, walking down a hall, or in the teacher's lounge or cafeteria, listen carefully to conversations around you. You may hear comments such as "He is so dumb!" "I hate her, she is so stupid," "You're weird," "That is so lame," "What a nerd," or "Drop dead." Children are obvious and to the point with their put-downs. As we grow older we become more subtle and sophisticated, but are equally cutting: "I would never think of doing that . . .", "He is nice, but . . .". Sexual harassment, bigotry, bullying, giving the silent treatment, and excluding people are also pervasive forms of put-down behavior.

Why do we spend so much time and energy trying to undermine each other? We put others down in a futile effort to raise our own insecure sense of worth. This behavior can be visually depicted with a teeter-totter or see-saw (Figure 1-2.) It is as though we are sitting on a teeter-totter and looking for someone to sit on the other end. If we put that individual down, we feel "up," or on a higher level. Feeling superior to others is a false "high" and very short lived. After a few moments, the person who has been put down leaves the teeter-totter and we come crashing down. We then look around for someone else to put down, to once again raise our relative sense of worth. This behavior can have addictive qualities and become so pervasive that one's teeter-totter moves with fanlike rapidity. Adolescence is typically a time of rapid change and insecurity. As a result, this stage of life is particularly vulnerable to frequent **"teeter-tottering."**

Teeter-tottering can easily become epidemic in the classroom—and teachers are not immune. This type of behavior naturally occurs in schools because we have become a society that is very proficient at put-downs. TV programs often glamorize put-down behaviors, and "putting someone in

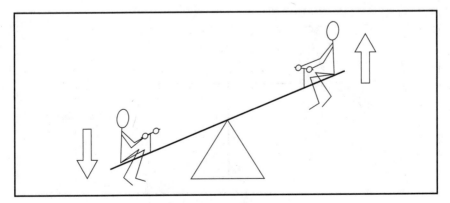

**FIGURE 1-2  Teeter-tottering**
Teeter-tottering is putting another down in an effort to feel better about yourself.

their place" is depicted as very "cool." Young people mimic being "cool" by gossiping, spreading malicious rumors, writing nasty e-mails, and excluding the "noncool." In too many homes put-downs are the predominant form of communication. Some children have become so calloused by this type of behavior that they don't even recognize its harmful effects.

How do we break out of the **teeter-totter syndrome**? First, we have to realize when we are caught up in it. Just as we take our temperature to see if we are ill, so we can check our emotional health by observing how often we teeter-totter. Students can easily monitor their own put-down behaviors when taught the principle depicted in Figure 1-2. Draw this simple diagram on the board and discuss how teeter-tottering works, or, more accurately, how it does not work. Once students understand the principle, classrooms can be designated as teeter-totter-free, much like tobacco-free environments have been established in buildings. Students don't appreciate being put down and are very willing to give up teeter-tottering to create a classroom where they feel emotionally safe and accepted. Once students accept this principle, a teacher can just say "Let's not have any teeter-tottering," or simply make a teeter-totter hand motion whenever she or he overhears a put-down.

Sociologists say that to successfully eliminate a behavior it is important to substitute another behavior. As we work at eliminating put-downs it is helpful to replace teeter-tottering with **hydraulic lifts** (Figure 1-3). A hydraulic lift is the act of raising someone else with kind acts or comments. When we are kind to another person we cannot help but feel better about ourselves. It is as if we were sitting on a hydraulic lift. As kindness is shown, we rise along with whomever we are trying to lift. This positive action creates a genuine "high" and a more lasting sense of self-worth. Helping children learn self-control by replacing teeter-totters with hydraulic lifts greatly enhances the emotional climate of any classroom and alleviates

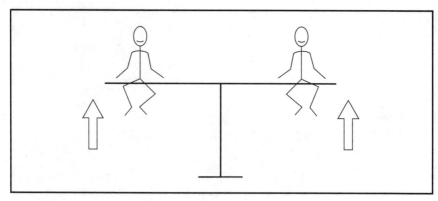

**FIGURE 1-3    Hydraulic lift**
When you lift another, you too are lifted.

many discipline problems as well. There are many ways teachers can assign students to practice being kind. For example, you can wrap your door with construction paper and invite the students to write on it every kind act they "catch" someone doing. This gives students an opportunity to do positive "tattletaling." (Additional hydraulic-lift-type activities are found in the Relationship Building section in Chapter 2. Chapter 7 discusses bullying in greater depth.)

## Sensitivity to Multicultural Diversity

We live in an exciting world where diversity of peoples and cultures abounds. Truly, no one culture is superior or inferior to another. As educators, we must strive to view individuals from various cultures from *their* perspectives rather than from *our* perspectives. This creates classroom climates of understanding and sensitivity to diverse cultures, ethnicities, and races.

Ethnocentric, racist, or stereotypic attitudes held by teachers and students serve as critical barriers to establishing sensitivity toward various cultures and ethnic groups. **Ethnocentricity** involves an attitude that one's own ethnic group or culture is better than others, or failure to recognize the existence or validity of other ethnic/cultural groups and their customs, values, beliefs, and norms. **Racism** expresses an attitude that defines certain cultural or ethnic groups as inherently inferior to others and legitimately subject to exploitation, discrimination, and various types of abuse. **Stereotypes** reflect conscious or unconscious attribution of exaggerated characteristics and/or oversimplified opinions, attitudes, or judgments regarding members of a given ethnic group or culture. A **prejudice** is a negative attitude toward a specific group based on comparison using the individual's own group as a positive reference point. Teachers have a professional responsibility to not let personal attitudes, stereotypes, and prejudices interfere with their teaching. For example, a teacher raised in one cultural group may have stereotypes or prejudices against another cultural group. This teacher would need to overcome these stereotypes and prejudices to successfully teach students of this cultural group. Of course, stereotypes and prejudices are not confined to cultural or ethnic groups. For example, some may have stereotypes and prejudices for impaired individuals, the aged, or for a variety of conditions or types of people.

Teachers can build cultural and ethnic sensitivity in a variety of ways. Teachers should strive to display appropriate personal skills, including showing warmth, respect, sincerity, concern, and caring for people of all cultures. Beyond this, it is critical to develop cross-cultural understanding in the communities where we serve and live. Recognizing culturally determined viewpoints and standards of behavior, including specific knowledge of and respect for differences, is important. Beyond developing personal cross-cultural understanding, emphasis should be given in the curriculum for cross-cultural competency for students.

It is also important to pay attention to culturally/ethnically appropriate learning and problem-solving styles. This involves recognition that a variety of strategies and approaches can complete a given task. To an extent, learning and problem-solving styles are culturally determined. A variety of approaches should be encouraged. Learning is also facilitated by appropriate style, manner, and content of communication for a particular cultural group. This includes the use of ethnically and culturally appropriate nonverbal skills such as eye contact, body language, and physical closeness.

## Working with Children with Special Needs

It is easy to become overwhelmed while working with the many students who have special needs. Many of these needs are complex problems that pose multiple difficulties in the lives of the affected children and for the school systems of which they are a part. Schools often have various staff in place to help students with special needs, such as guidance counselors, psychologists, learning specialists, social workers, special education teachers, and school nurses. A key to success in working with students with special needs seems to be the ability of these personnel to work together in a supportive team approach.

An example of a supportive team approach can be found at Francis Scott Key Elementary and Middle School in Baltimore, Maryland, where Melissa Grady works as a mental health therapist.

> Grady sees four-dozen children every week, some for the first time, others she's been counseling for years. Some are victims of sexual or physical abuse, have witnessed domestic violence or have dysfunctional parents who suffer from drug addiction or alcoholism. Others have been traumatized by family disruptions such as divorce or unstable living arrangements.
> "The huge thing is a lack of parental guidance," says Grady. "Its symptomatic of society. The children are not getting enough of what they need at home, they're not being taught the coping skills, the social skills. So, of course, all that's spilling out into the school system and the children are unavailable to learn or are disrupting others.[9]

Melissa Grady set up a student support team consisting of herself, a school psychologist, a counselor, a social worker, and teachers representing the elementary and middle schools. The team meets once a week to review the academic performance and special needs of the student body. They are proactive in looking out for students in need, such as those who are acting out, depressed, withdrawn, or displaying sudden changes in behavior or significant decline in grades or attendance. When a child with a special need is identified, the student support team arranges one-on-one sessions with the student, parent meetings and counseling, and adequate follow-up. This consistent, vigilant student support team effort is responsible for helping students improve their grades and cope with a variety of special needs. Teachers at the schools are thrilled that the student support team is in place and have seen a reduction in the severity of discipline problems. A seasoned teacher at the school, who has taught at seven other schools, commented, "You can really teach here."

The rest of this section of the chapter discusses some of the special needs that teachers face in their teaching career—children with chronic health conditions, learning disabilities, and attention deficit hyperactivity disorder (ADHD). Hopefully, you will be able to set up student support teams with other school staff in the schools you teach.

## Children with Chronic Health Conditions

Most teachers will have children with chronic health conditions in their classroom, because more than 5 million school-age youth are affected by chronic health conditions.[10] The chronic health conditions most commonly seen in students are asthma, diabetes, epilepsy, cerebral palsy, heart disease, cancer, and spina bifida. Another chronic health condition of concern in children is HIV/AIDS.

Children with chronic health conditions have special challenges and concerns. They want to be like everyone else and worry about being rejected by their classmates. They worry about being teased and excluded. In addition to these worries, they must cope with the effects of the illness and the treatments that they undergo. Often these symptoms make it difficult to put all of their energy into schoolwork. On the other hand, teachers worry about these students and about their own competence in responding appropriately to any medical emergencies that might arise in the classroom. What should I do if an epileptic child has a seizure in my classroom? What should I do if a diabetic child has a diabetic emergency?

Schools are often unprepared to deal with children with chronic health conditions, because of the burden placed on teachers and other school staff. Some students with chronic health conditions attending elementary or secondary school have an **individual education plan (IEP)** or **section 504 plan** that specifies how to manage these concerns in the school setting. Parents are entitled to these plans because of a federal law that promises all children a free and appropriate education in the least restrictive environment. However, there are also many young people with health conditions whose parents have not disclosed this fact to the school for fear of stigma or that the children will be treated differently. Unfortunately, this signals to a child that his or her condition is something to be ashamed of.

It is critical, then, that school personnel working with students with chronic health conditions have an understanding of the various health conditions and emergency management procedures of their students. A resource that teachers and students should be aware of is "Band-Aides and Blackboards" (www.faculty.fairfield.edu/fleitas/sitemap.html). This website contains a wealth of information on things that teachers and other adults can do to help children with chronic health conditions. The following are some tips that Joan Fleitas, developer of the website, gives to teachers:

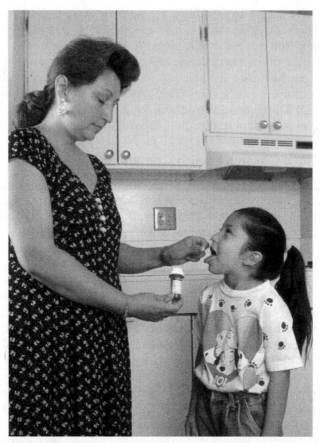

Many children have chronic health conditions that require taking medication at home and at school.

❖ Your attitude of kindness, empathy, and acceptance toward others has been found to generate similar attitudes in the classroom. That's how children learn attitudes. They watch the adults they care about, and model their behavior.

❖ You should know the protocol for emergencies and acute illnesses, so make sure that the school nurse has provided you with sufficient information about the medical conditions of the children in your classroom. It's important to communicate reassurance to both the child and the class if acute illness does occur.

❖ Be sensitive to when *not* to show concern, like when a child with cystic fibrosis is coughing. The cough is important to clear the lungs. Paying too much attention to a symptom often makes it worse and reinforces a child's sense of shame.

❖ Children with medical problems are often overly sensitive. Don't perceive their behavior as babyish or immature or a serious emotional problem. By reinforcing positive age-appropriate behavior, you are most likely to increase it.

When school personnel, parents, and health professionals work together in partnership and in a creative manner, having children with chronic health conditions in the classroom can be a stimulus for the growth of everyone in the classroom environment. An example of this is a second-grade student with spina bifida who asked for classmates to receive orientation about his disease after classmates teased him when he had urine leakage. During the session classmates asked many questions, including whether he would have children and whether he would live. Because of the careful preparation and support, he was not surprised by the questions and could answer them honestly.

## Children with Learning Disabilities

It is important for educators to have a basic understanding of learning disabilities in order to recognize symptoms and help students with them. A **learning disability** is a disorder that affects a person's ability to either interpret what he or she sees and hears or to link information from different parts of the brain. These limitations can show up in many ways—as specific difficulties with spoken and written language, coordination, self-control, or attention. They can impede learning to read or write, do math, or learn other important skills.

It is not exactly clear how many students experience learning disabilities. Some experts estimate about 1 in every 100; others estimate that almost one-third of children in school have some form of learning disability. What is clear is that many more boys than girls are affected. There are many kinds of learning disabilities and many causes for them. In some cases the brain is believed to have been harmed before birth or by a difficult birth, childhood head injury, or illness. Some learning disabled (LD) children have siblings and/or parents with the same problem, indicating that they may have inherited their learning disability. This is particularly true for dyslexia.

Many experts believe that learning disabilities are the result of a malfunction in the central nervous system that causes a breakdown in auditory, visual, or motor perceptions. These breakdowns in turn affect the way an individual learns. Learning is believed to take place through a five-step process:

1. We take in information through our senses.

2. We process the information for its meaning.

3. We file the information in our memory.

4. We later withdraw it from our memory and "remember" it.

5. We feed the information back to the outside world.

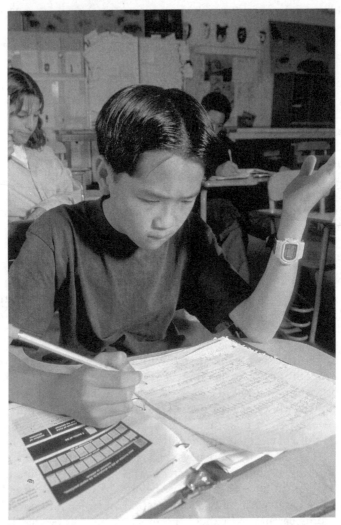

Students with learning disabilities are likely to feel stress and frustration while doing schoolwork.

Individuals with learning disabilities have a breakdown in one or more of these steps. Their eyes and ears may work fine, but something happens to the messages that tell the brain what they are seeing or hearing. Letters may seem to reverse themselves, or the same word on two lines of print may appear dissimilar. Some people cannot tell if sounds are alike or different, and a sentence such as "Put the cap on the pen" may come through as "Butt the cat on the pin."

Students who have trouble with the second learning process step may be able to perfectly and quickly read aloud from a text only to have none of it make any sense unless they reread it several times. Some LD students find lectures totally frustrating because the information is coming too fast for them. Taping lectures can help this problem.

The third and fourth steps of the learning process involve short- and long-term memory. A student with short-term memory problems might quickly forget instructions. Long-term memory problems are exhibited on exams where the student knew the information just a few days before. Math is especially difficult for memory disabled students.

The fifth step of learning concerns presenting the information that has been retrieved from memory. Many LD people have difficulty expressing themselves either orally or on paper. Ideas are often expressed out of order, such as a punch line coming in the middle of a story instead of at the end. Writing projects can be filled with sentences that either run on or are incomplete, and with common words misspelled in a variety of ways.

An individual may have one or many learning disabilities. Each problem may be mild, causing little trouble, or so pronounced that it is difficult to compensate for. Many learning disabilities are language oriented, such as reading, talking, spelling, or writing. Some children have problems listening, thinking, or remembering, and some have trouble learning the order of things. Other problems include the following: trouble smoothly moving small or large muscles (poor handwriting or trouble cutting along a line); trouble telling directions (knowing left from right, reading a map); mixing up or reversing numbers (reading "26" as "62"), letters ("b" for "d"), or words ("was" for "saw"); trouble talking clearly; hyperactivity; short interest span/easily distracted; and impulsivity, "leaping before they look."

Teachers can help children with learning disabilities by first recognizing the problem. All too often LD children are labeled dumb or unmotivated. It is essential that LD children be identified early, before they begin to see themselves as stupid and failing. Be suspicious if a fairly bright child has trouble learning certain skills. A referral can be made to a school counselor or special education instructor. Every school district has its policy for screening learning disabilities. Often a team works together to study the child. This team may consist of a physician, special education teacher, psychologist, and other school personnel. They should review the child's preschool learning patterns and health history. The child should be tested to see how he or she thinks, moves, and solves problems, for intelligence, and for reading, spelling, writing, and arithmetic skills. The child should also be tested to see how he or she sees and hears, for hand–eye coordination, and for memory retention. Most of all, the testing should discover what the child can do well. With this information an IEP can be designed. An IEP outlines the specific skills a student needs to develop and appropriate learning activities that will build on the student's strengths. With the right help, most LD children overcome their learning disabilities. It is helpful to remember the following famous people who had learning disabilities: Albert Einstein, Thomas Edison, Nelson Rockefeller, Ludwig van Beethoven, Winston Churchill, Bruce Jenner, George Patton, Leonardo da Vinci, and Woodrow Wilson.

As an instructor, you may have to show extra patience and give extra help to LD students. You can also help your students understand that almost every child has trouble learning something. Some have trouble with music, others find sports difficult, and others have a hard time drawing. Compassion and understanding for LD individuals can be fostered by the following activities:

1. Have students try to write a sentence with the hand they normally don't use for writing.

2. Have students hold a piece of paper up to a mirror and try to write their names by looking only in the mirror.

3. Take a story or text page and retype it switching all the "b's" for "d's" and all the "d's" for "b's." Have the students try to make sense of it.

If one of your students has a learning disability, find an activity for the class that will let the LD child use his or her strong points.

## Children with Attention Deficit Hyperactivity Disorder

**Attention deficit hyperactivity disorder (ADHD)** often interferes with academic and social functioning. It is a major cause of learning disorders. The primary signs of ADHD are inattention, impulsivity, and hyperactivity. *Inattention* is described as failure to finish tasks started, easy distractibility, seeming lack of attention, and difficulty concentrating on tasks requiring sustained attention. *Impulsivity* is described as acting before thinking, difficulty taking turns, problems organizing work, and constant shifting from one activity to another. *Hyperactivity* is described as difficulty staying seated and sitting still, and excessive running or climbing. ADHD is usually diagnosed when these signs become obvious and they are inconsistent with a child's developmental level.

ADHD has become the most common childhood psychiatric disorder. It is estimated that 3% to 5% of all school-age children have ADHD. On average, at least one child in each classroom needs help for this disorder. It is diagnosed three times more frequently in boys than girls. The cause of ADHD is unknown. There is some evidence, however, that ADHD is the result of a developmental failure in the brain circuitry that controls attention, inhibition, and self-control. There is no known cure for ADHD, and it often persists into adulthood. It can cause a lifetime of frustration and emotional pain.

*Classroom Needs and Help for Children with ADHD*   Children with ADHD have a variety of needs.\* Some children are too hyperactive or inattentive to function in a regular classroom, even with medication and a behavior management plan. Such children may be placed in a special education class for all or part of the day. In some schools, the special education teacher teams with the classroom teacher to meet each child's unique needs. However, most children are able to stay in the regular classroom. Whenever possible, educators prefer not to segregate children, but to let them learn along with their peers.

Children with ADHD often need some special accommodations to help them learn. For example, the teacher may seat the child in an area with few distractions, provide an area where the child can move around and release excess energy, or establish a clearly posted system of rules and reward appropriate behavior. Sometimes just keeping a card or a picture on the desk can serve as a visual reminder to use the right school behavior, like raising a hand instead of shouting out, or staying in a seat instead of wandering around the room. Giving an ADHD child extra time on tests can make the difference between passing and failing, and gives a fairer chance to show what's learned. Reviewing instructions or writing assignments on the board, and even listing the books and materials they will need for the task, may make it possible for disorganized, inattentive children to complete the work.

Many of the strategies of special education are simply good teaching methods. Telling students in advance what they will learn, providing visual aids, and giving written as well as oral instructions are all ways to help students focus and remember the key parts of the lesson.

Students with ADHD often need to learn techniques for monitoring and controlling their own attention and behavior. For example, students can be taught alternatives for what do when they lose track of what they are supposed to be doing—look for instructions on the blackboard, raise their hand, or quietly ask another child. The process of finding alternatives to interrupting the teacher makes a student more self-sufficient and cooperative. And because there is less interrupting, a student begins to get more praise than reprimands.

The teacher can frequently stop to ask ADHD students to notice whether they are paying attention to the lesson or if they are thinking about something else. The students can record their answer on a chart. As students become more consciously aware of their attention, they begin to see progress and feel good about staying better focused. This process helps make students aware of when their attention is drifting off, so they can

---

\* This section is adapted from National Institute of Mental Health, *Attention Deficit Hyperactivity Disorder* (NIH Publication No. 96-3572), 2002. Available at http://www.nimh.nih.gov/publicat/adhd.cfm.

return their attention to what is going on in the classroom. It can help ADHD students became more productive and help the quality of their work to improve.

Because schools demand that children sit still, wait for a turn, pay attention, and stick with a task, it's no surprise that many children with ADHD have problems in class. Their minds are fully capable of learning, but their hyperactivity and inattention make learning difficult. As a result, many students with ADHD repeat a grade or drop out of school early. Fortunately, with the right combination of appropriate educational practices, medication, and counseling, these outcomes can be avoided.

***Controversies in Treating ADHD with Stimulant Drugs***   Diverse and conflicting opinions exist concerning ADHD. As a result, it is a very controversial educational and health issue. A recent consensus statement from the National Institutes of Health notes that the controversy concerns the literal existence of the disorder, whether it can be reliably diagnosed, and, if treated, what interventions are the most effective.

Perhaps the major controversy concerns the prevalent use of stimulant drugs to treat ADHD, often in the absence of behavioral treatments. Concerns have intensified over potential overuse and abuse of stimulant drug treatment of ADHD. Stimulant drugs are more readily available and are prescribed much more frequently now than in the past. In the past decade prescriptions for stimulant medication among children have increased several-fold, even among preschool-age children. The Drug Enforcement Administration (DEA) reports that 90% of the world's methylphenidate (Ritalin), a drug commonly used to treat ADHD, is consumed in the United States. There are significant variations among regions of the country in the amount of stimulants prescribed by doctors to treat ADHD.

Stimulants such as **Ritalin** and **Dexedrine** (dextroamphetamine) have been used for some time in the treatment of ADHD. Newer drug formulations, such as **Adderall** (a combination of four amphetamines, including Dexedrine) and **Concerta,** are becoming more popular because of their longer-acting properties. As a result, these pills can be taken by a child or adolescent once a day, instead of two or three times a day, eliminating the need for a dose to be taken at school. Concerta is a controlled-release form of Ritalin that has a special coating that allows the medication to be slowly released for up to 12 hours. Avoiding having to take medication at school is an important benefit because it eliminates the need for a child to bring medicine to school and takes the burden of administering the medication to the child off of school nurses or other school personnel (see Box 1-4). One pharmaceutical company plans on releasing a methylphenidate skin patch in the future. The patch, worn under the clothes, will deliver the stimulant directly through the skin into the bloodstream. Many new drugs for the treatment of ADHD will probably appear in the near future because of the high demand for them.

IN THE
CLASSROOM

*1-4*

## "Mother's Little Helper"

It is another medication morning at Winnebago Elementary School in the middle-class Chicago suburb of Bloomingdale. Three pings sound precisely over the intercom at 11:45 A.M. Principal Mark Wagener opens a locked file cabinet and withdraws a giant Tupperware container filled with plastic prescription vials. Nearly a dozen students scramble to the office for their Ritalin, a drug that calms the agitated by stimulating the brain. These children—all ages, mostly boys—have been diagnosed with Attention Deficit Hyperactivity Disorder, a complex neurological impairment that takes the brakes off and derails concentration. The school nurse places the pills, one by one, in the children's mouths, a rite of safe passage before lunch. "Let me see . . . ," says nurse Pat Nazos, as she checks under each child's tongue for a stray, unswallowed capsule.

Source: L. Hancock, "Mother's Little Helper," *Newsweek,* March 18, 1996, pg. 51.

As with all medications, there is the potential for side effects. While on these medications, some children may lose weight, have less appetite, and temporarily grow more slowly. Others may have problems falling asleep. It is possible that stimulants may make the symptoms of Tourette's syndrome worse, but this is not known for sure. Other side effects can include irritability, agitation, nervousness, and periods of sadness. Serious side effects include facial tics and muscle twitching. Most of the side effects that do occur can often be handled by reducing the dosage.

One important concern about stimulant drugs is their potential for abuse. When these powerful stimulant drugs are abused, abusers have suffered psychotic episodes, violent behavior, and severe psychological dependence on the stimulant. Stimulants used to treat ADHD are classified by the DEA as Schedule II drugs, the most highly addictive drugs that are still legal. According to the DEA, drugs to treat ADHD rank among today's most-stolen prescriptions and most-abused legal drugs. Most abusers, DEA officials say, are kids. Most dealers are kids who are prescribed the drugs to treat ADHD. Parents of ADHD children have also been found to abuse the stimulant drugs.

Some experts believe that the use of stimulant drugs in treating ADHD can hamper a young person's self-esteem. Stimulant drugs often produce marked improvements in a child's schoolwork and behavior after starting medication. As a result, the child, parents, and teachers credit the drug for causing the improvement instead of crediting the child's own strengths and natural abilities. A child may feel less competent as a result. Instead, children, parents, and teachers should understand that the medication makes these changes possible, but that improvements can only come about if the child supplies the effort and ability. Parents and teachers need to praise the child, not the drug, for improvements.

## Key Terms

circle of concern   4
circle of influence   5
proactive people   5
reactive people   5
pyramid of influence   6
self-fulfilling prophecies   10
discipline   12
teeter-tottering   15
teeter-totter syndrome   16
hydraulic lifts   16
ethnocentricity   17
racism   17

stereotypes   17
prejudice   17
individual education
   plan (IEP)   19
section 504 plan   19
learning disability   21
attention deficit hyperactivity
   disorder (ADHD)   24
Ritalin   26
Dexedrine   26
Adderall   26
Concerta   26

## Review Questions

1. What is the circle of concern? How does it differ from the circle of influence? Within which circle do you spend most of your time? What can you do to become more circle-of-influence focused?
2. What are three major areas of a teacher's pyramid of influence?
3. What are the characteristics of effective teachers? Which of these characteristics do you exemplify? How did you score on the Emotional Health Inventory? As you reflect on your pyramid of influence, what positive and negative behaviors will you likely model in the classroom? How can you prepare to be a more positive role model?
4. Give several examples from the chapter of how teacher expectations can affect student performance in the classroom. Give several personal examples of positive and negative labeling you have observed in the classroom and discuss the effects of those labels. What are some measures you can take to become more positive toward all the students in your classroom?
5. What three common characteristics were found to exist in exemplary classrooms?
6. Identify the Ten Commandments for creating a positive emotional climate in the classroom and give examples of how you can incorporate these suggestions in your teaching.

7. Discuss the need for classroom rules and how to develop and enforce them.

8. Explain the teeter-totter syndrome and the hydraulic-lift principle. Discuss ways teachers can diminish put-downs and encourage kindness in the classroom.

9. Discuss ways teachers can build cultural and ethnic sensitivity.

10. Explain what a student support team is and identify the various professionals that can make up a team.

11. Identify the chronic health conditions most likely to be seen in students, and things that teachers can do to help children with chronic health problems.

12. Describe the various problems that individuals with learning disabilities can have. Discuss ways teachers can help children with learning disabilities.

13. Explain what ADHD is, its symptoms, and the needs and helps for children with ADHD.

14. Discuss the controversies in treating ADHD with stimulant drugs. Discuss the prevalence of use, benefits, and side effects of Ritalin, Dexedrine, Adderall, and Concerta.

## References

1. Covey, S. R. (1990). *The Seven Habits of Highly Effective People.* New York: Fireside.

2. Steinem, G. (1993). "The Royal Knights of Harlem." In J. Canfield and M. Hansen, eds. *Chicken Soup for the Soul.* Deerfield Beach, FL: Health Communications, 134–139.

3. Woodward, K. L. (1998, October 21). "The Life of a Great Teacher." *Newsweek,* 60.

4. Glasser, W. (1998). *The Quality School: Managing Students Without Coercion.* New York: HarperPerennial.

5. Bennett, W. J. (1994). *The Devaluing of America: Fight for Our Culture and Our Children.* Colorado Springs: Focus on the Family.

6. Rosenthal, R., and L. Jacobson (1968). *Pygmalion in the Classroom.* New York: Holt, Rinehart and Winston.

7. Hamachek, D. E. (1978). *Encounters with the Self.* New York: Holt, Rinehart and Winston.

8. Dobson, J. (1974). *Hide or Seek.* Old Tappan, NJ: Fleming H. Revell.

9. O'Conner, H. J. (1999). "The Cleavers Don't Live Here Anymore: Some Schools Are Facing up to Their Students' Mental Health Problems." ABCNEWS.com. Retrieved May 24, 1999, at http://www.abcnews.go.com:80/sections/livingdailyNews/nightline_teenviolence990520.html.

10. Fitzgeral, S. (2002, January 27). "For Teens with Diseases, Growing up Is Even Harder." *Philadelphia Inquirer.* Available at http://www.mtio.com/sitboard/messages/872.html.

# 2

## Skills for Emotional Well-Being

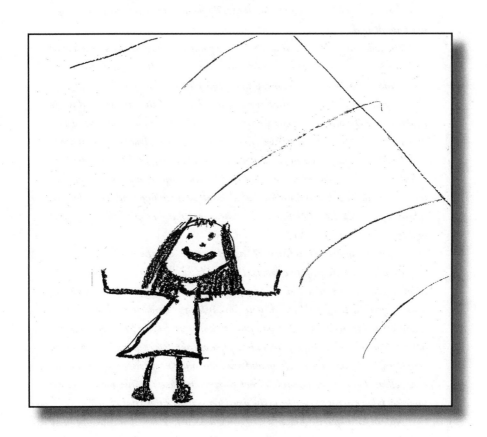

## Making a Difference

On my very first day of teaching a fight broke out. It was just before sixth period sophomore slow track English. As I entered my room I found two boys tussling on the floor. "Listen, you retard!" yelled the kid on the bottom. "I didn't take your stuff!"

The fight was quickly broken up. After class I detained Joe, who had apparently started the fight. With a flat voice and dead eyes he said, "Teach, don't waste your time on us. We're the retards of the school."

That entire night I couldn't get Joe's face and comment out of my mind. I tossed and turned in bed wondering if I really wanted to be a teacher. Finally, I knew what to do.

The following day I stood at the front of my sixth period class and looked each student in the eye. I then turned and wrote DRAHCIR on the board.

I said, "That's my first name. Can anyone please tell me what it is?"

They laughed and said I had a really weird name. I then turned and wrote RICHARD on the board. A couple of students blurted out my name and several gave me a funny look. They were suspicious and wondered if I was playing a joke on them.

I said, "Yes, Richard is my first name. I have a learning disability—something called dyslexia. In elementary school I had trouble writing my own name correctly. I couldn't spell and numbers got all jumbled up in my head. I was labeled retarded—RICKY RETARDED. I can clearly remember people calling me that and the way it made me feel."

"So how'd ya become a teacher?" asked a student in the front row.

I replied, "I hate negative labels. I love to learn and I'm not stupid. That's what my classes are all about, discovering just how smart you are and loving to learn. If you like the label 'retard,' you don't belong in here. Go see the guidance councilor and transfer out. But you have to know that I don't see any 'retards' in here. Now, this class isn't going to be a piece of cake. We're going to work hard, very hard. You're going to catch up and graduate and I'm sure some of you will go onto college. I'm not joking, and I'm not threatening you. I'm just making you a promise. I don't want to ever hear the word 'retard' again! Is that clear?"

No one transferred out and it wasn't long before the students began to believe more in themselves. As they came to expect more of themselves, they worked harder and harder, pushing themselves to catch up to their peers. We all learned a great deal about English literature that year, but so much more about life. While studying classics like <u>The Grapes of Wrath</u> and <u>To Kill a Mockingbird</u>, we discussed the need for taking responsibility for our actions, choices and consequences, and the need for setting life goals. We likened the characters'

*situations to similar problems they faced and talked about problem-solving meth-*
*ods, how to resolve conflicts, and other communication and relationship-building*
*skills. We discussed various labels people carry, how those labels affect people's*
*behavior, and how negative labels can be overcome.*

*All of them did graduate and five of them, including Joe, earned scholar-*
*ships to college. I'm now in my twenty-third year of teaching. I laugh whenever*
*I think back on my first day in the classroom and how, for a night, I wondered if*
*I really wanted to be a teacher. What could I possibly do that would be more*
*rewarding than trying to make a difference in young people's lives by teaching*
*them things that really matter?*

Source: Based on J. Connolly, "Don't Waste Your Time with Those Kids," in P. R. Kane, ed.,
*The First Year of Teaching: Real World Stories from America's Teachers.* New York: Walker, 1991.

We are certain that a major motive for your decision to enter the teaching profession is the sincere desire to be a positive influence in the lives of your students. You want your students to be successful in dealing with the pressures, concerns, and problems they confront during youth and later in adulthood. For this reason, it is imperative that you are optimally prepared to guide your students in developing essential life skills that foster healthy development and emotional well-being. Students acquiring these skills will be better equipped to deal with life challenges and avert problems.

As a teacher you can have an enormous positive impact upon the emotional well-being of students. **Emotional well-being** is one's ability to feel comfortable with self, to relate to other people, cope with disappointments and stress, solve problems, celebrate successes, and make decisions. We firmly believe that emotional well-being provides the foundation for the healthy development of youth. Emotional well-being gives young people the inner resources to withstand pressures to engage in risky behavior (e.g., alcohol and other drug abuse, early sexual activity). Youth with emotional well-being are more likely to be successful in life because they are able to make responsible decisions, set and achieve goals, solve problems, cope with disappointments and stress, and effectively communicate feelings.

The focus of this chapter is on the life skills that foster emotional well-being. We have divided these skills into nine areas: self-esteem, proactivity, emotional intelligence, resilience/asset building, relationship building, communication skills, goal setting, problem solving and decision making, and media literacy. We have also included activities that you can use in teaching these skills to students. You can easily modify these activities to fit the needs of your students and subject area. These skills and the provided teaching activities can be taught in health courses as well as in most subject areas (e.g., English, mathematics, social studies, history, family life, physical education, science). We are confident that as you become more familiar with these skills you will want to incorporate them into every course and subject area you teach in the curriculum. Emotional well-being should be promoted in every classroom!

## Self-Esteem

Self-esteem is viewed by many mental health professionals as the foundation of positive emotional well-being. Branden summarizes this perspective:

> Apart from problems that are biological in origin, I cannot think of a single psychological difficulty—from anxiety and depression, to fear of intimacy or of success, to alcohol or drug abuse, to underachievement at school or at work, to spouse battering or child molestation, to sexual dysfunctions or emotional immaturity, to suicide or crimes of violence—that is not traceable to poor self-esteem. Of all the judgments we pass, none is as important as the one we pass on ourselves. Positive self-esteem is a cardinal requirement of a fulfilling life. (pg. 5)[1]

Most schools have made major efforts to improve the self-esteem of students in an attempt to avoid the psychological difficulties mentioned above. Through these efforts, however, many misconceptions about self-esteem have arisen. One of the prominent myths concerning self-esteem is that it can be "injected" into students like a vaccination. Other self-esteem myths include the notions that self-esteem comes before accomplishment, that narcissism and self-centeredness are self-esteem, and that one should always feel good about oneself. These notions are responsible for what some have termed "The Self-Esteem Fraud." Efforts to enhance self-esteem that incorporate these myths fail.

Before we can successfully nurture self-esteem in our classrooms, we must first have a clear understanding of what it is. **Self-esteem** is the evaluative component of self-image, or the positive or negative manner in which a person judges herself or himself. It is a product of what we perceive ourselves to be (**self-image**), how we want to be (**ideal-self**), and the expectations that we perceive others have for us (**pygmalion-self**). Our senses of competency, worthiness, and belonging are formed by the combination of these three "selves." Figure 2-1 diagrams how all these factors combine to form self-esteem. Notice that the waves in the social mirror represent perceptions of reality. At times our perceptions are more distorted than at other times, such as on "blue days." Consequently, our self-esteem, how we judge ourself, is dynamic and ever-changing.

Negative self-perceptions can adversely affect a child's performance in school. This fact has prompted some educators to try to "inject" self-esteem into students to raise scholastic performance. Injection efforts include generously praising students for any effort they make and having students chant self-affirming statements such as "I'm great!" This approach can

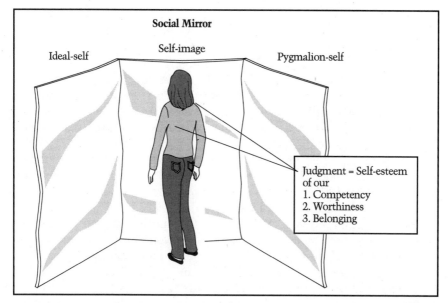

**FIGURE 2-1    Determinants of self-esteem**

produce students who feel good about mediocre performance but who do not experience a true lift in self-esteem. True self-esteem is experienced when we do our very best work—not from lowering the standards by which we judge ourselves.

Self-esteem is best nurtured by teachers when students are helped to achieve academic success and acquire emotional skills, and through establishing an emotionally warm classroom where students feel capable, competent, and accepted. Throughout the rest of this chapter, we provide you with insight and strategies to help students gain true self-esteem—the type that will facilitate their successes in life.

We will now look at factors influencing the development of the ideal-self and pygmalion-self. We examine how ideal-self and pygmalion-self reflections affect self-evaluation and feelings of self-worth, and how to rise above negative self-image scripting.

## Ideal-Self

*Ideal-self* is our perception of what we want to be. Ideal-self involves every aspect of our being, including physical characteristics, mental abilities, emotional and social skills, and moral standards. Ideal-self is based on the expectations that we have for ourselves. These expectations are shaped through relationships and interactions with family members, peers, and others. The media also affect ideal-self through the messages and images to which we are exposed.

The aspect of ideal-self that we tend to focus on most is our physical characteristics. This is particularly true for teenagers. Our physical ideal is what we perceive as the perfect body—our image of what we believe is the perfect height, weight, body build, coloring, facial features, and so forth. This ideal is tremendously shaped by the numerous media images we see of beautiful people, airbrushed to perfection, on television, in movies, in magazines, and on billboards. If we do not look like these people, it is easy to form the impression that we are less than ideal. Yet, the truth is that very few are capable of living up to these ideals. Even models report that there are things they don't like about their bodies. Cindy Crawford is reported to have said, "I wish I looked like Cindy Crawford." Therefore, the ideal that should be stressed is having a physically fit and healthy body. This is a healthy, achievable physical ideal.

While certain physical characteristics cannot be changed, moral characteristics can be attained. For example, everyone has the capacity to be honest, respectful, responsible, hard-working, and compassionate. These characteristics are not usually aspired to or sought after unless a person receives guidance and nurturing from adults. Too many youth idealize low moral characteristics (e.g., disrespect, disregard for the law, cruelty). In other words, the ideal-self of many young persons (what they aspire to be) includes low moral character. How can we help youth to want to incorporate moral characteristics into their ideal-self? The next sections on hero identification and character and values education address this question.

***Hero Identification***    Heroes are simply people that we admire. The people we choose to admire shape our perception of what we want to be (ideal-self). They provide a standard against which to measure ourselves. Thus, identifying one's heroes gives great insight into one's ideal-self. Think about who you truly admire. What is it that you admire about them? You will probably think of several heroes. Some may be people that you know personally. Others are people you know only from a distance or through the image portrayed through the media. Consider how your heroes affect your life. How much do you attempt to emulate the traits you find desirable?

How much do you think children and adolescents emulate the people they admire? If you ask children and adolescents who their heroes are, many will report celebrities—sports figures, actors, musicians, or other media stars. We tend to be a culture fixated on celebrity status. After September 11, 2001, New York firefighters and police officers became national heroes. In addition to celebrities and firefighters, some children will name family members, such as a parent, older sibling, aunt or uncle, or grandparent, as their heroes.

Young people need to be exposed to heroes of high moral character in history, literature, and in our neighborhoods and communities. There are many heroes in our communities with whom our young people should become acquainted (e.g., people who give community service). Being exposed to many different types of heroes helps youth form ideal-selves with high character qualities. It prompts young people to ask themselves if they have the various traits exemplified and inspires them to develop these traits.

Share your heroes with your students. Highlight the admired characteristics of the heroes you discuss with your students. Explain why the characteristics are important to you and how the hero may have developed these characteristics. Ask your students to interview adults, such as parents, relatives, neighbors, or others, about their heroes. Instruct your students to listen carefully and identify the admirable qualities these adults' heroes demonstrate. You can also have your students search local newspapers for articles that might identify some individuals who have acted in admirable ways and could be termed "heroes." As you do these activities have the class make a large lettered list of admirable character traits. Display this list in a prominent location for several months. In class discussions continue to highlight admirable character traits you encounter in history, literature, and elsewhere as the semester proceeds. The more exposure students have to examples of high character, the more likely they are to make those characteristics part of their ideal.

Many students have media heroes who do not display high moral character. We should help students identify the good qualities of these heroes. This helps put the focus on the positive aspects of the hero. It is also appropriate to discuss how the media hero's negative behavior can lead to problems for the hero himself or herself and for those who emulate this behavior.

***Character Education***   **Character education** is the deliberate effort to help people understand, care about, and act upon core ethical values. Many schools include aspects of character education in their curricula in hopes of curtailing societal problems such as violence, vandalism, stealing, cheating, disrespect for authority and peers, sexual promiscuity, and abusive and self-destructive behaviors. People who display these problem behaviors do not exemplify good character and lack moral elements in their ideal-selves. For this reason, character education holds promise as a solution for these problems. Thomas Lickona explains that good character "consists of knowing the good, desiring the good, and doing the good—habits of the mind, habits of the heart, and habits of action. All three are necessary for leading a moral life; all three make up moral maturity. When we think about the kind of character we want for our children, it's clear that we want them to be able to judge what is right, care deeply about what is right, and then do what they believe to be right—even in the face of pressure from without and temptation from within" (pg. 51).[2]

Therefore, character education consists of teaching students "the good," motivating them to desire "the good," and inspiring actions of good character. Lickona labels these three components of character education as *moral knowing, moral feeling, and moral action.* Effective character education programs require intentional, proactive, and comprehensive approaches that promote core values in all aspects of school life. Schools that take a comprehensive approach to character education do the following:[3]

❖ Publicly stand for core ethical values, including respect, responsibility, trustworthiness, fairness, diligence, self-control, caring, and courage

❖ Define these values in terms of observable behavior

❖ Model these values at every opportunity

❖ Celebrate their occurrence in and outside of school

❖ Study them and teach their application to everyday life, including all parts of the school environment (e.g., classrooms, corridors, cafeteria, playing field, school bus)

❖ Hold all school members, adults and students alike, accountable to standards of conduct consistent with the school's professed core values

Schools with effective character education programs provide students with repeated opportunities for moral action geared to help them develop their intrinsic motivation. To be successful, character education must take place in a school environment that is caring and academically challenging and supportive of all students. Parents and community members must be recruited by the school and made full partners in the character-building effort.

***Values Education***   **Values education** is very similar to character education, and like character education, schools offer it as a solution to problem behaviors. The values education in today's schools differs significantly from **values clarification.** In the 1960s and 1970s, there was considerable sentiment that schools should not teach values because of concern over which values would be taught. In an effort to avoid teaching specific values, schools taught "values clarification," which focuses on having students identify and clarify their personal values. In values clarification, teachers were instructed to not influence students' values by imposing their values. However, it became apparent that some students lacked moral values. Today we recognize that, even with vast diversities in our population, there are many values all of us share. Currently in values education, values are taught rather than "clarified."

Which values do schools teach? Values education centers on the foundational moral values of respect and responsibility. All cultures and societies universally affirm these values in one way or another. Other values, such as honesty, fairness, tolerance, prudence, self-discipline, helpfulness, compassion, cooperation, courage, civic virtue, and citizenship, assist one in acting respectfully and responsibly. Effective values education inspires students to incorporate these values into their ideal-self.

## Pygmalion-Self

You may be familiar with the Greek myth of Pygmalion, a sculptor who created an ivory statue of a beautiful young maiden. His creation was so realistic and beautiful that he fell in love with it. In recognition of Pygmalion's strong affection for the ivory maiden, Aphrodite, the goddess of love, turned the statue into a live maiden. Using the theme from this myth, George Bernard Shaw wrote a play entitled *Pygmalion*, upon which the film *My Fair Lady* is based. The play and film portray the relationship between a young flower girl, Eliza Dolittle, and a professor. Professor Higgins's determination and expectations transform Eliza from a flower girl into a lovely lady of high society. The powerful influence of expectations of others on behavior and self-esteem has been dubbed the **Pygmalion effect.** A common expression illustrating the power of the Pygmalion effect goes like this:

I am not what I think I am.
I am not what you think I am.
I am what I think you think I am.

*Pygmalion-self* is our perception of what we believe other people think of us. Thus, pygmalion-self is precisely what the expression above exclaims: "I am what I think you think I am." Eliza Dolittle became the lady Professor Higgins thought she could be. Take a moment to consider your pygmalion-self. What perceptions do significant people in your life have of you? How are you affected and shaped by these perceptions? Pygmalion-self-perceptions can be negative, positive, or even neutral. Can you think of ways in which you have been negatively and positively affected by your pygmalion-self-perceptions?

Relationships and interactions from several individuals contribute to a young person's sense of pygmalion-self, including family, teachers, peers, friends, coaches, and neighbors. However, pygmalion-self is also highly specific to each relationship and interaction. For example, it is common for a teenager to feel low regard from certain peers and yet feel high regard from other peers.

Pygmalion-self-perceptions are prone to inaccuracy. Consider the following case. Melissa wholly believes that one of her teachers thinks she is "dumb" and incorporates this perception into her pygmalion-self. In reality, the teacher considers Melissa as a slightly above-average student. Melissa's perception affects her schoolwork and her relationship with the teacher. Misperceiving the perceptions of others is a common problem associated with pygmalion-self. For this reason, the next section of this chapter addresses how to help students accurately evaluate their pygmalion-self. Too often individuals accept certain labels as reality when in fact they are unfounded, an issue we address later in this chapter. While labels are usually difficult to overcome, it is possible to develop unconditional worth and high personal regard. (We discussed pygmalion-self as it relates to teacher-student expectations in Chapter 1.)

## Accurate Self-Evaluation

Forming an accurate sense of who we are is important to high self-esteem. Therefore, the manner in which we evaluate ourselves has a profound affect on self-esteem. Self-evaluation is helpful because it allows us to scrutinize the various aspects of our ideal-self and pygmalion-self. When our ideal-self or pygmalion-self is distorted, our self-esteem is affected (see Figure 2-1). The key to forming a "true picture" of who we are is the ability to take a nonemotive third-person view of ourselves. What we mean by this is seeing ourselves through the eyes of another person while maintaining a nonjudgmental state. This is a skill that can be learned. It takes time, patience, and effort to develop the skills necessary for accurate self-evaluation. Therefore, it is best to start training in childhood. The following examples illustrate the need for more accurate self-evaluation.

Marie works hard in school and recently earned a 94% on a test. Upon reviewing her corrected test she remarked, "I really messed up on the test!" Jennifer is a very attractive 14-year-old with what her friends consider an enviably slender figure. Jennifer feels that she is at least 15 pounds overweight and sometimes even refers to herself as "Thunder thighs," the nickname given to her by her younger brother. This nickname is unwarranted because her thighs are rather slender. Michael is very agile and proficient in sports, the "athlete of the family." He does moderately well in school but not as well as his older brother, the "brain of the family." Therefore, he feels that he is dumb. These three young people have trouble evaluating themselves accurately. Being able to see oneself accurately is not an easy task, but it is an important component of emotional well-being.

Teachers can assist students in evaluating themselves more realistically by first helping them develop an awareness of their self-image, ideal-self, and pygmalion-self. A variety of activities can help students realize how they see themselves, including their physical and psychological traits, talents, shortcomings, roles, and labels. Other activities can help students answer the questions "How do I wish I were?" (ideal-self) and "How do others see me?" (pygmalion-self).

The second step to realistic self-evaluation is reviewing these three selves to see how they have been influenced over the years by the media, peers, parents, siblings, and teachers. Teachers can be especially effective in providing this kind of insight through lecture, discussion, and learning activities. Once students recognize all of these influences upon self-esteem, it is easier for them to evaluate the accuracy of their own self-image. They can also determine whether their ideal-self is what they really want it to be, and if they care to accept the pygmalion-self imposed on them by others.

In the earlier example, Marie was able to accurately identify that she earned a high score on a test, but unrealistically evaluated her efforts as a failure because her ideal-self demanded perfection. Perfection is an unrealistic foundation for self-evaluation. One of the general characteristics of individuals with negative self-concepts is that they make unrealistically high demands of themselves. People with low self-esteem tend to judge themselves on the basis of unattainable goals of perfection. Even though Marie is a very competent student, her negative self-evaluations have undermined the positive self-esteem that her achievements should have helped to develop. If Marie could be helped to see how her ideal-self has demanded perfection, she might be able to make the conscious choice to change her ideal-self.

In the cases of Jennifer and Michael, both had accepted labels as part of their identity. Jennifer had generalized the label of "thunder thighs" to mean, in her self-image, that she was very overweight. Focusing on one part of her body blurred her view of the rest of her figure. Even though her friends had tried to help her see herself in a more realistic light, she held to the label and perception of being overweight. Focusing on one negative physical characteristic and allowing it to adversely affect self-esteem is common, especially during adolescence. Jennifer needs help to see how she has accepted the label of "thunder thighs," generalized it, and incorporated it in her self-image. This insight might help her question the validity of the label and to listen to her friends' positive feedback concerning her figure and weight.

Michael accurately assessed himself as talented in athletics but inaccurately believed he could not be both athletic and intellectual. Assigning labels and roles to relatives is common in families. Parents often place labels such as "the musician," "the brain," or "the athlete" on their children in an effort to reinforce talents they see in them. Unfortunately, parents don't realize that placing the label on one child sometimes discourages siblings from developing potential in the same area. Another unfortunate consequence of labeling is that it makes the labeled person focus on the labeled trait to the exclusion of other talents or interests that he or she might have. By coming to realize how his family label has affected his self-image, Michael is not likely to suddenly perceive himself as being smart. However, he might wonder if he could be smarter than he had thought. He may challenge himself to see if he is capable of more than he had once believed.

Teachers are not in a position to counsel each student and individually review the student's assessment of the three "selves" for accuracy. However, teachers can help students become more aware of their "selves" and realize the influences of media, parents, peers, siblings, and teachers on the formation of self-image, ideal-self, and pygmalion-self (see Box 2-1). Then students can change inaccurate negative evaluations to positive ones, accept those things that they cannot change, and acknowledge their inadequacies as well as recognize their strengths. When students see their shortcomings in a balanced context with their strengths, they can then feel secure and competent enough to try to change.

# Teaching Activities for Self-Evaluation

The following teaching activities are for guiding students to more accurately evaluate themselves. Many of these activities help students identify positive character traits in others as well as in themselves. Each activity indicates its appropriate grade level.

> P = primary, K–3rd grade
> I = intermediate, 4th–6th grade
> J = junior high
> H = high school

In these and all other teaching activities remember that you are dealing with sensitive personal issues. Never pry, force a student to divulge information, or put him or her on the spot.

## "This Is Me" Folder

When students have completed the following activities, place the activities in personalized folders that the students can keep.   (P)

## Picture How I Look

Have students draw a self-portrait. Then have partners draw pictures of each other. Trace silhouettes of each student's shadow to show how the students actually look. Discuss as a class the differences in these three portraits.   (P)

## Describe How I Look

In writing, have students (I) describe each of their physical features in detail, beginning at the head and progressing to the feet, and (2) evaluate how they feel about each feature. When steps I and 2 are completed, have students write a summary of how they see their body as a whole and how they feel about that self-image.   (I, J, H)

## Positive Portraits

Have each student draw a classmate's name out of a hat. Have students draw a picture of that person, then under the picture write five positive characteristics they perceive that student possesses. Then have students share their pictures and the positive attributes they wrote.   (P, I)

*continued*

### Partner's Personality Recipe

Assign each student a partner to get to know over the course of a few weeks. Have them then write a recipe for their partner's personality (I cup athletic, ½ cup generous, etc.).   (I)

### Coat of Arms

On drawing paper, ask students to draw a large shield and then design a personal coat of arms with symbols representing personal talents, traits, values, and aspirations. Give reassurance that this activity is not an evaluation of artistic ability, but is an exercise to build awareness and allow exploration of their self-image.   (I, J, H)

### Getting to Know Me

Have students write endings to complete statements like the following. Encourage depth and honesty by assuring them their answers are for their eyes only.   (I, J, H)

 1. I hate ...
 2. I wish ...
 3. I fear ...
 4. I love ...
 5. I hope ...
 6. I'm embarrassed when ...
 7. The thing that bothers me most is ...
 8. The thing I am most afraid of is ...
 9. I want most to be ...
10. Regarding myself, I feel ...
11. I am most cheerful when ...
12. My greatest interest in life is ...
13. The person who means the most to me is ...
14. The person I would most like to be like is ...
15. I have great respect for ...
16. When bullied, I ...
17. When I am the center of attention, I ...
18. When I am late, I ...
19. When I feel awkward, I ...
20. When given responsibility, I ...
21. When I am embarrassed, I ...
22. When I want to show I like someone, I ...
23. When I am angry, I ...

*continued*

*continued*

24. When others put me down, I ...
25. Four of my greatest pressure points are ...
26. When I am under a lot of stress, I ...

## What Article of Clothing Am I?

Ask each student to draw an article of clothing that symbolizes herself or himself. Students should think about the color, texture, style, and function of the clothing before deciding what article would best describe them. Partners could also draw how they see the other person. Discuss in small groups.    (J, H)

## Strengths and Weaknesses

Discuss the Wiseman's Prayer:

"God grant me the strength to accept the things I cannot change, the courage to change the things I can, and the wisdom to know the difference."

Assign students to write a paper finishing the following sentences. (I, J, H,)

1. My most important strengths are ... (Consider health, creativity, common sense, good habits, natural ability, integrity, skills, etc.)
2. My most serious handicaps are ... (Consider bad habits, bad temper, moodiness, antisocial tendencies, poor ways of problem solving, etc.)
3. Things I can change for the better are ...
4. Things I am going to have to accept are ...

## The Person I Admire Most

Have students write papers on whom they admire most in this world and why. (I, J, H)

## If You Could Have Your Wish

Have students answer the following questions.

1. If you could have your wish for talent, what would it be?
2. If you could have your wish for a change in looks, what would you change?
3. If you could have your wish for money, how much would you want and for what?
4. If you could have your wish for a change in intelligence, what would you wish for and why?
5. If you had to rank your wishes, how would you do it? Does this help you see your ideal-self better?    (I, J, H)

*continued*

### Pygmalion-Self

Have students complete each of the following phrases with at least two answers, preferably in paragraph form.    (I, J, H)

1. My closest friend truly thinks I am ...
2. My classmates think I am ...
3. My parents honestly think I am ...
4. A stranger's first impression of me might include ...

### Roles I Play

After discussing how differently different people can perceive one person, have students complete the following sentences.    (I, J, H)

1. To me, I am ...
2. To my family, I am ...
3. To my peers, I am ...
4. To a special friend, I am ...

## Self-Worth

Feelings of self-worth come from both external and internal factors. Some external factors that contribute to self-worth are appearance, group approval, and social achievements. Thoughts such as "Buy some new clothes (or a sporty car) and you'll feel like a million bucks" or "Make the team, get the lead in the school play, or get a high GPA and *then* you'll be somebody" illustrate how appearance and personal achievements can affect feelings of self-worth. Another term for externally generated self-worth is **conditional worth.** Conditional worth is the concept that self-worth is conditional upon physical appearance, achievements, or competence. On the other hand, internally generated self-worth emanates from feelings that one is an important person regardless of performance or appearance, simply because one is a unique human being with infinite potential. Internal self-worth is also referred to as **unconditional self-worth.**

Most people see themselves and the world around them in external terms. If asked to play word association with names of individuals, people usually answer with external labels: cute, joker, sexy, athletic, skinny, fat, black, white, smart, old, rich, dentist, teacher, and so on. When we base our self-worth solely on external factors, life's challenges can be intensely painful. Consider what happens to the beautiful when beauty fades, is blemished, or altered. Plastic surgery is currently used as a form of psychotherapy for individuals whose self-worth depends on their appearance.

The suicides resulting from the stock market crash of 1929 attest to the loss of self-worth founded on the accumulation of wealth.

A common denominator among children and adolescents likely to attempt or commit suicide is a very low sense of self-worth. Young people basing their self-worth on conditional factors are vulnerable to feelings of worthlessness when there is failure or disappointment. Self-love and self-esteem for these individuals results from their performance or their capacity to feel worthy of it (conditional worth). They derive their esteem from conditions or situations. It is typical for many parents, teachers, and even society as a whole to espouse self-esteem in this manner. As a result of this tendency, we advocate that educational programs emphasize the unconditional worth of students and de-emphasize the conditional worth.

With unconditional self-worth there is diminished emphasis on the externally evident factors that we have discussed in this section (e.g., beauty, wealth, intelligence). You may recall the experience of Jim Brady, who was shot during the attempted assassination of former President Reagan. His injuries left him partially paralyzed and slightly brain-damaged at the height of his career. The shooting altered his personal appearance and slightly diminished his intellect. Nevertheless, Jim Brady demonstrated incredible determination, courage, and unconditional self-worth in making a new life for himself. Unconditional self-worth served as an anchor, and he approached his challenges and new life with enthusiasm, humor, and positive self-esteem.

Another classic example demonstrating unconditional self-worth is Ann Jillian. Ann is a celebrated actress and singer who developed breast cancer. She was one of the first celebrities to publically discuss her battle with breast cancer and she did so in order to help others suffering from cancer or other life calamities. It took great courage to disclose the loss of her breasts from the cancer, especially when you consider that she works in an occupation where a woman's figure is often deemed as important as talent. This demonstrates a high degree of unconditional self-regard. Internal self-worth helps us meet life's challenges and gives us a firm foundation that allows us to work at achieving without fear of failure.

There are many ways that you can boost students' feelings of self-worth. Box 2-2 provides several suggestions that you can use in your teaching career. We also want to stress that although external self-worth is conditional, it is still integral to one's sense of worth. You can help your students develop this type of self-worth by helping them gain skills that improve scholastic performance and emotional well-being. You will find that self-esteem is enhanced when students increase skills in emotion identification and appropriate expression, goal setting, problem solving, media literacy, communication, and relationship development. These skills serve students by fostering a sense of competence and belonging as they find their own special place in the world.

The manner in which teachers and other adults interact with students is critical in forming unconditional self-worth. Positive interactions demonstrating that students are unique, lovable, and important regardless of appearance or performance nurture a strong sense of internal (unconditional) self-worth. Chapter 1 discussed this at length in the section entitled "Interacting with Students."

Having and offering unconditional regard for every student is one of the most difficult, but most powerful, attributes a teacher can develop. It is a sad fact that among all the varieties of at-risk students (e.g., those with low educational aspirations, low self-esteem, low internal locus of control, negative attitudes toward school, history of academic failure, fractured family structure, and/or substance abuse problems), Kagan reports that "the single and most frequent consistent perception" is "that their teachers do not care about them" (pg. 106).[4]

IN THE
CLASSROOM
*2-2*

## Self-Worth Activities

These activities are for building accurate self-images, enhancing positive self-worth, and identifying admirable character traits in self and others.

### I Am Unique

Have students draw pictures or write words that show how they are unique as well as how they are similar to other members in the class. Discuss why people are different (e.g., family traditions, heredity, beliefs, environment, free choice). (P, I, J, H)

### Look at Me!

Place on the floor a large sheet of paper that is folded so it is double thick. Instruct students to lie down on the paper and then have someone trace around them. Cut out the figure. Have students color their figures to show how they look, both front and back. Put the two pictures together and staple around the figure, leaving part of one leg open. Stuff newspaper into the "big picture" and staple the leg shut. The paper dolls will be complete. Dolls can be displayed and then taken home to share with parents. (P)

*continued*

*continued*

### Fingerprints

Help each child make a set of fingerprints. Have them compare fingerprints with three other children. Point out the differences and discuss how each person is unique.   (P, I)

For variation, have students draw eyes, ears, hair, and so forth on their fingerprints and then compare with classmates. Explain that even though two people may look alike (such as identical twins), their fingerprints are different. Have students frame their fingerprints and keep them on their desks as a reminder of their uniqueness.   (P, I)

### Classroom Stars

Make a bulletin board of dark blue paper with a yellow moon in one corner. Have each student make a star, sign it, and write a positive personal quality. You may have to help them identify these qualities. Display all of the students' stars on the bulletin board.   (P, I)

### Sun Spots

Prepare or have students prepare one paper or cardboard sun (circle with perimeter lines for rays) for each student. Cut a hole in the center of each sun and have each student place one of their school pictures in their "frame." Then you, the student, or classmates write special things about each individual on the sun's rays.   (P, I)

### Show-and-Tell Hobbies

Schedule a day for students to share their hobbies with the class. Allow students the opportunity to teach their hobbies to interested classmates. (P, I)

### King/Queen for a Day

On birthdays or some other day, honor each student by having him or her wear a crown and cape and sit in front of the class. Have the other students write and/or illustrate something nice about the honored student. Make these writings and drawings into a "book" and place each student's book in the classroom library to be read by the class during free reading time. In time, have students take their books home.   (P, I)

*continued*

## I Am Good at . . .

Have each student draw a picture to complete this sentence, "I am good at . . .". Ask students to show and explain their drawings to the class. (P, I, J)

## Self-Talk

Introduce the idea that our thoughts affect our emotions, including feelings of self-worth. Ask the class for self-put-downs and self-praise comments and list them on the board. Have students keep a journal of their negative and positive thoughts about themselves, such as "Are you ever going to learn?" "How stupid can you be?" "Hey, you did all right on that!" and "I'm proud of that." Have them note the ratio of positive to negative thoughts and challenge them to a conscious effort to increase the positive.   (J, H)

## Eggs of Praise

At Easter time, give every student in the class a plastic egg with a message in it that recognizes talents, abilities, or positive behavior you have observed. (P, I)

## Fortune Cookies

At Chinese New Year, give every student a fortune cookie that contains positive messages.   (P, I)

## Spotlighting

Place a baby picture of a student on a bulletin board with the caption, "Who is this important person?" Highlight information about this student—place of birth, hobbies, number of siblings, favorite foods, and so on. Make efforts to spotlight students who need recognition or spotlight each throughout the school year.   (P, I, J)

## Slide Show

Throughout the school year, take photographs of the students as they engage in various learning activities. Toward the end of the year, set aside time for students to view the slides, to give and receive comments (positive), and to recall shared experiences.   (P, I)

## Responsibility:  Are We Proactive or Reactive?

Taking responsibility for our life, for our actions and choices, is another key element of emotional well-being. Three prominent theories of determinism—genetic, psychic, and environmental—state that factors beyond our control are responsible for our behavior. Genetic determinism basically says that "It's your grandpa's fault"; it's in your DNA, it's in your nature. Psychic determinism says "It's your parents fault"; it's your upbringing, your childhood experiences, or emotional scripting that makes you who you are. Environmental determinism says "It's your boss's, spouse's, or the economy's fault." In other words, someone or something in the environment is responsible for your situation.

We do not deny the influence that genetic, psychic, and environmental factors have on human behavior. However, we want to bring to your attention the concept of **proactivity,** which rejects the view that people and organizations are *controlled* by genetic, historical, or environmental forces. Covey explains: "As human beings, we are responsible for our own lives. Our behavior is a function of our decisions, not our conditions. We can subordinate feelings to values."[5] Highly proactive people "do not blame circumstances, conditions, or conditioning for their behavior. Their behavior is a product of their own conscious choice, based on values, rather than a product of their conditions, based on feelings" (pg. 71). The concept of proactivity emphasizes taking personal responsibility for behavior.

A classic example comes from the life of Victor Frankl, a Jewish psychologist incarcerated in Auschwitz during World War II. While standing naked, alone, and stripped of all his earthly possessions and family, Frankl envisioned that he had only one freedom left, the freedom to choose his responses. This realization led to the choice to forgive his captors. His forgiveness was not the result of benevolence; rather, he knew that holding on to hatred and resentment would destroy him. He continued to develop his freedom of response as the weeks and months dragged on. While digging ditches, marching, and enduring countless persecutions, he envisioned himself in the future, lecturing to university students on the lessons he learned in the concentration camp. In time, Frankl developed more freedom than his captors. Although they had more liberty, he had more freedom.

Christopher Reeve starred in the movies as Superman and in several other roles. In 1995 he was fully paralyzed as a result of a tragic accident suffered during an equestrian competition. Rather than allowing this situation to control him, he chose to take control over his life and to be happy. You can imagine how much anguish he feels upon awaking in the morning after a night of dreaming of walking, sailing, and playing with his children as the reality of his paralysis becomes evident. He reports that when this happens he "shakes it off" and focuses on what he can do. Although he does not have the freedom to move, he has been the major force mobilizing scientists to find a way of reversing paralysis, something most people thought impossible until Christopher Reeve joined the effort. You can see why Christopher Reeve is viewed by those who know his story as a real "Superman."

In every circumstance in life we have the choice to be reactive or proactive. **Reactive** people are more or less controlled by circumstance or the environment. If they are treated well, they tend to feel and act "good." If they are treated badly, they feel bad and are defensive. Reactive people build their emotional lives around the behavior of others, believing that love is a feeling, bestowed upon them like cupids' arrows. On the other hand, proactive people, such as Victor Frankl and Christopher Reeve, "carry their own weather" with them. This means that they choose, to a large extent, how they are going to respond. They are value driven, having a carefully selected and internalized value code. Proactive people have the ability to subordinate an impulse to a value. This is the essence of proactivity—choosing how to act rather than being acted upon by circumstance, environment, or even impulse. Proactive people also think love is a verb, something they do rather than something that happens to them. To be proactive is to be empowered.

We urge you to emphasize this powerful principle as you teach students. Individuals do not happen to just "fall into" proactive thinking. It takes self-awareness, effort, and the building of character to achieve this way of thinking and living. You can help your students develop proactive living through modeling this behavior in your interactions with them. Insist that they take responsibility for their own actions; do not allow them to blame their behavior on someone else. Help your students develop a proactive thinking and speaking style (see Box 2-3.) If you want to gauge your proactive versus reactive thinking, observe patterns in what you say to others. Reactive language contains statements such as "There's nothing I can do," "She makes me so mad," "That's just the way I am," "I have to do it," "I can't," and "If only . . . ". Proactive thinking is identified with statements such as "I can . . . ," "I control . . . ," "I choose . . . ," and "I will . . . ". You can help students substitute their "I can'ts" with "I will" and their "I have to's" with "I choose to."

---

IN THE
CLASSROOM

*2-3*

## Proactive Teaching Activity

Have each student list their "I can'ts" on a sheet of paper. Give students time to think and write until they have filled their paper with comments such as "I can't do long division," "I can't sit still very long," "I can't do a cartwheel,"

*continued*

*continued*

"I can't stand vegetables," "I can't stay up late." Be sure and do this activity along with your students: "I can't get the school to give me more funding," "I can't get Justin to complete his homework," "I can't get Jennifer's mother to come in for a conference."

After 10 or so minutes have the students put their pieces of paper into a shoe box that has been decorated to look like a coffin. Add your sheet of "I can'ts" to the box.

Lead your students out to the school yard and dig a grave for "I Can't." At the graveside read the eulogy provided below. If it is not possible to bury the box with your students present, modify this activity to meet your circumstances.

### Eulogy

We have gathered here today to honor the memory of "I Can't." While he was with us on earth, he touched the lives of everyone, some more than others. His name, unfortunately, has been spoken in every public building—schools, city halls, state capitols and yes, even the White House. We have provided "I Can't" with a final resting place and a headstone that includes his epitaph. He is survived by his brothers and sister, "I Can," "I Will," and "I'm Going to Right Away." They are not as well known as their famous relative and are certainly not as strong and powerful yet. Perhaps some day, with your help, they will make an even bigger mark on the world. May "I Can't" rest in peace and may everyone present pick up their lives and move forward in his absence. Amen.

After the funeral, cut out a large tombstone from butcher paper and write "I Can't" at the top, put RIP in the middle, and write the date at the bottom. Display this tombstone all year as a reminder for when a student forgets and says "I can't." When this happens, simply point to the tombstone and have your student rephrase his or her statement.    (P, I, J, H)

Source: Adapted from C. Moorman, "Rest in Peace: The 'I Can't' Funeral," in *Chicken Soup for the Soul.* Deerfield Beach, FL: Health Communications, 1993.

## Emotional Intelligence

In education classes you hear quite a bit about mental intelligence (IQ) and how it relates to success in academics and other aspects of life. Another type of intelligence that plays a prominent role in healthy development is **emotional intelligence.** Daniel Goleman explains in his widely sold book, *Emotional Intelligence: Why It Can Matter More Than IQ,* how essential emotional intelligence is to success in life.[6] He relates that success is difficult even for those who have high mental intelligence, if they lack emotional intelligence. On the other hand, those with modest mental intelligence but who have high emotional intelligence usually do quite well in schooling and career, social life, and family life. Goleman identifies the following as aspects of emotional intelligence:

1. *Knowing what you are currently feeling.* Developing this type of self-awareness takes time and practice and is crucial in making many of life's choices, such as choosing a career or marriage partner.

2. *Recognizing emotions in others.* Empathy is the fundamental people skill. People who are empathetic are more tuned to the subtle social signals of others. They have, so to speak, a social antenna. Individuals who can "read" others are often identified as "star" employees by coworkers. They are able to work well with others, cooperatively solving problems and creating synergistic energy. Conversely, those who have a hard time tuning into others find establishing and maintaining relationships difficult. They can become loners or bullies.

3. *Impulse control and delayed gratification.* These two key elements of managing emotions are the foundation of every accomplishment, from staying on a diet to pursuing a medical degree. Conversely, those having problems with impulse control and delayed gratification are more likely to drop out of school, become pregnant as teenagers, abuse drugs, and end up in jail.

4. *Being able to calm oneself.* We all experience anger, frustration, insecurity and other negative emotions from time to time. Knowing how to deal with these emotions and appropriately calm ourselves are critical aspects of emotional intelligence.

While mental intelligence is thought to be fixed, something we are born with, emotional intelligence can be developed. It can be nurtured and strengthened as children become experienced in various emotional situations. It is believed by Goleman that these learning experiences actually change the brain by creating new "circuitry" patterns that increase one's emotional intelligence. Educators play an integral role in the development of emotional literacy among students.

## Recognizing Emotions

You can facilitate the emotional intelligence of students by first teaching them to identify their feelings and the feelings of those around them (see Box 2-4). Young children especially find it difficult to articulate what they are feeling, other than to say they feel good or bad. Older students usually are not much more adept at identifying and articulating their emotions. Yet, once students are able to label an emotion, they can more easily verbalize their feelings and appropriately communicate their needs to others.

The ability to recognize and appropriately express emotions is especially important in adolescence. This is typically a very emotionally charged time of life, with many contributing factors, including hormones.

Teenagers need to know that it is normal for them to experience wide mood swings, to learn not to take these mood swings too seriously, and to develop appropriate ways of sharing their feelings with others. Group discussions help adolescents come to see that they are not alone in their experiences.

## Empathy

**Empathy** is the ability to understand the feelings of others, to recognize emotions and have the sensitivity to understand how those emotions can make someone feel. Another person's emotions are often displayed through body language, which serves as a means of communicating feelings. For example, in your mind you can probably picture the body language of someone who is sad or depressed. Other emotions invoke discernible body responses. Teach your students to recognize these responses. Through the use of video clips and pictures, students can learn to interpret the facial expressions and body movements of characters. You can also teach these concepts by having students role-play different emotions. Or, have students play charades in which different emotions are acted out and the students guess the emotion that is displayed. You can also teach empathy by discussing what people might have felt in historical settings, in fictional settings, or in real-life situations observed on the news or in daily interactions. Recognizing emotions and empathizing with others are skills some children learn quickly, whereas others need considerably more help.

## Impulse Control and Delayed Gratification

We live in a world saturated with advertisements whose messages tell us that we can have what we want *now*, that we *deserve it*, that we *should* have it. Educational efforts need to counterbalance these messages and pressures. Children can learn **impulse control** and **delayed gratification** through simple classroom structure. For example, these skills can be learned through very simple means, such as not getting a drink of water until a designated time, not speaking in class until called upon, and staying seated until the bell rings. Delayed gratification is learned when students achieve a reward that requires work and effort. Goal-setting activities help students learn the satisfaction of aiming for a goal, working to achieve the goal, and succeeding in reaching the goal. In the process, students learn delayed gratification.

## Calming Oneself

Part of knowing how to deal with emotions and how to calm ourselves is understanding what contributes to the intensity of our negative feelings.

Not getting enough sleep can magnify negative feelings, decrease coping skills, and create warped perceptions of reality. Children often stay up late watching TV and miss out on much-needed rest. Adolescents also lose sleep due to staying up late for such activities as watching TV, extracurricular activities, or studying. The need for sleep during adolescence is great because it is a time of rapid growth, but encouraging students to get more sleep can be difficult because a later bedtime is often thought to be a right of age. Class discussions on the emotional effects of sleep deprivation may persuade students to take a good look at their own sleep needs, especially if it is clear that healthy, mature people take responsibility for such needs.

Recognizing our negative thinking patterns can also be a powerful means of gaining control over our emotions and soothing ourselves. By changing our thinking patterns, we can change what we feel. Take the example of Ann, a very conscientious young driver who drives her parent's new car to school. Ann is in the habit of swearing under her breath at inconsiderate drivers on the road. As a result, she often arrives at her destination exasperated, tense, and angry. In class she learns how negative thoughts can produce negative emotions and takes the challenge to think positively of those she perceives to have wronged her. On her way home, a car pulls out in front of her and she has to slam on the brakes in order to avoid a collision. Just as she is about to burst forth with colorful language, she remembers her resolve and, instead, says out loud, "I . . . I . . . I . . . I bless you to get wherever you are going safely!" Immediately she starts laughing, feeling relaxed, calm, and even happy. Ann had been in the habit of thinking others were thoughtless, self-centered, reckless drivers out to put a ding in her parents' new car and get her in trouble. In actuality, poor drivers like the one who pulled out in front of her might be confused, distracted, or ill. When Ann blessed the other driver she in effect blessed herself.

There are several techniques for gaining control over negative emotions and being able to sooth ourselves. The old advice of counting to 10 in a frustrating situation can be very helpful, especially if during that time we evaluate why we are frustrated, check any thinking patterns that add to our frustration, and determine if the situation is worth getting upset over. Is there anything we can do about it? Distracting ourselves can also help minimize negative emotions. Ann distracted herself when she took time to think of the blessing she gave to the other driver. We can distract ourselves by turning on a radio, reading something, engaging in a physical activity, or by looking for something humorous in the frustrating situation. One family has a rule that they can argue about anything, but when doing so they must lie down beside each other and sing their hostilities to one another. This family has discovered that arguments handled in this way soon turn into giggling sessions.

# Teaching Activities for Emotions

Additional activities dealing with emotions, including empathy, are located in Box 2-5: Relationship-Building Activities.

## Emotional Charades

Have students act out different emotions, utilizing only nonverbal language. This activity can be used to help younger children identify and then label different emotions, demonstrate how emotions affect behavior, and demonstrate concepts in nonverbal communication.   (P, I, J, H)

## Sentence Completion

Have students complete sentences such as the following, to help them see that feelings are universal.   (I, J, H)

> When nothing seems to go right, I feel . . .
> When someone laughs at me, I feel . . .
> When I do a good job on something, I feel . . .
> When I am afraid, I feel . . .

## Show-and-Tell Emotions

For show-and-tell, have everyone explore topics such as my most frightening experience, my most embarrassing experience, or what makes me really angry. Sharing can help them realize that others sometimes feel as they do and can help them cope.   (P)

## Pictures

Have students cut out pictures of people showing various emotions. Make a bulletin board. Discuss possible reasons for the feelings that are expressed. Animal pictures may also be included.   (P)

## Faces of Emotions

Have students try to match these pictures with the following emotions.

| | | | |
|---|---|---|---|
| • Anger | • Distrust | • Frustration | • Pride |
| • Confusion | • Embarrassment | • Happiness | • Sadness |
| • Contentment | • Excitement | • Indifference | • Satisfaction |
| • Determination | • Fear | • Love | • Worry |

*continued*

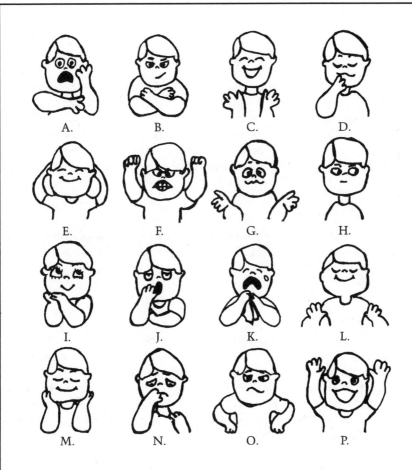

A.    B.    C.    D.
E.    F.    G.    H.
I.    J.    K.    L.
M.    N.    O.    P.

## Drawing How I Feel

Ask students to draw a picture of how they feel right now. When the pictures are completed, discuss the following questions: What colors did you use and why? What is the size of the picture in relation to the paper? What were you thinking about as you were drawing? Have your feelings changed since completing the picture? If so, why?   (P, I, J)

## Fear and Shadow Games

Using ordinary objects, turn out the lights and use a spotlight to show the frightening shadows these objects can make. Involve students by asking them to suggest other objects that cast shadows. Discuss fear of the dark and how they have or might be able to overcome their fear.   (P)

*continued*

*continued*

### What Am I Feeling?

Break students into groups of three. Have them discuss for a few minutes how they remember feeling in the distant past (e.g., in kindergarten, two Christmases ago). Then ask them to discuss in their small groups how they felt on a particular day last week. Finally, ask them to discuss how they are feeling right now. Gently push them beyond one-word answers such as "bored" or "tired." Tuning into present feelings is more difficult than identifying emotions felt in the past.   (J, H)

### Emotional Crisis

Ask each student to collect newspaper articles that describe how individuals have reacted to an emotional crisis. Discuss the emotional need the person may have been trying to satisfy. In what other ways might the emotional need have been met?   (I, J, H)

### Letting off Steam

As a class, define what emotional "steam" is, discuss where it comes from, and the proper and improper times and means of "letting it off." Have students make a simple poster illustrating both destructive and constructive methods of letting off steam. Discuss posters and any unaddressed methods. Display posters on the wall. *Object lesson:* Introduce the concept by demonstrating how real steam can be both harmful (burn) and beneficial (fuel a steam engine).   (P, I, J, H)

### Emotional Log

Have students keep a two-day log of the emotional reactions displayed by people around them. Discuss in class and/or have students write a report of the effect these reactions had on them and other people who were present.   (I, J, H)

### Influence of Emotions

Discuss how emotions can influence routine activities and make them unsafe (e.g., driving a car, baby-sitting). Ask students to relate personal experiences. (J, H)

### Thoughts on Thoughts

Make bulletin boards of the following quotes and discuss how our thoughts influence our feelings.   (I, J, H)

*continued*

> *Shakespeare:* "There is nothing either good or bad, but thinking makes it so."
>
> *Milton:* "The mind is its own place, and in itself can make a heaven of hell, a hell of heaven."
>
> *Ralph Waldo Emerson:* "A man is what he thinks about all day long."
>
> *Norman Vincent Peale:* "It has been said that thoughts are things, that they actually possess dynamic power. You can actually think yourself into or out of situations. Conditions are created by thoughts far more powerfully than conditions create thoughts."
>
> *Dale Carnegie:* "Our thoughts make us what we are."
>
> *David O. McKay:* "Happiness is not an external condition, it is a state of the spirit and an attitude of the mind."
>
> *Hugh B. Brown:* "You can't think crooked and walk straight."
>
> *Source unknown:* "The city of happiness is found in the state of mind."

## Resilience and Asset Development

**Resilience** can be defined as succeeding in spite of serious challenges and adverse circumstances (e.g., neglect; maltreatment; dysfunctional, alcoholic or drug-dependent families; high levels of family conflict; poverty; physical disability; trauma). Although resilience means success in terms of healthy human development and well-being, it does not mean that resilient youth remain unaffected, invulnerable, or unscathed. We can learn a great deal from resilient children and youth. Studies have been conducted to discover how these children thrive in spite of difficult circumstances. Researchers have looked to find what resilient children have in common. The characteristics they found have been called **protective factors.** Masten points out that results from longitudinal studies of resilient children and youth show that the most important of all protective factors is a strong relationship with a competent, caring, prosocial adult.[7] She also lists the following as critical protective factors: normal cognitive development (e.g., average or better IQ scores, good attention skills, and "street smarts"), feelings of self-worth and self-efficacy, feelings of hope and meaningfulness of life, attractiveness to others (in personality or appearance), talents valued by self and others, and faith and religious affiliations.

If a high-risk environment is the family itself (e.g., children are growing up in an alcoholic or drug-abusing family), studies suggest that children have a better chance of growing into healthy adulthood if they meet the following criteria.[8]

❖ Can learn to do one thing well that is valued by themselves, their friends, or their community

❖ Are required to be helpful as they grow up

❖ Are able to ask for help for themselves

❖ Are able to elicit positive responses from others in their environment

❖ Are able to distance themselves from their dysfunctional families so that the family is not their sole frame of reference

❖ Are able to bond with some socially valued, positive entity such as school, community group, church, or another family

❖ Are able to interact with a caring adult who provides consistent caring responses

**Asset development** focuses on naming and increasing the positive building blocks in young people's lives. It has become a movement supported by government, communities, and school districts. More than 500,000 students from sixth to twelfth grade helped the Search Institute identify 40 developmental assets that act as protective factors for youth.[9] These assets have been organized into eight categories: support (family support, caring school climate), empowerment (service, safety), boundaries and expectations (family and school boundaries, positive peer influence), constructive use of time (youth programs, religious community), commitment to learning (homework, reading for pleasure), positive values (integrity, restraint), social (planning and decision making, cultural competence), and positive identity (sense of purpose, positive view of personal future). A detailed listing and explanation of the 40 assets can be found at www.search-institute.org.

Research has shown that the more assets youth have, the fewer the risk patterns and the more positive behaviors youth experience. Asset-rich young people are much less likely to abuse alcohol or to experience negative behaviors. The average young person has less than one-half of the 40 assets. Only 8% of youth are asset rich, that is, having 31 to 40 assets. One in five young people are asset poor, experiencing as few as 0 to 10 assets. Youth have fewer assets as they get older. The least common assets experienced by youth (just 19% to 25%) are a caring school, being treated as valuable resources, reading for pleasure, having their community value youth, and spending time in creative activities.

Asset development endeavors to emphasize the informal relationships and opportunities that all adults can provide for young people in their everyday lives. Often Americans fail to do something about children's problems because they feel overwhelmed as they hear, see, and read about the extent of the problems facing young people today. Asset building says to everyone that we have a role to play, that we can say hello to a teenager, ask youth to help us help others, thank media when positive messages are broadcast about youth, and just smile more at young people. Those working in schools can have a direct impact on about one-half of the assets and an indirect effect on most of the rest. School professionals can help create a caring school climate, ensure there are plentiful after-school programs with lots of physical activity for all children, ensure that young people develop good goal-setting and decision-making skills, and provide opportunities for youth to contribute service and help others.

## Relationship Building

Relationship-building skills are vital to emotional well-being. Positive interpersonal relationships form the basis for many human needs. Relationships with significant others can alleviate loneliness, secure stimulation, establish contact for self-knowledge, and provide a means of sharing joy and pain. Young people often lack the skills to initiate and maintain satisfying relationships, resolve conflict, and deal with the deterioration or dissolution of relationships.

Intimate friendships do not develop immediately, but are built as they progress gradually through a series of stages. Understanding these stages and the skills necessary for their development and maintenance can help students build meaningful friendships. It can also help them strengthen family bonds.

In the first stage, initial **contact** is made and basic information is exchanged ("Hi, my name is Brittany"). Physical appearance often plays an important initial role. Other important factors are personal qualities such as friendliness, warmth, and openness. Classroom activities can help students develop and refine skills in initiating conversation and relationships. Students should learn about their tendencies to label and make premature judgments based on physical appearance. This knowledge will help them to develop greater empathy and appreciation for their classmates and others. Learning about the processes of nonverbal communication helps students to analyze and interpret the messages they send and receive during the contact stage.

The **acquaintance stage** entails a commitment to get to know another person better and to become more open with this person. Feelings and emotions are shared, but only in a preliminary way. Relationships often abort during this stage when one person is unable to open up to the other, or opens up too much too soon. It is helpful for students to be aware of levels of communication. Communication ranges from a level of small talk ("That's a great shirt you're wearing") to the sharing of ideas ("Why don't we try doing it this way?") to self-disclosure ("I'm having trouble getting along with my mom").

The **intimacy stage** is characterized by a further commitment to another person. Becoming a best friend, boyfriend, or girlfriend are examples of this type of relationship. Intimacy is reserved for very few people at any one time. Children, for example, often have best friends to the exclusion of playing with others. Deep feelings and emotions are exchanged by intimates that are not shared with others outside this bond.

Having a best friend helps children learn intimacy skills. However, such strong bonding should not and does not mean excluding all others. Students can be taught how harmful cliques can be to the self-esteem of others and to themselves. Charity can be fostered for all class members as they are encouraged to interact with each other.

The **deterioration stage** is experienced when individuals begin to feel that the relationship may not be as important as they once thought, or when the parties grow apart. Less time is spent together, awkward silences may occur, communication is not as open, and physical contact is not as frequent. Conflicts are more likely and reconciliation more difficult than earlier in the relationship. Conflicts often go unresolved because there is an inclination not to bother with reconciliation. When efforts are not taken to alter these events, deterioration can progress to dissolution of the relationship.

Deterioration is sometimes a natural, healthy way for individuals to grow apart. Children and adolescents need to learn how to gracefully stop being a best friend with someone or to "break up" with a girlfriend or boyfriend. Unfortunately, all too often youth become cruel in their efforts. Role-playing and effective communication skills (discussed later in this chapter) can help students learn to be kind in this stage.

Even though the deterioration stage is sometimes healthy, there are times when relationships crumble that could and should have been maintained. Family ties and relationships are especially vulnerable if left in the deterioration stage. Coming to understand mixed messages by appropriately using "I" messages, engaging in active listening, and being appropriately assertive can assist individuals in resolving conflicts. Students can be asked to take a good, long look at the health of some of their most important interpersonal relationships. They can ask themselves, "What needs to be improved? How can *I* make it better?" See Box 2-5 for more ideas on maintaining and rebuilding a relationship.

A relationship **dissolves** when bonds are severed that once united individuals. Sometimes roles are redefined, such as from boyfriend or girlfriend to "just friends." At other times, so many negative emotions are present between individuals that they purposely avoid each another. Divorce is the outcome of a marriage that has reached this stage. Pain, bitterness, anger, rage, frustration, betrayal, and hurt are a few of the negative emotions that can result when a relationship dissolves. Many students have experienced some of these negative emotions due to dissolved relationships with peers or family members. Discussions of how to handle these negative emotions or avoid them in future experiences can be helpful.

Covey gives great insight into how we can develop and maintain strong relationships.[5] He likens personal relationships to bank accounts. We have a different "bank account" with everyone we know, and we need to consciously make many deposits in accounts if we want them to remain "fiscally sound." Whether our relationship with another is at the low- or high-quality end of the relationship continuum depends on the amount of deposits and withdrawals we have made in that account. High-quality relationships have accounts with abundant funds. When a person makes an occasional withdrawal, such as being unsympathetic, not keeping a promise, or disciplining a child, the relationship survives fine because there were enough "funds" to cover the withdrawal. Relationships at the low-quality end of the relationship continuum have minimal funds or have been run into bankruptcy. Such relationships are full of conflict and animosity. The only way to correct such accounts is to minimize withdrawals and make steady generous deposits over time. Covey identifies six major types of deposits we can make: understanding the individual, small courtesies and kindnesses, keeping commitments, showing personal integrity, clarifying expectations, and apologizing sincerely. We will now take a closer look at each type of deposit.

*Understanding the individual* entails recognizing what is important to that person and taking interest in it. A teenage boy may not be interested in the stock market, but occasionally reading the financial section of the newspaper and discussing it with his father who is a stockbroker will make large deposits in their joint intimacy account.

*Small courtesies and kindnesses* are often underrated, but the relationship funds banked by notes, winks, hugs, tired-feet massages, opening doors, and saying thank you quickly add up. These small acts demonstrate appreciation and that the other person's physical and emotional state are important to us.

*Keeping our commitments* means doing what we say we will when we say we will. A boy who promises to attend his girlfriend's game but doesn't makes a withdrawal. A 12-year-old boy who promises to mow the yard when he comes home from school and does so without further reminders makes a deposit. A teacher who takes promised disciplinary action makes both a withdrawal and a deposit, thus breaking even.

*Clarifying expectations* is critically important in avoiding contention and hurt feelings. We can easily encounter daily conflicts when we try to read others' minds or expect them to read ours. A mother's idea of a clean room may be much different from that of her child's. A newly wed woman's perception of sharing the housecleaning chores may be different from her husband's. A father picking up his daughter at the mall may expect her to be waiting somewhere different from where she is. A teacher's perception of an A-quality report may be different from his students. Clearly communicating our expectations helps us strengthen our relationships.

*Showing personal integrity* means demonstrating character in all our actions and relationships. For instance, if a person speaks ill of someone not present, we may wonder what that person says about us behind our back. How we treat one person can affect our relationship with 30. A young man once said to his youth leader, "You know how you are always telling us you love us? I didn't believe you until today." The leader asked what had made the difference. The young man replied, "I've always tried to be real good around you. I figured if you knew the real me you wouldn't love me. Today Johnny messed up real bad and you wouldn't let the rest of us crawl all over him. You loved Johnny even when he didn't deserve it. That's when I knew you loved me."

*Apologizing sincerely* when we have intentionally or unintentionally made a mistake is one of the surest and fastest ways of strengthening a relationship. Unfortunately, our pride often holds us back from saying, "I'm sorry . . .". Our mistake turns into a relationship deficit when it could have easily become a relationship asset.

---

IN THE
CLASSROOM
*2–5*

## Relationship-Building Activities

### Relationship Bank Accounts

Make a relationship bank by wrapping a cereal box in paper and putting a slit in the top of the box. Place a picture of a person on the front of the bank to represent who the account is with. Use the items pictured below to help students identify and remember the various kinds of relationship deposits. Create a deposit slip for each type of relationship deposit and then make six copies of each type of slip. Divide the class into six groups. Give each group a set of deposit slips. Instruct the groups to write real-life examples on each of their slips. Have group representatives take turns sharing with the class what is written on their slips and placing their slips in the relationship bank.    (P, I, J, H)

Showing **interest**

Small **change**—acts of kindness

Good **credit**—keeping commitments

*continued*

**Checking** expectations

Pure **gold**—showing integrity

**Cash**—apologizing

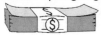

## A Pat on the Back

Have students pin a blank piece of paper on their backs. Every student is to write one positive thing about each classmate on his or her back. You should participate as well. When everyone has written on everyone else's backs, have the students return to their seats, take the papers off their backs, and quietly read the comments. Discuss how it felt to have others write on their backs and how the comments make them feel. (Comments may be shallow and superficial, such as "nice shoes.")

Ask the class to help you come up with a list of admirable characteristics (e.g., hard working, honest, loyal). Make a permanent copy of this list and display it in the classroom. Tell the students that they will be repeating this activity in a couple of months. Challenge the students to look for these characteristics in one another and be ready to write even more meaningful comments on each others' backs. Be sure to follow through and repeat the activity.   (I, J, H)

## Catch Somebody Doing Something Good

1. Have students draw and display posters showing good things they catch somebody doing.
2. Chart every time a student describes something nice he or she caught someone else doing, and encourage sharing such comments with the entire class. Or, place a large sheet of paper on or near the door for the students to record who they caught doing something nice and what the person was doing.
3. Post a tally sheet next to the door for marking down every time the students felt like tattling on others' bad behavior but didn't.

*continued*

*continued*

4. Evaluate class progress by keeping weekly records of the number of positive comments and negative tallies.
5. Include parents through letters, phone calls, or parent night. Encourage catching children doing good things at home.   (P, I)

### Label Headbands

Create a list of positive and negative character traits (e.g., beautiful, athletic, smart, creative, sensitive, ugly, stupid, smelly, rude). Place a headband labeled with one of the characteristics on each student, taking care that they don't see what the labels say. Instruct students not to tell each other what their labels say. Give them a small group activity to complete with instructions to treat every person in the group according to his or her label. After the assigned activity, and before the students have removed the headbands, have them guess what their labels say. Discuss how they treated each other according to the labels and how it made them feel.   (I, J, H)

### Secret Pals

Have each student draw the name of a classmate for whom he or she is to do something special, for example, draw a picture, write a poem, give a special little treat. Make sure each child receives something from a secret pal, even if one has to be you.   (P, I)

### I Do Care

Have the students individually make a list of the most important people in their lives. Have them write down ways to show these people that they care about them (e.g., inquire about their activities, listen carefully, apologize when wrong, compromise, show appreciation, respect their ideas, show affection) and a list of things the students do that might make these people feel they do not care (don't listen, talk only about self, interrupt, act uninterested, criticize, break promises, never show appreciation or affection). Have each student choose one person from the list and keep a log of his or her interactions with that individual for a week. Challenge students to make a conscious effort to increase the ways they show this individual that they care.   (J, H)

### A "Fuzzy" Activity

**Part One:** Read the short story "A Fuzzy Tale" on p. 67 and discuss these questions:

*continued*

1. What is a "warm fuzzy"?
2. Why don't people give away more warm fuzzies?
3. Can someone really die from the lack of warm fuzzies?
4. What are "cold pricklies"?
5. What kind of potions and salves do people really buy?
6. Why do people spend so much money on these products?
7. How can people buy warm fuzzies?
8. What are plastic fuzzies?
9. How do you tell the difference between a warm fuzzy and a plastic fuzzy?

**Part Two:** Practice giving warm fuzzies (see other activities on giving compliments and communication skills). Have students make "live" (acrylic pom-pons) or paper warm fuzzies they can exchange with each other as they exchange emotional warm fuzzies.

**Part Three:** Have students draw a picture of their favorite warm, fuzzy experiences.   (P, I, J, H; higher grades need modifications)

### A Fuzzy Tale

Once upon a time, not far from here, lived a very happy couple called Tyler and Megan. They had two children named Michael and Emily. To realize how happy this family was, you have to understand how things were in their day. You see, at birth everyone was given a small, soft, fuzzy bag. Whenever a person reached into this bag he or she could pull out a warm fuzzy.

Warm fuzzies were in great demand because whenever you received one it made you feel warm and fuzzy all over. Getting enough warm fuzzies was never a problem. Whenever someone felt like it, he or she could walk up to you and say, "I'd like to have a warm fuzzy." You would then reach into your bag, pull out a fuzzy the size of a newborn kitten, and place it on the person's shoulder, head, or lap. The warm fuzzy would cuddle against the person's skin and melt, spreading the warm feeling from head to toe. There were plenty of warm fuzzies to go around, and as a result, everyone felt warm and fuzzy most of the time.

One day a bad witch became angry because everyone was so happy and no one was buying her potions and salves. The wicked witch devised a fiendish and very clever plan. One beautiful spring morning she crept up to Tyler while Megan was playing with their daughter and whispered in his ear, "Look there, Tyler. See all the fuzzies Megan is giving to Emily? You know, don't you, that if she keeps this up, she's going to eventually run out and there won't be any left for you!"

Tyler was shocked. He wheeled on the witch and said, "Do you mean to tell me that there won't be a warm fuzzy in our bag every time we reach into it?"

*continued*

*continued*

The witch slyly answered, "That's right! And once you run out, buster, that's it. You can't get any more." She then sped away on her broom, cackling hysterically.

Tyler took the witch's warning to heart and began to notice every time Megan gave a warm fuzzy to someone else. He eventually became very worried and upset because he adored Megan's warm fuzzies and didn't want to give them up. He certainly didn't think it was right for Megan to spend all her warm fuzzies on the children and on other people. He began to complain every time he saw Megan give a warm fuzzy to someone else. Because Megan didn't like to see Tyler upset, she stopped giving warm fuzzies to other people so often, and reserved them for him.

The children observed this and soon got the idea that it was wrong to give up warm fuzzies any time they were asked or felt like it. They too became very careful. They would watch their parents very closely, and object whenever they felt that one of their parents was giving too many fuzzies to others. They also began to worry whenever they themselves gave away too many warm fuzzies. Even though they found a warm fuzzy every time they reached into their bags, they reached in less and less often, and became more and more stingy.

People soon began to notice the lack of warm fuzzies, and they began to feel less warm and fuzzy. They began to shrivel up and, occasionally, people would die from the lack of warm fuzzies. More and more people went to the witch to buy her potions and salves even though they didn't seem to work.

The wicked witch was delighted at her increased sales but was distressed by the deaths due to the lack of warm fuzzies, because dead people don't buy potions and salves. So, the witch came up with a new plan. She saw to it that everyone was given a bag that was very similar to a fuzzy bag, except this one was cold while the fuzzy bag was warm. Inside the new bag were cold pricklies. These cold pricklies did not make people feel warm and fuzzy, but cold and prickly instead. The cold pricklies, however, did prevent people from shriveling up and dying.

From then on, whenever someone said, "I want a warm fuzzy," people who were worried about depleting their supply would say, "I can't give you a warm fuzzy, but I can give you a cold prickly." Sometimes two people would walk up to each other, thinking they could get a warm fuzzy, but one or the other would change his or her mind, and they'd end up giving each other cold pricklies. The result was that while very few people were dying, a lot of people were feeling very cold, prickly, and unhappy.

The situation got very, very complicated. Since people were no longer freely exchanging warm fuzzies, there were fewer and fewer to go around.

Warm fuzzies, which used to be thought as plentiful as air, became very valuable. This caused people to do all sorts of things to obtain them. Before the witch appeared, people used to gather in groups of three, four, or five, never caring too much who was giving warm fuzzies to whom. After the coming of the witch, people began to pair off and reserve all their warm

*continued*

fuzzies exclusively for each other. People who forgot themselves and gave a warm fuzzy to someone other than their partner would immediately feel guilty. People who could not find a generous partner had to buy their warm fuzzies. Some people somehow became "popular" and got a lot of warm fuzzies without having to return them. These people would then sell their warm fuzzies to people who were "unpopular."

A further complication was that some people would take the easily available cold pricklies, coat them white and fluffy, and pass them off as warm fuzzies. These counterfeit warm fuzzies were really plastic fuzzies, and they caused additional difficulties. For instance, two people would freely exchange plastic fuzzies presuming the fuzzies would make them feel good, but they felt hollow and bad instead. Since they thought they had been exchanging warm fuzzies, people grew very confused about this, never realizing their cold prickly feelings were the result of having been given a lot of plastic fuzzies.

And so, you see, the situation was very, very dismal and it all started because of the witch who made people believe that some day, when least expected, they might reach into their warm fuzzy bag and find it empty.

Source: Adapted from the Idaho State Health Education Guide Grades K–3, 1977.

## Communication Skills

Understanding the principles of effective communication is helpful in developing and maintaining interpersonal relationships. Communication skills include understanding the dynamics of how messages are sent and received, listening skills, and communication styles. Artwork can also be a powerful means of communicating ideas and emotions.

### Sending and Interpreting Messages

We communicate in many ways. The saying "Actions speak louder than words" refers to the importance of **body language** in communication. Actors understand the importance of body language in communicating emotion. When happiness, disappointment, disbelief, or other emotions are displayed on the screen, they are done so primarily through body language. Body language includes facial expressions, posture while standing, sitting, and walking, how close we are to others, and the amount and type of eye contact made.

The tone of voice used is also an important part of sending and interpreting messages. Take a simple statement such as "You are really good at math" and see how many messages you can express changing your voice and inflection. Can you express praise, ridicule, and scorn without changing the wording of the statement?

When we send mixed messages others have trouble interpreting our message. **Mixed messages** are sent when spoken words and body language or tone of voice do not match. For instance, a little boy said to his teacher, "You don't like fourth-grade boys, do you?" His teacher responded, "I love fourth-grade boys." The little guy then said, "I wish you would tell your face that." When we receive a mixed message we tend to believe the non-verbal over the spoken message.

## "I" Messages

Effective communication is enhanced when we take responsibility for our feelings. All too often we convey blame to others for our feelings ("You make me so mad!"). Instead, we should take responsibility for our emotions and convey them as such. For example, a student who is upset with his father for forgetting to come to his soccer game shouts out in frustration, "You're so wrapped up in your work that you don't care for anybody else in this family!" The father may resent such a strong statement and an argument may ensue. Instead, assume that this student takes responsibility for his feelings and says, "Dad, when you didn't come to my game, I felt like you didn't care about me." This statement would encourage open communication because it describes true feelings and because the father is more likely to respond positively without becoming defensive. When we own our feelings and thoughts we use **"I" messages** and say, "This is how *I* feel," "This is how *I* see it," "This is what *I* think."

## Listening Skills

Listening is the most powerful communication skill that most of us don't even consider. After all, we were blessed with two ears and only one mouth. Listening can be passive or active. In **passive listening,** an individual attentively listens without talking and without directing the speaker in any nonverbal way. Passive listening can be effective when you want the speakers to feel free to develop and express thoughts without concern for evaluation or intrusion from you as a listener.

**Active listening** requires a great deal more mental and physical effort and energy than passive listening. It involves giving complete attention to what an individual is communicating. Through active listening, a listener conveys understanding and caring to another person, using either verbal or nonverbal means. Active listening requires that you not think about the experiences and insights you want to add to a conversation, but instead "listen" with your eyes, ears, and heart. Verbal responses focus on what the other is saying and convey sympathy, respect, acceptance, and encouragement; for example: "I understand," "What happened then?" "Is that right?" and "That's wonderful!" You can also show you care and understand by using **reflective listening.** Reflective listening consists of paraphrasing ("Are you saying that . . . ?"), comparing ("Was it like . . . ?"), verbalizing unexpressed feelings ("Did it make you feel . . . ?"), and by seeking more information ("Tell me more about . . .").

## Communication Styles

People tend to express opinions and feelings in one of three communication styles: passive, aggressive, or assertive (see Figure 2-2). We act according to each of these three styles on certain occasions, depending on our situations. However, if we generally respond in one of these styles then we can be classified as either passive, aggressive, or assertive. Those who are **passive** tend to hold back their true feelings and go along with the other person or persons. They are timid, reserved, and unable to assert their rights. **Aggressive** individuals take charge of almost all situations and express their opinions, beliefs, and values with little or no regard for others. Their messages may be threatening or disrespectful. **Assertive** persons carefully express their true feelings in ways that do not threaten or make others feel anxious. They speak their minds and invite others to do likewise. Assertive individuals are especially skilled at using "I" messages and reflective listening. They demonstrate greater emotion intelligence skills than assertive or passive individuals.

| | Assertive | Passive | Aggressive |
|---|---|---|---|
| **Speaking Behaviors** | Speaks clearly and confidently with eye contact | Mumbles, nervous, avoids eye contact | Yells or refuses to speak; points finger, glares, uses physical force |
| **Evaluations** | Expresses appreciation and respect | Criticizes self and is always apologizing | Criticizes, never compliments |
| **Focus** | Uses "I" messages to communicate | Hopes the other person will guess his or her feelings | Uses "you" messages to blame |
| **Problem Solving** | Seeks compromise | Gives in to others | Wants his or her own way |
| **Listening Behaviors** | Uses active listening skills | Silent, rarely speaks | Interrupts, is sarcastic |
| **Emotions** | Tries to understand other's feelings | Denies own feelings and makes excuses | Makes fun of others, uses name-calling |

**FIGURE 2-2   Communication styles**

## Communication Through Artwork

Drawing, painting, and other artwork are very useful communication techniques for expressing thoughts, feelings, and perceptions. Artwork is a particularly helpful means of expression for children. As children draw or paint their mental perceptions of school experiences, family experiences, or themselves, they draw what they know and feel, rather than what they see. Art can be a useful tool for self-expression and a means for teachers to see what their students are thinking and feeling.

We cannot really understand another's drawing until the artist explains it. This provides an account of the picture's meaning and gives us insight into the artist's thoughts and feelings. When you have students draw, do not praise any completed work (praise implies judgment of the worth or value of the student) but instead say something like, "You've worked hard on this drawing" (to convey acceptance of feelings) and "Tell me about your drawing" (to gain insight). As a student responds, note what each part of the drawing represents according to what the student communicates about it (verbally and nonverbally).

After you have talked with an artist about his or her work, examine the drawing for any of the indicators of feelings delineated in Table 2-1. You can compare the impression obtained from the student's discussion with the impression obtained by comparing it to the table guidelines. Usually, these interpretations validate each other. If not, you should either repeat the art experience or validate her or his impression through other communication techniques. If a student draws a disturbing picture or pattern of pictures, and your impressions are supported by interactions with the student, relay your concerns to a school counselor or psychologist.

**TABLE 2-1    Guidelines for interpreting artwork**

| Characteristics | Feeling Indicated |
| --- | --- |
| *Overall General Impression* | |
| Lightly or hesitantly drawn | Inadequacy |
| Darkly or heavily lined drawing | Unexpressed anger |
| Compartmentalized picture | Isolation, insecurity |
| Scribbling over or erasing part or all of drawing | Anxiety over what was revealed |
| Figures tiny in comparison to paper | Insecurity, withdrawal |
| Figures large | Competence, security |
| One or more figures oversized for rest of picture | Aggression toward or feeling overwhelmed by person or thing (powerful, important) |
| Name of child always added or never added to picture | Correlates with decreased recognition or too much criticism of child at home, inadequacy |

**TABLE 2-1**   *continued*

| Characteristics | Feeling Indicated |
| --- | --- |
| Colors predominately used (if child has choice): | |
| White or purple | Overwhelming object or experience |
| Black | Depressed feeling |
| Purple | Depressed feeling |
| Warm, light colors | Happy mood |
| Yellow | Cheerful |
| Red | Excited or anxious |
| Orange | Excited or anxious |
| Green | Refreshed |
| Blue | Calm |
| Darker colors | Unhappy, sad |
| ***Significance of Figures or Parts of Drawing*** | |
| Shaded or omitted part(s) | Anxiety over function or symbolic importance of part(s) |
| Exaggerated or oversized part(s) | Feeling (e.g., power or lack of power) proportional to person or object drawn exaggerated or oversized; exaggerated or oversized object or person is more powerful |
| Omitted hands or legs | Painful or worrisome anxiety, inadequacy, insecurity |
| Stick figure (after developmentally appropriate age) | Immaturity, anxiety |
| Slanted figure | Instability |
| Fragmented, scattered, without boundaries | Gross personality disorganization |
| Facial expression of person with whom child identifies | Reflection of child's inner feelings |
| Transparency of body (older school-age, adolescents) | Acute anxiety, conflict about body image |
| Gross asymmetry | Confusion, distortion of outlook on life |
| ***Indication of Family Relations*** | |
| Size of each member and order in which members drawn | Largest denotes most powerful |
| Position of members in relation to each other | Those closest to each other denote those with closest relationship |
| Omission of self or placement of one member far away from others | Does not feel part of family |
| Similarity of expressions or clothes of members | The more similar, the stronger the relationship |
| Family members without hands and/or not standing firmly on ground | Helpless or ineffective |

Source: J. Servonsky and S. R. Opas, *Nursing Management of Children*. Boston, MA: Jones and Bartlett, 1987.

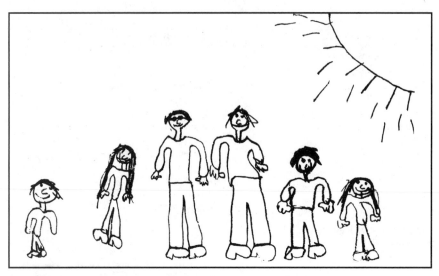

**FIGURE 2-3**
This drawing shows how a happy, adjusted 8-year-old boy saw his family.

Psychological and emotional evaluation through art is very complex. Table 2-1 will help teachers be aware of what to look for in general. Figures 2-3 to 2-5 provide examples of children's artwork for inspection. Box 2-6 provides teaching activities for developing communication skills.

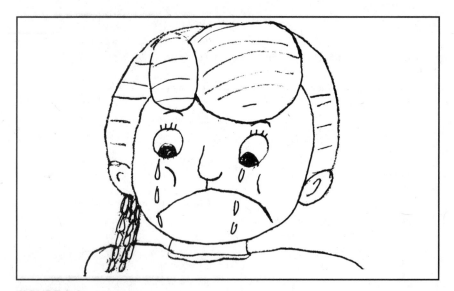

**FIGURE 2-4**
A 10-year-old girl drew this picture when she was "feeling sad" one day. Note the detail and largeness of the figure.

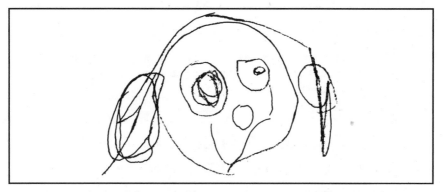

**FIGURE 2-5**
A self-portrait of "Tadpole Man" drawn by a 5-year-old. The child was very happy yet chose to draw with black and brown colors, stating, "I like these colors on this paper. They show up!"

IN THE
CLASSROOM
*2-6*

# Communication Activities

## Understanding with Feedback

Draw a geometric diagram on a three-by-five card. Give the card to one student and have him or her describe the diagram to the class without using hand gestures or allowing for clarifying questions. Have the class members try to draw what they think was described to them. Compare the students' drawings with the original. Repeat the exercise with a different diagram and student describer. This time encourage students to ask clarifying questions.   (I, J, H)

## Gossip

Whisper a message into a student's ear. Have that student repeat the message by whispering it in another student's ear. Continue this process until the message has been passed through the class. Have the last student to hear the message repeat it out loud and check to see if it is the original message. (P, I)

## Body Language

With the students, identify various types of nonverbal communication (e.g., arms crossed, sitting forward or lounging back, palms opened or clenched,

*continued*

*continued*

direct or indirect eye contact, amount of space between participants, voice inflections). Discuss how mixed messages can be given when verbal and non-verbal language do not agree.   (I, J, H)

### Concentration

Have students mentally do a lengthy dictated arithmetic problem:

$$(5 + 2, - 3, + 8, + 10, - 11, + 4, + 25, - 10, + 50 = ?)$$

Make the point that listening in conversations takes concentration as well.

Have students pair up, then have one person listen while the other discusses a topic such as "the happiest moment of my life" or "the most important person in the world." Ask the listener to summarize what the speaker said.   (I, J, H)

### Sociogram

Have the class break into groups of five to eight persons. Have the groups discuss a question (e.g., Why are some people constantly putting down others? or What are some things that cause communication to fail?). As the group discusses the topic, a ball of string is passed from one speaker to the next, unraveling as it goes. Only the person holding the ball of string can speak. When another person wants to speak, the ball is passed and the string unravels more. After a few minutes, a sociogram will be revealed to the group. Group members can see who is dominating the conversation and they can include those who have not yet spoken. Repeat the exercise with another topic and challenge the students to do a better job of including everyone who wants to speak.   (I, J, H)

## Goal Setting

Setting and reaching goals are key skills needed for emotional well-being. Even very young children can be taught how to set and achieve realistic goals and thus realize the joy that comes from these experiences. Four-year-olds naturally set goals such as learning to tie their shoes and dressing themselves. As children grow and mature they need direction in the kinds of goals they should set and in how to reach long-term goals.

Students can learn to see their academic progress in terms of goal setting and achievement rather than reactions to assignments given by teachers. All too often students are not involved in the setting of their academic goals. Teachers, curriculum committees, and others set standards for students to achieve. If students do not feel ownership for these standards they can easily rationalize their lack of accomplishment (e.g., "The teacher expected too much," "The goal was set too high," or "No one should be required to do so much"). When students are involved in the goal-setting process, however, using such defense mechanisms is more difficult and accomplishments are personally felt, generating new motivation and enthusiasm.

Students can benefit by learning different types of goals to set, how to set them, and the process of reaching them. A key to setting goals is to base them on past performance and to differentiate between long-term and short-term goals. Individuals with negative self-concepts tend to set their goals either unrealistically low or unrealistically high. Either way, the results are perceived as failure. Children also tend to set unrealistically high goals; they don't feel comfortable with low goals. Teachers who have worked on goal-setting techniques have reported that children, when asked how many times they will try to respond correctly, usually set goals that are high in relation to past performance. The most reasonable type of goal setting is to make the goal slightly higher than previous performances. For many students, this may be at a level far below the long-term goal for which they and their teacher are aiming, but this shorter-term goal is attainable. Goals that are not attainable do not contribute to long-term commitment and performance. One way teachers can handle this tendency to set unrealistically high goals is by charting a child's goal as long-term with smaller, more easily achieved short-term goals identified as stepping-stones. As the child focuses on and obtains the first short-term goal, a sense of competency is felt along with motivation for taking the next step.

As students work toward goals they have set, they need to evaluate their progress and deal with any failures. Students can be helped to see failure to meet a goal as an opportunity to learn more about how to set goals. Students can ask and answer "Was the goal unrealistic?" and "Should the goal have been set lower, and if so, what are some shorter-term goals that would lead up to it?" with a teacher's help. Students' efforts toward obtaining goals should also be part of the evaluation process. See Box 2-7 for teaching activities related to goal setting.

The following six steps are involved in the goal-setting process:

1. Identify your goal in writing. If it is not written, it is just a wish.

2. Identify any short-range goals or steps necessary to achieve the major goal.

3. Identify all resources that can assist you in achieving the goal.

4. Identify alternative plans and solutions for any foreseeable conflicts.

5. Implement, and as you progress, continue to improve and refine your plan, reviewing steps 2 and 3. If you don't achieve success with the first plan, begin another.

6. Evaluate. What went well? What could you improve on when pursuing a similar goal in the future?

# Activities for Goal Setting

## Thoughts on Goals

Display the following thoughts on bulletin boards to stimulate class discussions.   (J, H)

◆ The poor man is not he who is without a cent, but he who is without a dream.

◆ What will I wish a month, a year, or five years from now that I had done today?

◆ No man has become a failure without his own consent.

◆ No man has ever climbed the ladder of success with his hands in his pockets.

◆ There are two kinds of people that never amount to much. Those who can't do what they are told, and those who can do nothing else.

◆ Too many people itch for what they want without scratching for it.

◆ You can eat an elephant if you just eat him one bite at a time.

◆ Life by the inch is a cinch, but life by the yard is hard.

◆ Success comes in cans, not in can'ts.

◆ Success consists of getting up just one more time than you fall.

## Wishes to Reality

Have students write five things they wish to accomplish in the next three months. Ask them to choose one wish and work that wish through the first four of the six goal-setting steps contained in this chapter. When they are finished, have students break into small groups and review each other's work for help in identifying aspects they may have overlooked. Challenge students to work on goals. Occasionally have the small groups review progress that individuals are making toward their goals. At the end of three months, have students turn in a paper regarding the project.   (I, J, H)

## Class Goal

As a class, set one or more class goals. These can be academic or behavioral. Help students write the goal, based on past performance, and have it be short-range. Work through the goal-setting steps with the students, being sure to evaluate and then follow up with additional goals.   (I, J, H)

*continued*

### Individual Academic Goal

Have each student, in conference or in writing, set a goal relevant to the class subject material. Review the goals set to see that they are based on past performance and that they are short-range. If any goal does not meet these standards, help the student modify it. This is imperative if the student is to achieve the goal.   (P, I, J, H)

### Teach Study Skills

Sometimes the difference between the good student and the poor student isn't the amount of time spent studying, but the amount of effective time spent. Take time in class to teach study skills such as skimming, scanning, using parts of the text, previewing reading material, outlining, notetaking, identifying key concepts, memorization techniques, and test taking.   (P, I, J, H)

## Problem Solving and Decision Making

Problem solving and decision making are very closely related. In essence, decision making is one of the steps in problem solving. We will first discuss problem solving as a whole and then take a closer look at decision making.

Problem-solving skills are, unfortunately, seldom seen modeled by young people. On television they see complex problems easily resolved (often with violence) in a 30-minute to 2-hour program. Advertisements are everywhere, convincing them that life should be pain-free and enjoyed without any thought of the cost. Today few families eat dinner together more than one or two times per week. With so little family time, children are not in a position to observe their parents confront, handle, and overcome everyday problems. And sadly, in some homes, young people are told that they *are* the problem, not that they *have* a problem.

It is important for students to realize that life is filled with problems for people in all walks of life. Often youth feel they are the only ones with the burdens they carry. Simply discussing the universality of conflicts in people's lives can help students feel less isolated and overwhelmed by their problems. Such discussions help put one's own trials in proper perspective. Looking at other individuals' lives and how they have overcome difficulties can help young people learn to solve problems and overcome obstacles.

Problem-solving steps are quite simple. The difficulty comes in focusing on the problem. Our impulse is to become sidetracked and waste a great deal of time and energy bemoaning the "realities" of a problem and blaming others for its existence. For instance, how often do we yell about "spilled milk"? The milk on the floor is a reality. How to clean it up is the problem—something that can be solved. Being a pregnant teenager is a reality. Securing the welfare of the mother and unborn child is a solvable problem. Once we clearly see what the problem is, we must decide to do something about it. Successful problem solving is accomplished by following these steps:

1. Identify the problem. (Address the cause and how it can be avoided later.)

2. Identify possible resources and solutions.

3. Identify probable consequences for each possible solution.

4. Decide on one of the solutions.

5. Act on it—solve the problem according to this plan.

6. Evaluate the result of your actions.

Now we will take a closer look at decision making. It is a problem-solving step, and much more. We make decisions everyday without really considering them to be part of problem solving. What we eat, wear, say, and do are all examples. In effect these decisions create or avoid problems in our lives. Young people need help in recognizing how small and major decisions affect their lives.

There is also a moral aspect of decision making. Too often choices are made based on what feels good, what others will think of us, or on what everyone else appears to be doing. It is important to consider the moral right or wrong of a decision. Reviewing expectations set by parents, school, church, and community members can help children make morally correct decisions. Asking "What would happen if everyone in the world did this?" can also identify the moral implications of a decision.

It is helpful for students to see the thought processes that go into the countless decisions teachers make and the problems they solve each day in the classroom. Teachers can model problem-solving and decision-making skills by sharing with students some of the problems they face and the decisions they must make. Teachers can identify the steps they take in solving their problems and making their decisions. They can also ask their students to help them identify possible solutions and choices. Student involvement in this way helps them feel more responsible, capable, and part of the solution rather than the problem. Box 2-8 contains more suggestions for problem-solving and decision-making activities.

## Activities for Problem Solving and Decision Making

### Apollo 13

Watch the movie *Apollo 13* and have students take note of the following:
1. The realities—things that have happened that cannot be changed
2. The problems
3. How people act/react to realities and problems
4. How problems are solved    (I, J, H)

### Kids' Court

Have students brainstorm scenarios of problems that youth often face. From this list, select cases (scenarios) to try in kid's court. Select students to play the roles of the accused, defendant, prosecutor, witnesses, jury, and judge. The teacher serves as moderator to assist students in their various roles. The jury decides the solution to the problem based on the evidence presented. (I, J, H)

### What Would You Do?

Ask students to suggest common problems, such as one they might have at home or school with peers, brothers, or sisters. Assign students to role-play different problems without providing the solution. Discuss or have different students enact possible solutions. A variation of this activity is to collect newspaper articles about people who have made choices with negative effects (e.g., robberies, assaults, cheating, playing with guns). Discuss what early choices might have led to the major decision that resulted in tragedy. Discuss appropriate choices that could have prevented the negative outcome.    (P, I, J, H)

### "Dear Abby"

Have each student write a "Dear Abby" letter expressing a personal problem or one bothering a friend. As a class, discuss the problem, alternative solutions, and the advantages and disadvantages of each solution. Or, assign

*continued*

*continued*

students to answer the letters in small groups. Later read and discuss the original letter and answers as a class.   (I, J, H)

### Worry Solutions

Have each student anonymously compile a list of things that worry him or her. Compile a master for the class indicating the most common worries. Propose solutions.   (I, J, H)

### Cornflakes

Prepare a place setting including a bowl, spoon, milk, sugar, and cold cereal. Review problem-solving steps as a demonstration. Which should go into the bowl first, the milk, cereal, or sugar? Why? What should go second, third? Why? In effect the class is identifying alternatives and possible results. Then take other common problems and work out solutions as a class, identifying the steps as you go.   (I, J, H)

### Recall

Have each student write down one decision he or she made during the past three months. Have them list the alternatives and identify the decision. Have them evaluate the decision and rethink whether it is the same decision they would make today.   (J, H)

## Media Literacy

There are many different forms of media: movies, television, radio, the World Wide Web, video games, billboards, magazines, newspapers, CDs, bumper stickers, T-shirts and caps, and packaging all bring us messages. These messages from media tell us how to act, what to think, what our roles and expectations in life should be, and what we should buy. Many of the messages conveyed through media do not promote good health and safety. The media often depict, promote, condone, and glamorize violence, alcohol and other drug use, unrealistic expectations about physical appearance and body image, unhealthy eating habits, and sexual promiscuity. Women's and men's bodies are used to sell almost any kind of product. People of color are stereotyped. Young people are exposed to hundreds of thousands of advertisements telling them that they don't measure up unless they look or act in a certain way.

One tool to help young people living in our media-saturated environment is media literacy. **Media literacy** refers to the skills and knowledge needed to question, analyze, interpret, and evaluate media messages. To be media literate is to understand that media messages are produced by someone with an agenda to sell, persuade, or change behavior. A message is constructed very carefully to maximize the agenda. To be media literate is to be able to critically interpret one's media environment. Young people who are media literate are able to **deconstruct** media messages to understand a messenger's motives so that they are not manipulated by them. Today's youth most certainly need to become media literate because they are constantly exposed to media messages specifically designed to influence their behavior. Youth are less likely to be influenced by media messages if they have developed skills to refute such messages. Youth are able to transfer the approaches and strategies of media literacy to address other independent living skills (substance abuse prevention, sexuality education, parenting skills, etc.).

According to the American Academy of Pediatrics, media-literate or media-educated people do the following:[10]

❖ Decipher the purpose and message of media rather than accepting them at face value

❖ Understand that all media messages are constructed

❖ Understand that media messages shape our understanding of the world

❖ Understand that individuals interpret media messages uniquely

❖ Limit use of media

❖ Make positive media choices

❖ Select creative alternatives to media consumption

❖ Develop critical thinking and viewing skills

❖ Understand the political, social, economic, and emotional implications of all forms of media

## Media Exposure

Exposure to several forms of media is widespread and pervasive. According to the American Academy of Pediatrics, the average American child or adolescent spends more than 21 hours per week viewing television.[11] This amount of time does not include time spent watching movies, listening to music or watching music videos, playing video or computer games, or surfing the Internet for recreational purposes. Time spent with electronic media often displaces involvement in creative, active, social, or physical activity pursuits.

The study *Kids & Media @ the New Millenium* by the Kaiser Family Foundation found that the typical American child spends an average of more than 38 hours a week consuming media outside of school.[12] This is nearly 5.5 hours a day using television, computers, video games, movies, music, and print media. Children 8 years and older spent more time each day on average (6 hours and 43 minutes) using media than children aged 2 to 7 years (3 hours and 34 minutes). The study showed that among kids 8 years old and over, nearly two-thirds have a TV set in their bedroom and say that the TV is usually on during meals in their home. Sixty-one percent say their parents have no rules about TV watching and that their parents watch TV with them only 5% of the time. Nearly one of every four children over the age of 8 (24%) spends more than 5 hours a day watching TV. Among children in the 2- to 7-year-old age range, one-third (32%) have a TV in their bedroom. Thirty-five percent of parents of children in this age range say the TV is on in their homes "most of the time," and 47% say it is usually on during meals. Parents watch TV with their young children only 19% of the time.

Young people spend an average of almost an hour and a half a day listening to CDs, tapes, or the radio. After TV, music is the medium of choice for most children, especially teenagers. Nearly 7 in 10 kids (69%) have a computer at home, and nearly 45% have Internet access from home. Although 82% of kids spend time reading for fun each day, this study showed that kids spend more than five times as much time in front of a TV, computer, or video screen each day than they do reading. See Table 2-2 for additional statistics on media use.

Susan Villani notes that TV viewing often begins before age 2 years.[13] Television shows such as *Teletubbies* have been specifically designed to appeal to infants and toddlers. This has caused considerable concern about the use of the television by parents and caretakers as an alternative to human interaction from parents, other adults, and other children. Another trend of concern that she notes is the rapid proliferation of videocassette recorders (VCRs) and the expansion of cable television and movie channels. This has increased the amount of programming available for young people to see and has blurred the distinction between television and movie programming. It has also made the viewing of extremely violent and sexually explicit movies accessible for millions of youth right in their own homes, often in their bedrooms because so many have their own TV sets.

It is interesting that medical associations such as the American Academy of Pediatrics advocate that health care professionals assess children's media exposure as part of routine medical practice. Susan Villani makes the following recommendations for health care professionals based on an extensive review of the literature on the impact of media on children and adolescents:

> Health care professionals, and particularly child and adolescent psychiatrists, should incorporate a media history into the standard evaluation of children and adolescents. With the growing evidence that certain media use is included as a risk factor for acting out violently, as well as for other

**TABLE 2-2    Media use in America**

- 98% of American households have at least one TV set; the average has 2.7.
- Televisions are on 7 hours a day in the typical home.
- The average American spends nearly 4 hours a day watching TV—almost 50 days per year. By the age of 65, he or she will have spent 9 years watching TV.
- 77% of families have cable/pay TV.

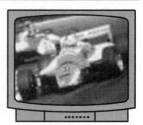

- People with low incomes watch more television than those with high incomes, and highly educated people watch less television than those with less formal education.
- 87% of homes with children have multiple television sets.
- Over the course of a year, the amount of time that children spend watching TV is twice as much as that they spend in school.
- 48% of children aged 2 to 17 have a TV set in their bedrooms.

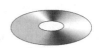

- Girls aged 11 to 19 watch MTV more than any other network.
- Teenagers spend an average of 4 hours per weekday watching TV.
- 78% of Americans consider watching TV with their children a family activity.
- The average child views 30,000 commercials each year.
- Teens aged 12 to 20 make up 16% of the population but purchase 26% of movie tickets.
- 90% of 12- to 20-year-olds report going to the movies frequently or occasionally.
- Moviegoing is considered an "in" activity among 92% of teens.
- 97.8% of families own a VCR.
- Watching a video is America's number one leisure activity.
- The average household buys more than 8 new videos a year.
- 62% of youth aged 9 to 17 say they watch a video at least once a week.
- The average age for first computer use among children is 2 years.
- Teens spend an average of 2 weekday hours online.
- 67% of homes with children own video game equipment.
- 90% of households with children either rent or own a video or computer game.
- Children who have home video games play with them about 90 minutes a day.
- 58% of teens say their parents do not have rules about playing video games.
- American teenagers listen to an estimated 10,500 hours of rock music between grades 7 and 12—just 500 fewer hours than they spend in school over 12 years.
- 87% of 13- to 17-year-olds report listening to music after school, and two-thirds name music as a hobby.
- Listening to music is students' number one nonschool activity.
- In the last three months, 71% of teens purchased at least one full-length music CD, 33% bought a CD single, and 35% bought a full-length cassette.
- 75% of 9- to 12-year-olds and 80% of 12- to 14-year-olds watch music videos.

Source: Mediascope, "Media Use in America: Issue Briefs." Studio City, CA: Mediascope Press, 2000. Available at http://www.mediascope.org/pubs/ibriefs/mua.htm.

high-risk behaviors, the standard of practice has evolved over the past decade to warrant incorporation of the media history into everyday clinical practice. For adolescents, this needs to include careful questioning about musical preferences and the meaning of the music to the adolescents. This should extend to actively educating parents about the potential dangers of the television as an "electronic baby-sitter" for young children, televisions in children's bedrooms, prolonged periods spent playing violent video games, and the risks of unsupervised Internet use.

The challenge to adults who deal with children, either personally as parents or professionally, will be to monitor media use in ways that foster curiosity and the positive aspects of the ability of media to teach, yet simultaneously protect children from spending too much time with media at the expense of human interactions, from being overexposed to material that cannot be adequately processed or understood, and from having their value systems shaped in negative ways by media content. The cost of ignoring the impact of the media on children and adolescents will be enormous, both in absolute dollars and the immeasurable cost of human pain and suffering. (pg. 399)[13]

***Limiting Media Exposure***    Considering such widespread access and exposure to media, youth need parameters on what they view, when they view it, and how much time they spend in front of a screen. Parents are ultimately responsible for monitoring and controlling their children's media use. However, teachers can help parents by providing them with information and by helping their students understand the importance of viewing guidelines such as these:

❖ Have a television (and computer, video game, etc.) allowance. Determine the appropriate total hours per week for viewing and develop a media time budget for these hours.

❖ Preselect programming. Look for age-appropriate programs that are fair in their treatment of people, are not violent, do not display sexual images or themes, do not use vulgar language, and do not display other inappropriate behavior or messages. Immediately turn the TV off at the end of the program. Do not allow yourself to be sucked in to watch the following program or to begin channel surfing.

❖ Finish homework and chores before watching TV.

❖ Don't eat in front of the television set. The increased rate of obesity in childhood and adolescence is closely correlated with sedentary activities such as watching TV and eating the advertised junk food. Eating while watching TV is a "double whammy" that contributes to overweight and obesity.

❖ Watch TV as a family and discuss the following: what is "real" and "unreal" on TV, choices characters made and the consequences of these choices, and the advertisements—their messages, why advertisers choose to run them during certain programs, and any underlying messages or morals, including those that might not have been intended by the writers.

❖ Encourage parents to be good role models by selectively using media and limiting their own choices, thereby allowing children to observe healthy use of media, such as reading a book or newspaper.

❖ Emphasize alternative activities such as physical activity, crafts, hobbies, and visits to museums.

❖ Avoid using television, video games, and computers as electronic baby-sitters.

❖ Encourage parents to create an "electronic media-free" environment in children's rooms.

The American Academy of Pediatrics recommends that parents avoid TV viewing for children under the age of 2 years.[11] They stress that research on early brain development shows that babies and toddlers have a critical need for direct interactions with parents and other significant caregivers for healthy brain growth and the development of optimal social, emotional, and cognitive skills. As a result, exposing young children to TV programs should be discouraged.

## Evaluating Media Messages

The various media are among the most pervasive influences in the lives of children and adolescents. Media don't just sell products, they also "sell" values, attitudes, and beliefs. Thousands of studies have shown a relationship between media violence and aggressive behavior. Many have also shown a cause-and-effect relationship between exposure to violence in media and violent behavior. The American Academy of Pediatrics states that more than 1,000 studies attest to a causal connection between media violence and aggressive behavior in children. The threat of children imitating the behavior they see on the screen is real and grave.

Another troubling aspect of media is exposure to ugly, consistently dysfunctional images and messages. Many programs on the air celebrate dysfunctionality by rejecting and making fun of the very things that make civilized life possible: discipline, self-control, hard work, delayed gratification, faith, and a commitment to family and spouse. All too often, television and movie writers and producers opt for the dollar-laden low road, competing to see who can get away with the most first and what old taboos can be broken. Media literacy involves not only scrutinizing the underlying messages of advertisements, but those of the programs one watches as well. Box 2-9 offers teaching activities to promote media literacy.

## The World of Advertising

We have been conditioned into believing that a media program (e.g., a television show) is brought to us by a sponsoring company ("today's game is brought to you by Brand X"). The truth is, however, that the program (television show, radio broadcast, magazine article, website) exists for the purpose of rounding up an audience to see and hear the advertisements. Thus, we, the potential consumers, are in reality the products being sold. The very reason that a television program or magazine exists is for the purpose of selling the products that are advertised through the medium. Have you ever examined the amount of advertisements in a magazine compared with its editorial content? What you will find for most magazines is that they are essentially catalogs of advertised products with a few stories sprinkled in. This is particularly true of teen and women's magazines. The stories contained in magazines are also influenced tremendously by the advertisers. Magazines that carry tobacco advertisements do not run stories about the health effects of cigarettes anymore than magazines bearing alcohol advertisements carry stories about the tragedies of alcohol abuse.

Noted advertising expert Jean Kilbourne explains more about how the very purpose of the media is to deliver us to the advertisers:

> Make no mistake: The primary purpose of the mass media is to sell audiences to advertisers. *We* are the product. Although people are much more sophisticated about advertising now than even a few years ago, most are still shocked to learn this.
>
> Magazines, newspapers, and radio and television programs round us up, rather like cattle, and producers and publishers then sell us to advertisers, usually through ads placed in advertising and industry publications. "The people you want, we've got all wrapped up for you," declares *The Chicago Tribune* in an ad placed in *Advertising Age*, the major publication of the advertising industry, which pictures several people, all neatly boxed according to income level.
>
> Although we like to think of advertising as unimportant, it is in fact the most important aspect of the mass media. It *is* the point. Advertising supports more than 60 percent of magazine and newspaper production and almost 100 percent of the electronic media. Over $40 billion a year in ad revenue is generated for television and radio and over $30 billion for magazines and newspapers. As one ABC executive said, "The network is paying affiliates to carry network commercials, not programs. What we are is a distribution system for Procter & Gamble." And the CEO of Westinghouse Electric, owner of CBS, said, "We're here to serve advertisers. That's our raison d'etre."(pg. 34–35)[14]

The average American is exposed to about 3,000 advertisements per day through television, radio, magazines, newspapers, and billboards. In this "ad-vironment," it is common to hear people say that they just ignore the ads. However, it is impossible to filter out the amount of advertising to which we are constantly exposed, especially when advertisements are carefully designed to affect us. Every minute detail of an advertisement is planned, researched, and pilot-tested. In response to advertisements, it is best to consciously recognize the underlying messages they contain and critically question the validity of those messages. "If I buy this product will imaginary playmates appear, making my life fun and exciting? Will it solve all my problems, make me popular, make me thin and beautiful? Does this toy really do all the things it is shown to do and do all the accessories come with it? Will using this product really help make people of the opposite sex find me more desirable or sexy?"

The power of advertising is evidenced by the fact that lots of people pay lots of money for numerous highly advertised products. Today's grocery stores stock about 24,000 items, up from about 9,000 a decade ago. Have you ever wondered why so many people are willing to buy a bottle of water worth two cents and pay $1.50 for it? More than buying the product itself (the water), they are buying the values that advertising has attached to the product (e.g., being hip). There is an old Madison Avenue saying that "You don't drink the beer; you drink the advertising."

Most advertising is based on two fundamental messages. First, you should be dissatisfied with yourself. Second, purchasing the product being pushed is the only way to resolve this dissatisfaction. We are bombarded with ads saying that our hair is too oily, our breath stinks, or that we have body odor. Purchasing shampoos, mouthwashes, and deodorants is the solution to this dissatisfaction. Ads make us feel insecure about our weight, appearance, and ability to attract lovers—the list goes on and on. Eating this cereal, taking this over-the-counter product, or drinking this beer are presented as solutions to these insecurities. Advertising has the capacity to influence people to believe that their life and worth are defined by what they possess. If you are feeling ugly, have a beer. If you think you are not sexy, buy the breath mint, perfume, designer clothing, or automobile that promises you the magical transformation that the product will make you sexy. People who feel empty or who suffer from a sense of low self-worth are most vulnerable to advertisements. If individuals harbor negative feelings about themselves, they are more likely to turn to products promising to resolve these feelings. It is a sad fact that teenagers raised in disrupted families exhibit higher levels of compulsive consumption than those raised in intact families.

**Targeting Kids**     To the corporate world, kids are big business. Advertisers aim not only at the billions of dollars kids spend each year, but also at the billions of dollars that adults spend on kids—an amount that might be ten times as high. The fact that kids influence between 25% and 40% of household purchases has made all kinds of companies—from automakers to airlines—aim their advertisements at youth. In a recent year, teenagers spent $141 billion of their own money in the retail market, and it is estimated that children under 12 control or influence the spending of almost

$500 billion. Marketers also know that when brand allegiances are formed in childhood, the customer usually remains loyal to the product for many years to come. Thus, marketers try to "win" a child so that they can enjoy that enduring loyalty. Children begin developing brand preferences in early childhood, even before entering school.

This lucrative "kids market" drives the development and marketing of products and services for children and teens. It has also spurred a proliferation of television channels (e.g., Nickelodeon, Fox Kids Network, the Disney Channel, and the Cartoon Network) to advertise these products and services. The online marketing of products and services to children and teens is growing at a tremendous pace. Many of the most popular websites visited by kids are those sponsored by companies with commercial marketing interests, such as McDonald's, Hasbro, Mattel, Frito-Lay, Lego, and numerous lines of clothing. These and other websites built around products offer a variety of appealing online activities, such as contests, games, and sending e-postcards. At the same time that kids are playing these games and contests, marketers are extracting information from them that can be used in future marketing pitches to the child and the child's family. Prizes or incentives are sometimes promised to children who share the e-mail addresses of their friends. Such sites also feature online stores or links to websites that are created to make direct sales. Some websites have created "digital wallets" that allow a parent to use a credit card to place a set amount of money into a child's online account. Many youth who surf the Web have no trouble finding the websites for alcohol and tobacco companies, which are appealing and enticing to young people.

**School-Based Advertising and Marketing** Advertisements are pervasive—they are even in our schools, where we see them on bulletin boards, scoreboards, book covers, and educational materials bearing corporate logos. Schools use curricular materials that are produced by the Coca-Cola Company and Pizza Hut. School buses and school athletic fields are "decorated" with ads. Incentives, promotions, and contests are other frequently used in-school marketing devices. Channel One, a daily ad-bearing TV news program containing 2 minutes of ads for every 12 minutes of programming, is aired in over 12,000 schools. Schools who participate in Channel One receive televisions and VCRs in exchange for the schools' commitment to show its news program, with advertisements aimed at students, at some point in each school day. Many parents and educators object to the Channel One program, but for schools with limited budgets it is difficult to pass up the offer of free TVs and VCRs in every classroom. Channel One promises its advertisers "the largest teen audience around" and "the undivided attention of millions of teenagers for 12 minutes a day."

Another school marketing program is Zap Me. Zap Me schools are provided with a computer lab with advanced computers loaded with Microsoft software. Each computer is equipped with a sophisticated Web browser and the capacity to download full-motion images. The computers are linked to a "netspace" for which corporations pay to provide content. Students can get to the Internet through this browser, but it requires their parents' permission to do so. Schools getting the Zap Me labs have to guarantee that students will use them for a set amount of time each day. Of course, the browser portal has advertising on it. Therefore, in order for a student to complete Internet assignments or homework, he or she must view the advertising. So, in essence, if a teacher makes an assignment requiring a student to use the Zap Me browser, the child is being required to view the commercials. Students participating in this program are being sold to the advertisers by the schools.

Kingsley Hammett, in his article "Cashing in on Kids," describes the commercial environment of many of today's schools:

> Look around any public school these days and it's not hard to detect the relentless creep of naked commercialism: McDonald's signs on the baseball fence, Coke machines in the hallway, students forced to watch blue-jeans commercials on Channel One. This endless stream of corporate messages is everywhere, and along with promoting sexuality, eating disorders, and inappropriate brand loyalty, it undermines the most fundamental of our democratic institutions: public education.
>
> The schools are now effectively integrated into the marketing machine and long-term planning of most corporations, where the school has become simply another part of corporate sales and public relations strategy. Corporate messages find their way into the schools through every means imaginable: Web browsers with ads, school voice mail systems with commercialized messages, credit cards tied into school promotions, corporate-sponsored educational materials, television programs with advertisements, the sale of school space to mount advertisements, sponsorship of activities, incentive programs, door-to-door sales promotions, and the naming of facilities, even classrooms. (pg. 27)[15]

Schools are vulnerable to allowing companies to "cash in on kids" in an attempt to solve financial difficulties. For example, Coca-Cola has entered into several "partnerships" with schools in which the company gives schools large sums of money in exchange for a long-term contract giving Coca-Cola exclusive rights to school vending machines. Tax monies can only be stretched so far, and so financially strapped schools are often willing to enter into ventures with generous commercial sponsors. These sponsors willingly provide numerous enhancements (e.g., computers, educational materials, TV monitors) that a school might not otherwise be able to afford. Sadly, in the process, children gain more access to vending machines selling fatty foods and sugary soft drinks, are exposed to an increasing number of advertisements and corporate logos, and learn from corporate-sponsored lessons and curricula. Is it any wonder that today's students drink twice as much soda as milk and that the diets of many are full of junk foods?

School children form a captive audience to school-based marketing, and the campaigns carry an implied school endorsement. Students are especially vulnerable to these marketing tactics because they believe that what they are exposed to at schools is good for them. School-based advertising creates a blurred line between education and propaganda. For this reason, students need to learn to analyze, interpret, and evaluate all of the messages contained in an advertisement, even those to which they are exposed at school. Hopefully, more schools will make efforts to become advertising-free schools. This requires a significant, ongoing community commitment and involvement. Parents and taxpayers have to support the effort to provide an advertising-free environment for school children. It requires a strict policy and replacing lost corporate contributions with large donations of time, talent, and money.

## Online Kids

Children and adolescents are increasingly using the Internet. According to a Georgia Institute of Technology study, about one-third of teenagers spend 10 to 20 hours a week online.[16] The teens in the study reported that 18.6% of this time is spent on entertainment, 17.1% on education, 16.3% on personal information, 16% on time wasting, 11.8% on communications, 8.2% on shopping, 7.8% on work, and 4.2% on other activities. Another study of children aged 2 to 12 showed that the most popular online activities are e-mail (46.4%), games (44%), surfing the Web (37.6%), and homework (30.4%).[17] Many kids have Internet access in their own homes. Many go online when they first come home from school and when their parents are not home. This means that they are unsupervised when surfing the Web.

***Online Safety Tips***　Cyberspace requires some media literacy of its own. Although its wealth of information makes the Internet a valuable resource, there are problems that students need to learn to avoid. For instance, some websites try to pry into young people's private lives by using games and special promotions as bait to capture names, ages, and addresses. Spending inordinate amounts of time online is another problem. Internet use can have addictive qualities, where hours seem like minutes and cause problems as relationships and responsibilities are ignored. Chat rooms are especially bad in this way. Teachers can aid in the development of students' media literacy by sharing the following online safety tips with students and their families:

❖ Establish clear ground rules for Internet use before subscribing to online services.

❖ Place computers in the family room or another open area of your home.

❖ Never give out personal information online, especially in chat rooms and bulletin boards.

❖ Never plan a face-to-face meeting with online acquaintances.

❖ Do not respond to offensive or dangerous e-mail, chat, or other communications.

❖ Immediately turn the computer off if a pornographic site is accidentally accessed. Some pornographic sites disable the user's ability to escape when using normal key functions such as ESC (escape) and bring up additional windows containing pornographic sites.

---

IN THE
CLASSROOM
*2-9*

# Teaching Activities for Media Literacy

## *Advertisement Appeals*

Discuss with students the following persuasive appeals that advertisers use to promote products. Have students identify examples of each they have seen. Sometimes promoters use two or more appeals in one advertisement. (P, I, J, H)

| | |
|---|---|
| Exaggerations: | The message has some truth but the benefits of the product are stretched, such as exaggerating a toy's performance. |
| False Images: | Subtle messages include "Cool people use this," "It will make you popular," "It will make you attractive and give you sex appeal." Another type of false image is when a product is shown with many accessories and the false impression is given that everything comes with the product. |
| Humor: | The product looks fun to use or the commercial makes you laugh so that you will feel good about the product. Jingles or cartoons are sometimes used. |
| Bandwagon: | "Everyone's doing it ..." |
| Testimonial: | A common person, celebrity, or supposed authority directly promotes a product or implies endorsement by using it. |
| Rewards: | Special prizes, gifts, or coupons are given if you buy the product. |
| Progress: | "New and improved ..." |
| Comparisons: | A specific brand is better than another. Brand loyalty is formed. |
| Snob: | The product may cost more than its competitors, but "You are worth it!" or "You deserve it!" |
| Underdog: | Appeals to the underachiever, the unattractive; the "geek" that many people can identify with. |
| Scientific Evidence: | Survey or laboratory results provide confidence in a product. "Nine out of ten doctors recommend ..." |

*continued*

*continued*

## Media "Apples"

Take a firm, shiny, attractive apple and insert a large nail into the center on the bottom side. Remove the nail and then expose the center of the apple to contamination so that it will bruise or begin to rot. This can be done by using microorganisms from decaying fruit or vegetables. Swab a contaminated item with the nail or a cotton swab and then insert it into the apple. A few days later, show the students the apple. Discuss the attractiveness of the apple: Is it pretty? Does it look good to eat? Cut the apple in half, exposing its unattractive insides. Ask the students, "How is this apple like some advertisements?" or, "How is this apple like some TV programs or movies?" Discuss the hidden negative messages contained in commercials and programs.    (P, I, J, H)

## Commercial Cynicism

1. Videotape television commercials. You might want to record only commercials aired after school, on Saturday mornings, during prime time, or during athletic events. Show these in class and discuss which industries choose to run their ads at these various times and why. Analyze each ad for the appeal(s) used. Discuss the validity of the information presented and any values, attitudes, or beliefs taught by each advertisement.    (P, I, J, H)
2. Collect magazines of varying types. (You can have students bring them in, collect them from doctors' offices, or retrieve them from recycling bins.) Have students analyze the types of products advertised in each of the various magazines as well as the appeals used by each ad. Have students look for mixed messages within a magazine, such as a magazine with an article on health while at the same time having smoking ads. Another example is a magazine with dieting tips in one article and fattening recipes in another. Check for magazines that consistently carry mixed messages. (Many do.) Discuss why magazines might consistently publish conflicting messages.    (I, J, H)
3. Have students create a list of all the billboards they see during a typical week. Make a chart or grid showing how many times each billboard is looked at by students in the class. Discuss the types of products advertised in this way in their community and why promoters might be choosing this form of advertising. Discuss the validity and persuasiveness of each billboard.    (P, I, J)

## Internet Cookies

A "cookie" on the Internet is a promotional gimmick, such as a game, song, or video clip, that can be accessed by providing personal information such as

*continued*

name, age, and address. Discuss with students the risks of giving out personal information on the Net as well as other Internet safety guidelines.   (P, I, J, H)

## Pull the Plug

Challenge students to give up TV for one week. (You might challenge them to give up video games as well.) Prepare by discussing TV alternatives. During the designated week provide motivation and encouragement. When the experiment is over, have students write essays on their experience. Discuss as a class.   (P, I, J, H)

## Money Management

Have students compare their money habits with other 9- to 14-year-olds who filled out a nationwide survey. Out of 100 surveyed:

> 74 bought food (mostly snacks)
> 17 bought clothes/accessories
> 14 bought magazines/comics, toys/stickers/games, movie tickets, arcade games
> 13 bought gifts
> 12 bought music, movie rentals
> 11 bought sneakers and footwear
> 11 bought grooming products

Have students notice how many kids *didn't* buy each item. An item not on the list meant hardly anyone spent money on it. Discuss how the survey revealed that 1 in 10 kids spent nothing at all, that almost 80% said they wished they hadn't spent so much, and more than half said they wished they had saved their money. Discuss budgeting and saving practices and benefits such as compounded interest. For instance, kids spend about $5 a week on food. If they saved that, how much would they have in five years? Discuss how money management relates to delayed gratification and impulse control.   (I, J)

*Source:* Data from "What Kids Buy," *Zillions Consumer Reports,* Nov/Dec 1997, 12–15.

## Key Terms

emotional well-being   33
self-esteem   34
self-image   34
ideal-self   34
pygmalion-self   34
character education   37

values clarification   38
values education   38
Pygmalion effect   39
conditional worth   45
unconditional self-worth   45
proactivity   50

## Review Questions

1. Paraphrase Branden's comments concerning the prominent role of self-esteem in emotional well-being. Do you agree with his point of view? Identify and explain prominent self-esteem myths.

2. Define and differentiate the terms *self-image, ideal-self,* and *pygmalion-self.* Describe what your three "selves" look like. Discuss how the three "selves" are formed from one's sense of competency, worthiness, and belonging.

3. Explain why physical traits tend to dominate one's ideal-self and how teachers can help students develop fuller, healthier ideal-selves?

4. Describe effective character education programs. Explain how you can incorporate value/character education into your classrooms?

5. What is the Pygmalion effect? Give examples of positive and negative Pygmalion experiences you have witnessed in the classroom.

6. Explain how students can be helped to more accurately evaluate themselves.

7. Differentiate between external/internal and conditional/unconditional self-worth. Explain how students can be helped to focus on their unconditional self-worth while working toward developing conditional aspects of self-worth.

8. Explain the difference between reactive and proactive people. Give examples of each. Explain how teachers can help students become more proactive in the classroom.

9. Identify the four major aspects of emotional intelligence and explain how they can be fostered within the classroom.

10. Explain the concepts of resilience and asset development. Describe how teachers can foster resilience and asset development.

11. Identify the various stages that relationships can go through. Explain the relationship bank account concept, including its various types of deposits.

12. Discuss the variables involved in sending and receiving messages such as body language, mixed messages, "I" and "you" messages, listening skills, and communication styles. Identify ways in which teachers can help students learn to better communicate.

13. How can artwork be a helpful form of communication in the classroom? What steps must a teacher take to ensure an accurate interpretation of a student's artful communication?

14. Explain the benefits of students setting and reaching goals. List the keys for effectively helping students set and reach goals.

15. What steps are included in problem solving? Identify a problem you are currently facing and identify a possible solution using these steps. Identify tools students can use for making morally correct choices.

16. Use statistics to describe the type and amount of media young people are exposed to. Discuss how advertising targets kids and "sells" them more than products. Explain how teachers can help students become media literate.

## References

1. Branden, N. (1988). *How to Raise Your Self-Esteem*. New York: Bantam Books.

2. Lickona, T. (1991). *Educating for Character: How Our Schools Can Teach Respect and Responsibility*. New York: Bantam Books.

3. Center for the 4th and 5th Rs (2002). "What Is a Comprehensive Approach to Character Education?" Available at http://www.cortland.edu/c4n5rs/comp_iv.htm.

4. Kagan, D. M. (1990). "How Schools Alienate Students at Risk: A Model for Examining Proximal Classroom Variables." *Educational Psychologist*, 25: 105–125.

5. Covey, S. R. (1990). *The Seven Habits of Highly Effective People*. New York: Fireside.

6. Goleman, D. (1995). *Emotional Intelligence*. New York: Bantam Books.

7. Masten, A. S. (1997, Spring). "Resilience in Children at Risk." *Research/Practice*, 5(1). Available at http://education.umn.edu/CAREI/Reports/Rpractice/Spring97/resilience.htm.

8. Center for Substance Abuse Prevention (1997). *Making Prevention Work*. Available at http://www.health.org/pubs/mpw-book/mpw.book.htm#power.

9. Scales, P. C. (1999). "Reducing Risks and Building Developmental Assets: Essential Actions for Promoting Adolescent Health." *Journal of School Health*, 69(3): 113–119.

10. Devito, J. A. (1986). *The Interpersonal Communication Book*, New York: Harper and Row.

11. American Academy of Pediatrics (1999). "Policy Statement—Media Education (RE9911)." *Pediatrics*, 104(2): 341–343.

12. Kaiser Family Foundation (1999). *Kids & Media @ the New Millennium: A Comprehensive National Analysis of Children's Media Use*. Available at http://www.kff.org/content/1999/1535/KidsReport%20FINAL.pdf.

13. Villani, S. (2001). "Impact of Media on Children and Adolescents: A 10-Year Review of the Research." *Journal of the American Academy of Child and Adolescent Psychiatry*, 40(4): 392–401.

14. Kilbourne, J. (1999). *Can't Buy My Love: How Advertising Changes the Way We Think and Feel*. New York: Touchstone.

15. Hammett, K. (2001). "Cashing in on Kids." *Designer/Builder: A Journal of the Human Environment*, 8(4): 27–31.

16. Graphics, Visualization, and Usability Center, Georgia Institute of Technology (1998, October). "GVU's 10th WWW User Survey." Available at http://www.gvu.gatech.edu/user_surveys-1998-10/graphs/use/q30.htm.

17. Jupiter Communications (1998). "Kids Evolving Revenue Models for the 2–12 Market." Available at http://www.jup.com/sps/briefs/9808/cc42/cc42.html.

# 3

## Dealing with Stress

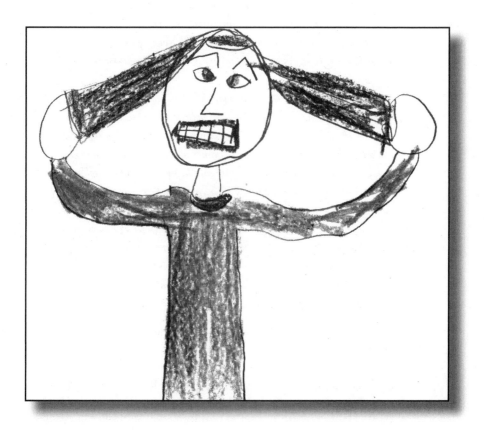

# What's Eating Ricky?

*"An ulcer? Doctor, I don't understand. How can Ricky have an ulcer? I mean, he is only nine years old. What can be so troubling for a fourth grader?"*

*"Well, Mrs. Rivera, is there anything in Ricky's home life right now that is hard for him?"*

*"Do you mean, like marital problems? No. My husband and I are happily married. We have our differences, but we don't fight or anything. My husband has a good job too and I don't work so I'm at home and take care of the kids. Ricky gets along OK with his brothers and sister. Our home life isn't perfect, but it is good."*

*"What about school? Has Ricky had any problems there?"*

*"No . . . Ricky gets good grades, almost all A's. He works real hard at school. Last week he finished second in an all-grade spelling bee. He is always studying for different contests they are having in his classroom. He is a bright kid. He does real well."*

*"Does he get along well with other kids?"*

*"As far as I know, he does. He plays on Little League baseball and soccer teams. He's not the greatest athlete, but he seems to do OK. His buddy, Jerome, comes over all the time and they play video games and watch movies in his bedroom. He hates the school bus, so I drive him and Jerome to and from school."*

*"Mrs. Rivera, ulcers can be caused by a virus. Ricky's isn't. The lining of Ricky's stomach could be genetically weak, but I don't think that is the reason he has an ulcer either. I have seen young kids come in with this problem before. There is usually something or many things in their life that are causing them a lot of stress. I suggest you take a second look at the stressors in Ricky's life. We can medically treat the ulcer, but it is best to understand what is causing it and, if possible, make changes at the root of the problem."*

Do you have some ideas about what might be "eating" Ricky? Look for clues in this chapter.

All children and adolescents have stress in their lives. Growth and maturation is partially brought about by encountering and effectively coping with stress. Unfortunately, many children and adolescents react to family, school, and other pressures and demands in unhealthy ways. This chapter gives insights into the many stressors young people face and offers suggestions for how teachers can help their students better deal with them. Additional stressors, such as pressure to be thin and violence, are discussed in other chapters.

# Understanding Stress

The term **stress** was first used in its current physiological and psychological sense by Hans Selye, a pioneer in the study of stress.[1] He defined stress as "the nonspecific response of the body to any demand made upon it." Selye coined the term **stressor** to refer to specific or nonspecific situations or demands that cause stress. Stressors may be specific (e.g., conflict between a child and teacher, giving an oral report in class, or nearly being hit by a car while crossing the street), but the response is a generalized physiological response. This generalized response is known as the **General Adaptation Syndrome (G.A.S.)**, which consists of the following three stages (see also Figure 3-1):

1. **Alarm** The body initially responds to a stressor (whether real or imagined) by preparing for a physiological emergency. This response has been referred to as the "fight-or-flight" response because the body is prepared for an emergency. Some of these physiological responses are increased respiration and heart rate, sweaty palms, muscle tension, pupil dilation, and an increase in blood flow to the heart and skeletal muscles (see Figure 3-2).

2. **Resistance** During this stage the body uses its energy reserves to attempt to return to normal internal activity, or **homeostasis.**

3. **Exhaustion** Long-term exposure to a specific stressor or a combination of stressors can lead to a depletion of the energy required to return to homeostasis. If this happens the signs of the alarm stage

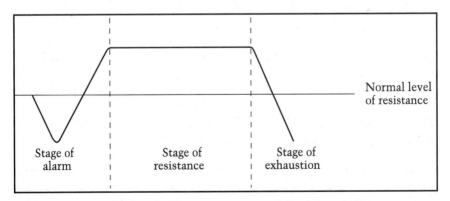

**FIGURE 3-1   Three phases of G.A.S.**
In the stage of alarm, the body's normal resistance to stress is lowered from the first interactions with the stressor; in the stage of resistance, the body adapts to the continued presence of the stressor and resistance increases; in the stage of exhaustion, the body loses its ability to resist the stressor and becomes exhausted.

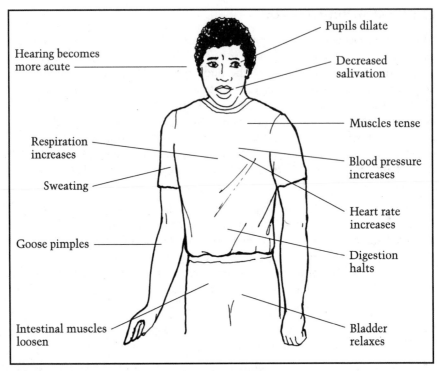

**FIGURE 3-2    The fight-or-flight response**

return. It is during this stage that physical or emotional disease may be initiated.

We have all experienced alarm from time to time. Imagine yourself carelessly crossing a street when you suddenly realize that a speeding car is coming right at you. Your heart pounds, your muscles flex, and you find yourself jumping farther and running faster than you ever thought possible. Your body is in motion before you really have time to think, as it utilizes all its energies for survival. Once you are safely out of the car's path, you take a deep breath and slowly your body returns to its former relaxed state.

The **fight-or-flight response** isn't as useful for us today as it was for our ancestors. The many stressors we experience today sometimes put us in a chronic state of alarm. All too often days, weeks, and even months pass without our relaxing—returning to a state of homeostasis. Stress then manifests itself in our bodies as tension headaches, backaches, or insomnia. Stress can also play a role in the onset or aggravation of migraine headaches, asthma, hay fever, ulcers, diarrhea, constipation, eczema, allergies, influenza, and even the common cold. Cardiovascular disorders, cancer, lupus, and diabetes have also been found to be linked to stress.

# Stress in Children and Youth

Although stress is a natural part of life and necessary for growth and development, there is growing concern about the role of stress in the lives of children and adolescents. Young people are exposed to a variety of stressors and may experience a wide range of reactions. These reactions include behavioral problems, depression, mental illness, and suicide. Some examples of less serious reactions are fatigue, headaches, stomach problems, mood swings, and poor attention span.

Life events create stress in the lives of youth. Some of the most serious life events that cause stress in children include the death of a parent, sibling, or grandparent; divorce of parents; remarriage of a parent and the merging of families; hospitalization of a family member; loss of employment by a parent; and birth of a sibling. Major transitions are also stressful, such as leaving home for the first time to enter school, meeting a new teacher, and moving from grade school to junior high or from junior high to high school. Many health conditions can also cause or contribute to stress, as listed in Table 3-1.

It is important that educators acknowledge that it is not only major life events, or highly stressful environments, that take a toll on the lives of

**TABLE 3-1  Health conditions that can be caused or aggravated by stress**

| | |
|---|---|
| Accident proneness | Musculoskeletal disorders |
| Cancer | Rheumatoid arthritis |
| Cardiovascular disorders | Low back pain |
| Coronary artery disease | Migraine headache |
| Essential hypertension | Muscle tension |
| Congestive heart failure | Pain |
| Gastrointestinal disorders | Psychological disorders |
| Constipation | Obsessive–compulsive behavior |
| Diarrhea | Depression |
| Duodenal ulcer | Phobias |
| Anorexia nervosa | Panic attacks |
| Bulimia | Schizophrenia |
| Obesity | Respiratory disorders |
| Ulcerative colitis | Asthma |
| Irritable bowel syndrome | Hay fever |
| Menstrual irregularities | Tuberculosis |
| Metabolic disorders | Skin disorders |
| Hyperthyroidism | Eczema |
| Hypothyroidism | Pruritus |
| Diabetes | Urticaria |
| | Psoriasis |

young people. Day-to-day problems and irritants have a cumulative effect and can be destructive as well. Examples of daily "hassles" that concern young people are physical appearance and peer acceptance, homework assignments and tests, and misplacing or losing things. Repeated minor hassles can add up to a major stress reaction.

## Stress and the Community and World Environments

The community climate in which young people grow up greatly affects the amount of stress they experience. Environmental factors that are highly stressful include living in poverty or crowded housing, being exposed to a pervasive drug culture and periodic street violence, attending poor schools, and having a dysfunctional family.

World events often cause children and adolescents stress. The amount of distress experienced is dependent on the extent of exposure and the degree to which a young person feels personally connected. Everyone was affected by the tragic events of September 11, 2001. Those living in or near New York City or Washington, D.C., or who knew individuals killed in the terrorist attacks, were the most affected. The New York City Board of Education conducted a survey to find what children were experiencing in the aftermath of 9/11, the subsequent anthrax attacks, and the plane crash in the Rockaways. The *New York Times* reported on the results of the survey, stating that 15% of the city's fourth through twelfth graders had fear of public places.[2] About 10% of the children suffered stress disorders with symptoms that included nightmares and other sleeping disorders, trouble concentrating, and obsessive thoughts.

### The Media

The media can cause stress in ways other than reporting disturbing news such as the terrorist attacks just mentioned. The amount and type of TV programming a young person watches influences the amount of stress he or she feels. Violent acts depicted on movies, TV shows, and video games can be distressful. Nightmares and night terrors can result from viewing troubling images. There is also evidence that heavy TV viewing is linked to depression, anxiety, and obesity.

### Sleep Deprivation

Many Americans, both children and adults, get less sleep than they need. On average we sleep 1 hour less than we need on weeknights and $1/2$ hour less than what we need on weekend nights.[3] By the end of the year we are short 338 hours. **Sleep deprivation** is the result, and the lack of sleep can be very stressful. Stress is experienced when we don't have the energy and alertness we need to concentrate and interact effectively with others. Lack of sleep also causes physical stress on the body, especially when sleep deprivation becomes a way of life.

Many adults and children become sleep deprived from staying up late at night watching TV programs or movies. Others become fixated on computer games or Internet surfing. Parents who let their children fall asleep in front of the television compound the problem. A study on the sleep and TV habits of children aged 5 through 10 reported that more than 76% of parents said TV viewing was a part of their child's regular bedtime routine, that 15.6% of children fell asleep in front of the TV at least two nights a week, that 26% of the children studied had a television in their bedroom, and that 40% of parents said their children had at least one sleep problem.[4]

Young people also become sleep deprived as they try to cram 28 hours of living into 24 hours. Many adolescents, in an effort to gain an edge in getting into a highly rated university, sign up for every possible school sport and activity while trying to earn top grades and give community service. When these youth finally try to go to bed they are often too wired to fall asleep.

Sleep experts say that elementary through high school aged kids need 9 to 11 hours of sleep a night, yet only 15% of adolescents say they sleep 8.5 hours or more on school nights, and 26% of students report typically sleeping 6.5 hours or less each school night.[5] School districts in a few states have shifted their schedules to give teens a little more time to sleep before school begins. Those who oppose such moves argue that a later starting time plays havoc on work, bus, after-school, and extracurricular activity schedules. The end result might be teenagers getting to bed even later, nullifying the desired outcome of more sleep.

## Overscheduling

The American lifestyle is often characterized as being "on the go," with the successful living "in the fast lane." It has almost become an American norm for parents to enlist their children in every extracurricular activity they can fit into their schedule. Some children are constantly on the go because their scheduled activities serve as baby-sitters for their working parents. From predawn until late at night, children and adolescents participate in team sports; take music, art, and dance lessons; attend school, scouting, and other youth group activities; and give community service.

Family life in the fast lane can leave both children and parents exhausted and irritable. Some schools have instituted "family nights" to try to give students and their parents time to relax and enjoy one another's company. On these family nights no homework is assigned and no school activities are scheduled. Parents have become proactive in some communities, stating that "enough is enough." These parents have organized themselves and taken petitions to local youth sports programs, schools, and community officials requesting these institutions to schedule their activities in a more family-friendly manner.

## Stress and the Home Environment

The home environment can give children a sense of belonging, provide appropriate role models, and teach communication and social skills, all of which buffer the degree of stress children experience. Changes in family structure and function, such as increases in the number of single-parent households, the increased proportion of two-parent households in which both parents work, and the growing number of "latchkey children," create additional demands for childhood adjustments. It is in the home that youngsters initially learn stress-coping techniques that are modeled by parents, other adults in the household, and older siblings. We will now look at some of the major home environment stressors.

### Home Alone

Being home alone can be stressful for children. The term **latchkey child** has been used to describe a child who is regularly left without direct adult supervision for a part of the day. The number of latchkey children has mushroomed in the last 20 years as the number of single-parent households and the number of families in which both parents are employed outside of the home have dramatically increased.

Latchkey children are at risk for a variety of problems. Sometimes children who are routinely left to care for themselves are more fearful than those who receive adult supervision. Two prevalent fears of latchkey children are that someone will break into their home and hurt them while they are alone or that older siblings will harm them. Latchkey children may also be more lonely and bored than supervised children. There is some indication that children who are unsupervised over large periods of time are at higher risk for having personality problems and depression during adolescence and adulthood. Children left unsupervised are also at increased risk of sexual abuse and accidents. Conversely, sometimes children who look after themselves achieve greater self-confidence and independence than those who are supervised.

You can help the latchkey children in your classroom in the following ways:

1. When you design homework, keep in mind that many of your students will not have adults at home to help them. Consider asking for parent volunteers or others to provide a telephone hotline for homework.

2. Schedule a few moments each day during which students can discuss personal concerns. Latchkey children especially need this time to just talk with an adult.

3. Be sure your school has clearly established procedures for contacting working parents in the case of an emergency and for providing for a child that becomes ill at school.

4. Encourage your school to provide extended day-care programs for before and after school. Some research indicates that children do better with continuous adult supervision in school-based programs than they do when left on their own.

## Parental Conflict, Separation, and Divorce

Parental conflict can arise from numerous situations, including financial problems, alcoholism, adultery, abuse, and selfishness. Rarely is a child responsible for marital discord, but children almost always feel somehow responsible. Children experience high levels of stress as they deal with their parents' fights and their own misplaced guilt.

Parental separation and divorce are traumatic and create stressful situations for children and adolescents. Whatever the reason for separation, psychological separation is more traumatic for a child than physical separation from a parent. Separation from siblings can also be significantly stressful. When a parent remarries, children have to contend with a new series of adjustments, such as having a new parental figure in the home, feeling conflicting loyalties between biological and stepparents, and dealing with new routines, responsibilities, and personal space issues. All of these adjustments are intensified when stepsiblings are involved. Children of parents granted joint custody must also make the monumental adjustments of living in two different households.

Approximately half the families in this country have undergone the pain of marital separation, with 60% of those partings affecting children. Parental divorce has been linked in children to delinquency, psychological disturbance, hostility and acting-out behavior, low self-esteem, low evaluation of families, early home leaving, and poor self-restraint and social adjustment. For many children of divorced families, school represents the only stable part of their environment. Educators and school personnel should be prepared to assess the student's behavior for signs of stress and recognize the signs of emotional problems.

The child's age at the time of the divorce directly influences his or her feelings and reactions. *Preschoolers* may become frightened about the divorce because they fear being deserted. As a result, they may be anxious about leaving their homes to attend school. Regression is also a common response to divorce among preschoolers. Lapses in accomplished developmental tasks, such as toilet training or self-dressing, may occur. Retreats to the use of security symbols, such as dolls and blankets, are likely to occur as well. In addition, children may blame themselves for causing the divorce and experience guilt as a result.

The most striking reaction among *young school-age children* is sadness, which is characterized by crying and sobbing. Fear is likely to be present, as are yearnings to be with the separated parent and feelings of conflict in loyalty to parents.

Intense anger is often a response to divorce among *older school-age children*. Interestingly, children in this age group are apt to respond to this anger with vigorous physical activity. This is quite unlike younger children, who become depressed and do not feel like participating in physical activity. Older children also have a shaken sense of identity and quite often will choose to ally themselves with one parent rather than the other.

## Dysfunctional Families

Children reared in **dysfunctional families** are exposed to many childhood stressors, such as parental alcoholism or drug dependency, mental illness, ineffective parenting skills, and poor communication patterns. Parental alcoholics often place unreasonable demands upon their children, such as the following: to keep secrecy about the alcoholic's behavior, to take responsibility for the alcoholic, to neither acknowledge nor express their own feelings, to accept the blame for their parent's drinking, and to provide emotional support and companionship for the alcoholic's spouse. (A detailed discussion of children of alcoholics is provided in Chapter 6.)

Family stress results when families are unable to openly discuss issues and reach mutually agreed-upon solutions. Healthy communication occurs when both parents and children learn to listen, honestly express feelings, remain nonjudgmental, and solve problems in a mutually beneficial manner. Parents and educators should use normal conversational tone when communicating with children and speak to children and adolescents in the same manner as they do adults. Communication with young people is furthered by asking open-ended questions, rather than questions with "yes" or "no" responses.

## Death of a Parent

The death of a parent or loved one represents a tremendously stressful life event for a child or adolescent. Acceptance of the death often takes many months to a few years. Reactions depend largely upon a child's age and developmental level. Fortunately, most children survive a parent's death with only minor emotional scars, but effective coping is assisted greatly by supportive adults. (A more detailed discussion of children and death is provided in Chapter 9.)

# Stress and the School Environment

The school environment presents a number of conditions and situations that can evoke stress in children and adolescents. Examples of stressors encountered in the school environment include teacher attitudes, behavior, personality, and mannerisms; peer pressures; harassment; homework;

grading and evaluation; competition and academic pressure; length of the school day; and extracurricular activities. Competitive stress occurs when teachers place emphasis upon competition in school situations, causing an individual to feel unable to perform up to expectations or demands. When teachers overemphasize competition and the need to finish first, unnecessary stress is created in the lives of students.

Children in kindergarten, first grade, and second grade often feel a great deal of stress about schoolwork, understanding work assignments, and completing creative projects correctly. After schoolwork stressors, the greatest source of worry to these youngsters is peer relationships. Peer relationship stressors include peer pressure, friendships, sharing, playing, and arguing. Other prominent stressors for this age are personal injury or loss (getting hurt, pushed or kicked, theft, emergency drills, destruction or loss of personal belongings) and loss of personal comfort, space, or time (school schedule, homework interfering with personal time, loss of recess time, noise in lunchroom, changing classes, teacher not present or absent).

Adolescents are seriously concerned about social rejection and fear of exposure in public. Losing friends, being ignored socially, feeling rejected, speaking in public, and making mistakes are examples of stress-provoking fears among adolescents. The resulting anxiety can lead to regressive and/or self-destructive behaviors, school phobia, academic difficulty, and withdrawal. As a result, parents, teachers, counselors, and school administrators should assist adolescents in identifying and coping with these fears.

Teachers can also experience stress in the school environment. Their stress is greatly intensified when they feel unsafe, unsupported, overworked, or out of control. Persistent long-term school-related stress can facilitate teacher "**burnout**"—a condition in which teachers become emotionally exhausted and ineffective. Chapter 1 gives insight into how to create a supportive school environment and effective classroom discipline. Chapter 7 discusses bullying and creating safe schools. Teachers can do the following things to reduce the amount of stress they and their students experience in school:

❖ Focus on speaking to children in a soft tone. Speaking or teaching in a loud or harsh voice or screaming creates stress.

❖ Listen to and respect students' thoughts and feelings.

❖ Recognize that a certain amount of talking, activity, and noise in the classroom is inevitable and positive.

❖ Establish classroom rules that are realistic for the appropriate age and grade level.

❖ Monitor schoolyard activities and track conflict resolution skills.

❖ Coordinate homework assignments with other teachers to avoid student overload.

❖ Be sure that demands placed on children are realistic and meaningful.

❖ Assign projects with children's ability and capacity in mind, allowing students the opportunity for success.

❖ Remember that a degree of stress enhances academic performance, but that too much anxiety impairs functioning.

❖ Have homework-free nights on which students' parents are encouraged to keep TVs turned off and to participate in family-based activities.

❖ Coordinate tests and test periods among teachers so students do not take multiple tests on the same day or during the same week.

❖ Before giving a test, explain its purpose, format, and focus.

❖ Be objective when grading, have grades serve as a positive reinforcement, and have cumulative grades take into account a variety of student work.

❖ Meet with students to explain why a certain grade was earned, convey that they are valued regardless of the grade, and help students set realistic goals for the next learning step.

❖ Help children understand that some failure is normal and acceptable.

## Managing Stress

Significant stressors in a young person's life are likely to cause problems with schoolwork. However, with appropriate support and assistance from school professionals, students can learn to effectively manage their stress by utilizing coping strategies and relaxation techniques. These students can then gradually make up missed work and return to their previous levels of academic achievement.

One of the first steps in helping children manage stress is getting them to recognize when they are experiencing it. Because children often lack the ability to express abstract feelings, they may have difficulty communicating the stress they feel. Therefore, educators should encourage students to talk about the stress they feel and should be alert for reactions to stress such as those noted in Box 3-1.

### Coping Strategies

Coping strategies can be used to reduce the amount of stress people experience in life. Children and young people can learn to be effective copers. Effective copers are likely to have role models whom they emulate and

## Assessing Stress in Students

The following checklist may help you identify students who are experiencing excessive stress. Students with several of these signs or symptoms may need referral to appropriate counseling professionals. These signs appear in children who have experienced a loss (e.g., parental separation or divorce, death of a loved one) or are having difficulty at home or school (e.g., rejection by classmates, difficulty with schoolwork, parental drug dependency). The more signs or symptoms a child has, the greater the likelihood of a stress-related or stress-induced problem. Children who are suffering great levels of stress exhibit it in their patterns of behavior. Often, they:

_____ Complain of headaches
_____ Complain frequently of an upset stomach
_____ Have out-of-control crying episodes
_____ Show evidence of not getting enough sleep
_____ Exhibit general tiredness
_____ Frequently appear irritable
_____ Appear restless
_____ Exhibit loss of appetite
_____ Have difficulty paying attention in class
_____ Tend to be physically aggressive with other children
_____ Easily become upset by changes
_____ Tend to quit tasks that are difficult
_____ Display difficulty concentrating
_____ Appear to lack emotion
_____ Seem depressed
_____ Lack self-confidence

from whom they learn specific coping skills. In addition, effective copers have people they can turn to for support, encouragement, and advice. They are able to trust and to maintain important interpersonal relationships and friendships.

Children with effective coping skills are able to enjoy play, smile and laugh, and have relaxed bodies. Successfully encountering and coping with stressful life situations brings about a sense of competence and enhances self-esteem. Optimism is a characteristic of those who effectively cope with stress. Teachers can do a number of things to help their students cope with stressful situations in the classroom (see Box 3-2). Some additional coping strategies are discussed in this section.

IN THE
CLASSROOM
3-2

## Helping Children Handle Stress

Teachers can help their students handle a stressful time by doing the following:

◆ *Mini vacation.* Have the student make a funny face or do a funny dance—anything for a distraction or to add humor to the situation. Taking a "mini vacation" will reduce the amount of anxiety the student feels and make it so he or she can better deal with whatever is stressing him or her.

◆ *Burn off energy.* Provide appropriate ways for students to release energy created by the adrenaline released during stressful situations. This could be running in place, taking a walk, playing a game in the gym, or having an early recess.

◆ *Relaxation techniques.* Have students do a relaxation technique, such as taking deep breaths and concentrating entirely on breathing from the diaphragm for a few minutes.

◆ *Talk.* Encourage students to talk about their stress by making statements such as "Talk to me about your stress," or "Tell me what worries you."

◆ *Check for thinking distortions.* Help students recognize cognitive distortions that are adding to their stress by asking questions such as "What is the worst thing that could happen if ...?"

The basic message to give children who are feeling a great deal of stress is to not give up, and to work through their stressors. Help them realize that we all encounter stress on a daily basis, and that stress can be minimized but not totally avoided. Help them realize that they can manage their stress by knowing how to deal with it.

***Play*** Play serves as an important stress management tool in the lives of children. Through play, problems are symbolically reenacted and solved. Tension is also relieved.

***Journal Writing*** Keeping a journal not only helps students develop writing skills, but also helps them identify and express their emotions. Encourage students to keep a stress journal of the stressors they encounter during the day. Writing such a journal can teach children to:

❖ Identify specific situations at home and school that are stressful

❖ Describe feelings and reactions to stressors

❖ Learn how to avoid certain stressors in their environment

❖ Give insight into how to cope or confront stressors

❖ Provide feedback about efforts to avoid and control stress

***Rest and Sleep***    Getting adequate rest and sleep reduces the amount of stress an individual experiences and helps a person better cope with everyday hassles. Inadequate rest and sleep can lead to chronic fatigue, inability to concentrate, nervousness, and irritability. Many young children stay up late watching TV, and the busy schedules of adolescents keep them from getting adequate rest. Stress reactions in young people are also often linked to sleeping problems or insomnia. Encourage your students to get the rest and sleep they need, especially during times of rapid growth.

***Cognitive Restructuring***    **Cognitive restructuring** is becoming aware of one's thinking patterns, evaluating them, and changing them when needed. We experience stress when we perceive something as stressful. For instance, having a "bad hair day" may be perceived as terribly embarrassing by one teenage girl and mildly annoying by another. Uncooperative hair doesn't cause stress, but thinking that one's hair must be perfect does.

Most people have some distorted thinking patterns that exacerbate the amount of stress they feel. Adolescents are particularly prone to **distorted thinking patterns.** Here are a few examples of various types of distorted thinking patterns:[6]

❖ *All-or-nothing thinking.* Anything less than perfection is a failure. Evaluating in extreme black-or-white categories. "I got a 93% on the test . . . I really messed up!" "I spilled my glass . . . the dinner was a disaster." "If part of me is bad, I'm all bad."

❖ *Jumping to conclusions.* Conclusions are not tested but are based on hunches, intuition, and experiences. There are two types: *mind reading*—"She did that on purpose!" "My teachers don't like me"— and *fortune telling*—"If I tried out I'd blow it." "She'd say no if I asked her to go out with me."

❖ *Overgeneralizing.* Thinking in a negative pattern. Key words are *always, never, all,* and *none.* "I always screw things up." "I never do well in math."

❖ *Filtering.* Dwelling on the negative details or aspects of a situation to the exclusion of all others and concluding that the whole situation is negative. "That guy ruined my whole day." "How can I concentrate when my hair looks terrible!"

❖ *Labeling.* Giving oneself or another a label based upon imperfections, as though a single word could completely describe a complex human being. "I'm so stupid." "He's an idiot."

❖ *Catastrophizing.* Thinking that something is so horrible or so awful that one cannot bear it. In the process one feels helpless and pathetic.

"I'd die if Johnny were to break up with me." "All hell will break loose if I don't catch that pass."

When we begin to feel stress, it is helpful to take a moment and try to discover what it is we are thinking that may be causing the stress response. Thinking patterns are so habitual that we are usually unaware of them unless we make an effort to notice them. Once we are aware of our thoughts, we can evaluate them for their validity and can reevaluate the situation with a broader perspective. We can also check and fine-tune our expectations. Teachers can help their students develop these cognitive restructuring skills.

**Humor**   Perhaps nothing dissipates the stress response more quickly than humor. Humor can reduce pain, diffuse anger and anxiety, buffer the amount of stress experienced, and give one a sense of power in the middle of chaos.[7] Learning to laugh at one's own shortcomings and to not take life too seriously are critical for effective stress management. People can enlarge their "funny bone" by studying the various types of humor (parody, slapstick, absurdity, irony, puns, and so forth) and by learning to look for humor in everyday situations. Whereas humor reduces stress, laughing at someone else's expense does not. It is helpful to remember the difference between humor and ridicule (see Figure 3-3 ).

**Time Management**   Students cope better with varied stressors at school if they are organized and self-disciplined in their use of time. Some schools provide students with day-planners that contain calendars for students to record dates of tests and when major assignments are due. These planners

---

## Humor Versus Ridicule

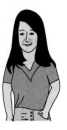

**Laughing with**
1. going for jocular
2. caring and empathy
3. builds confidence
4. involves people in fun
5. laughing at self
6. amusing
7. supportive
8. builds bridges
9. pokes fun at universal human foibles

**Laughing at**
1. going for jugular
2. contempt and insensitivity
3. destroys confidence
4. excludes some people
5. being the butt of a joke
6. abusing, offends
7. sarcastic
8. divides people
9. reinforces stereotypes by singling out a particular group as the "butt"

**FIGURE 3-3   Humor versus ridicule**

also provide students an organized means of keeping track of daily assignments and homework. When planners are not provided, teachers can help students develop their own. Teachers can also help students develop time management skills by teaching them how to break down a large assignment into steps with self-imposed due dates. This skill prevents the stress caused by rushing to complete an assignment at the last moment.

***Additional Coping Strategies***    Other essential coping strategies for managing stress include the life skills discussed in Chapter 2: self-evaluation, self-worth, proactivity, emotional IQ, relationship building, communication, goal setting, problem solving, and media literacy. Be sure to review the teaching activities in Chapter 2 for more ideas on addressing stress in your classroom.

## Relaxation Techniques

Relaxation techniques are activities that help the body return to a relaxed state—homeostasis. They can be used to effectively deal with an intense stressor or with the effects of cumulative stress. While some relaxation techniques require special training or equipment (e.g., yoga, tai chi, biofeedback), others are relatively easy to teach and are highly effective.

***Exercise***    One of the best ways to help students handle stress is to provide opportunities for regular physical exercise. Exercise can serve as a diversion from stressors. When students play hard they forget about other things that are bothering them. Exercise also helps students relax by releasing excess muscle tension, by causing fight-or-flight stress hormones to be metabolized, and by encouraging the body to release endorphins. Endorphins, which are chemicals produced by the body, are closely related to opium and create a feeling of well-being.

***Progressive Muscular Relaxation***    Progressive muscular relaxation is a technique used to help people become aware of the difference between relaxation and tension in body parts. Stress can cause muscle tension in various locations of the body, such as the neck, shoulders, or back. Young people can learn **progressive relaxation** by tensing and relaxing muscles in one set of muscles after another. See Box 3-3 for an example of a progressive relaxation exercise that can be used in the classroom.

***Mental Imagery***    **Mental imagery** allows children to forget about their stressors and achieve a relaxed state by visualizing a pleasant situation. Visualized scenes that induce relaxation are quiet, peaceful, and warm. Imagined water in the form of a mountain stream, lake, river, or ocean also encourages relaxation. Visualizing oneself performing a physical task such as an athletic move to perfection can be relaxing as well. It is often helpful

IN THE
CLASSROOM
*3-3*

# Progressive Relaxation

*I. Concentrate on Breathing.*    Instruct your students to sit quietly with their eyes closed and with one of their hands on their abdomen. Tell them to take a deep breath and try to completely fill their lungs by using their diaphragm muscle. Then, have them exhale slowly. Instruct them to concentrate on their breathing for a few minutes, noticing the rhythmic flow of air as it enters and leaves their body. Have your students visualize that the air coming into their lungs is white, clean, and pure, and that the air they are exhaling is dark and filled with any negative emotion they might be feeling.

*II. Go Limp.*    After students have concentrated solely on their breathing, instruct them to turn their attention to the amount of tension they feel in their back, shoulders, and neck. Ask them to try to relax the muscles in this area of the body. Remind them of how, as a small child, they went totally limp when they didn't want someone to pick them up. Have them try and duplicate this feeling of going totally limp.

*III. Progressive Exercise.*    Explain that we often do not realize the amount of muscle tension we have in our body. As we become more aware of it we can better relax. When we relax our body, our mind usually follows and relaxes as well. Follow the order outlined below to take your students through a progressive relaxation exercise. Instruct your students to tense the muscle group identified to 100% of their ability for about 5 seconds and to then relax for about 15 seconds. Then tense the same muscle group to 75% and relax, 30% and relax, 10% and relax. This will help the students identify the amount of tension they are experiencing in each muscle group and the difference between the various degrees of tension and relaxation. This type of relaxation technique is especially helpful for "hyper" individuals who find it difficult to relax by just sitting still.

Follow this sequence:

1.  Back, shoulders, and neck

2.  Face and scalp

3.  Arms and hands

4.  Chest and stomach

5.  Legs and feet

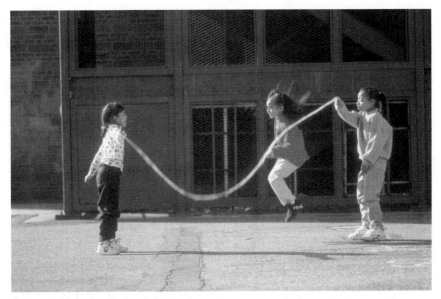

Recess and physical education classes can offer students a chance to release the stress that often builds up in an academic environment.

for students with persistent test anxiety to practice mental imagery. Have them get into a relaxed state and then imagine themselves taking a test while maintaining that relaxed state. They can also use mental imagery just before taking a test to help become relaxed. The following is an example of a mental imagery exercise that can be used in the classroom.

Very slowly, instruct the students as follows:

Close your eyes. Take a deep breath and let it out slowly. Imagine yourself lying someplace that is soft, quiet, and filled with sunlight. This sunlight is very yellow and pleasantly warm. Feel the warmth of the sunlight. Notice how this warm yellow light covers you like a blanket. The warm yellow rays warm your face, your arms, your body, your legs, and your feet. Stretch in the light and then totally relax. Your entire body is relaxed. You feel warm, heavy, and relaxed.

*Music*    Music can alter our moods and either relax or excite us. Have you ever noticed the type of music played in elevators? This acoustic slow-tempo music is piped into elevators to help people better cope with the stresses of being with strangers in a small confined space, while rapidly ascending or descending. Young people usually prefer fast-paced energizing music, but teachers can help students identify more tranquil forms of music to listen to while coping with stress.

## Key Terms

stress   101
stressor   101
General Adaptation Syndrome
  (G.A.S.)   101
alarm   101
resistance   101
homeostasis   101
exhaustion   101
fight-or-flight response   102

sleep deprivation   104
latchkey child   106
dysfunctional families   108
burnout   109
cognitive restructuring   113
distorted thinking patterns   113
progressive relaxation   115
mental imagery   115

## Review Questions

1. What do you think is "eating Ricky"? Give evidence for your answer from information you found in the chapter.
2. Define *stress* and *homeostasis*. Describe G.A.S. and the effects of stress on the body.
3. Identify the many sources of stress in the community and world environments.
4. Identify the many sources of stress coming from the home environment.
5. Identify things that educators can do to help latchkey children.
6. Identify what children in different age groups find stressful at school. Discuss the many ways teachers can reduce the amount of stress experienced at school.
7. Identify the signs that may indicate a child is suffering from excessive stress.
8. Explain what teachers can do to help students cope with stressful situations in the classroom.
9. Explain how play, rest, and sleep help people better cope with stress.
10. Identify several distorted thinking patterns and explain how they magnify the amount of stress a person experiences. Give examples of distorted thoughts you have had or observed within the last week.
11. Discuss how humor reduces stress, and explain the differences between humor and ridicule.
12. Discuss ways educators can help students become better time managers.
13. Explain how exercise helps reduce the amount of stress a student feels.
14. Explain what progressive muscular relaxation is and how it can help a student relax.
15. Describe a mental imagery exercise that could bring about relaxation.

16. Describe the types of music that can initiate a relaxation response. Give examples of how music could be used in the classroom to reduce stress.

## References

1. Selye, H. (1977). *Stress Without Distress.* New York: Signet Books.
2. Goodnough, A. (2002). "Post-9/11 Pain Found to Linger in Young Minds." *New York Times*, May 2. Available at http://www.nytimes.com.
3. Brink, S. (2000). "Sleepless Society." *U.S. News and World Report*, October 10. Available at http://www.usnews.com/usnews/issue/001016/nycu/sleep.htm.
4. Webber, T. (1999). "Watching TV May Cause Sleep Problems in Kids." ABC News, September 8. Available at http://www.abcnews.go.com/sections/living/DailyNews/tvkids990907.html.
5. National Sleep Foundation (2002). *Adolescent Sleep Needs and Patterns: Research Report and Resource Guide.* Available at http://www.sleepfoundation.org/publications/teensleep.html.
6. Schiaraldi, G. R. (1993). *Hope and Help for Depression: A Practical Guide.* Miami Beach: Healthy People.
7. Seaward, B. L. (1999). *Managing Stress.* Boston: Jones and Bartlett.

# 4

# HEALTHY EATING AND
# PHYSICAL ACTIVITY PATTERNS

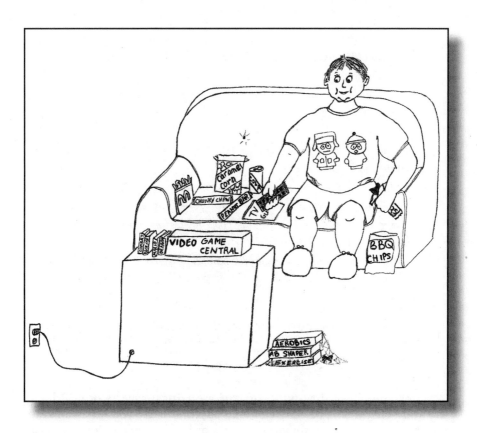

## Shirleisa and Too Many Other Children

*Shirleisa Rogers is 10 years old and weighs more than 200 pounds. Every morning, she slips a needle full of insulin into the fat on the back of her right arm. At lunch, she finds a spot on her left arm. Before she goes to bed, she pumps the syringe into her stomach.*

*The San Leandro girl has a kind of diabetes once so rare in children that doctors call it "adult-onset." A decade ago, the pediatricians treating Shirleisa would have been surprised to see such a case in a child. Now, they see two to five youngsters a day with it.*

*California public health experts say children like Shirleisa are ailing canaries in a coal mine—the early signs of a deeper problem. The state's kids are the fattest they have ever been.*

*Specialists at Children's Hospital Oakland, where severely obese Northern California children go for treatment, see teenage boys whose hip bones have popped from their sockets. They treat girls whose hormones have gone so haywire they're growing beards. They prescribe high blood pressure pills for 12-year-olds and worry that high school patients might have heart attacks or strokes.*

*"I'm looking 9-year-olds in the eye and talking to them about their bodies as if they are 50- or 60-year-olds," said Barbara King-Hopper, a nurse educator at the children's hospital.*

*More than a quarter of the state's children ages 9 to 17 are overweight, some by only 10 or 20 pounds, some by 100 pounds or more. Certain groups, such as African Americans, Latinos, and poor whites, are even heavier. And the fattest kids are getting fatter.*

*After decades of holding steady, the number of severely overweight children in the United States has doubled since 1980. The situation is so bad the surgeon general in January declared childhood obesity a national epidemic.*

Source: From K. Severson, and M. May, "Growing Up Too Fat: Kids Suffer Adult Ailments as More Become Dangerously Obese," *San Francisco Chronicle*, May 12, 2002. Available at http://www.sfgate.com/cgi-bin/article.cgi?file=/chronicle/archive/2002/05/12/MN237512.dtl.

Eating and physical activity patterns are critical aspects of health and well-being. These patterns not only contribute to a young person's current health but are also important to his or her future health status as an adult. Healthy eating patterns and regular physical activity promote optimal health, growth, and development in childhood and adolescence and reduce the risk for chronic disease in adulthood (e.g., coronary heart disease, cancer, and stroke). The eating and physical activity patterns established in youth often extend into adulthood. The purpose of this chapter is to help teachers recognize their potential in helping students adopt and establish lifelong healthy eating behaviors and physical activity patterns. This chapter examines how patterns of eating and physical activity contribute to health and well-being and explains what teachers can do to help young people establish these healthy habits.

## Needs and Concerns

School-age youth need to have a healthful diet and to enjoy a physically active lifestyle. A healthful diet contains the amounts of **essential nutrients** and **calories** needed to prevent nutritional deficiencies and excesses. Healthful diets also provide the right balance of **carbohydrate, fat,** and **protein** to reduce risks for chronic diseases (e.g., heart disease, certain cancers, diabetes, stroke, osteoporosis), and are a part of a full and productive lifestyle. Healthful diets help children grow, develop, and do well in school. Such diets are obtained from a variety of foods that are available, affordable, and enjoyable. Many youth need more physical activity, because a sedentary lifestyle is unhealthful. Increasing the calories burned in daily activities helps to maintain strength and a healthy outlook on life, and allows young people to eat a nutritious and enjoyable diet without fear of becoming overweight.

Young people need help from educators in developing lifelong eating and physical activity patterns that positively affect healthy growth and development. Many young people do not follow dietary and physical activity recommendations. On average, children and adolescents consume too much fat, saturated fat, simple sugars, and sodium, and not enough fruits, vegetables, or calcium. Also, many young people do not engage in moderate or vigorous physical activity at least three days a week. Physical activity among both boys and girls declines steadily during adolescence with increasing age.[1] Adolescent girls are more likely than boys to be sedentary. School-age youths are fatter now than were children in the 1960s and 1970s. This section of the chapter examines nutritional and physical activity concerns of young people.

### Poor Eating Habits

Today's children and adolescents frequently decide what to eat with little adult supervision. The increase in one-parent families or families having two working parents, along with the availability of convenience foods and fast-food restaurants in the community and in the school cafeteria, inhibit the ability of parents to monitor their childrens' eating habits. Yet, eating habits are important to a young person's health, weight, and emotional well-being. A high demand for nutrients and energy results from a large spurt in growth and development during adolescence. This physiological need combines with psychosocial changes such as the desire for independence and identity, concern for appearance and peer acceptance, and an active lifestyle. Family background, increased independence and mobility, and money for discretionary spending on food products also influence eating habits.

Some of the poor dietary habits often displayed by adolescents include the following:

❖ Skipping meals, especially breakfast

❖ Avoidance of nutritious foods, such as milk, fruits, or vegetables, out of dislike

❖ Frequent consumption of "fast food" and other low-nutritive, high-energy foods

❖ Dieting

Adolescent girls are at higher risk of failing to meet nutritional requirements than are boys. The overwhelming desire by many adolescent girls to be thin can create energy and nutritional inadequacies as well as lead to psychological problems, such as anorexia nervosa or bulimia. A high proportion of girls at normal weight believe that they are overweight and are dissatisfied with their body image. Adolescent boys on the whole consume greater amounts of food than girls and are less likely to suffer nutritional deficiencies. Figures 4-1, 4-2, and 4-3 provide additional information on the unhealthy eating patterns of youth.

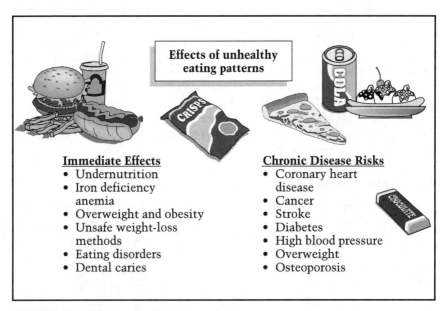

**Effects of unhealthy eating patterns**

**Immediate Effects**
• Undernutrition
• Iron deficiency anemia
• Overweight and obesity
• Unsafe weight-loss methods
• Eating disorders
• Dental caries

**Chronic Disease Risks**
• Coronary heart disease
• Cancer
• Stroke
• Diabetes
• High blood pressure
• Overweight
• Osteoporosis

**FIGURE 4-1    Effects of unhealthy eating patterns**

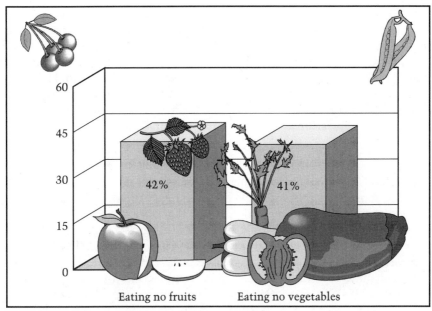

Source: Data from Youth Risk Behavior Survey, 1997.

**FIGURE 4-2** **Percentage of high school students not eating on the previous day**

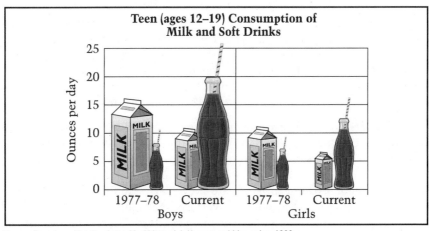

Source: Data from *Nutrition Action Healthletter*, July/August and November, 1998.

**FIGURE 4-3 Liquid candy**
Soda pop has become our drink of choice. The average teenage boy who drinks soda con-
sumes 42 ounces a day and only 10 ounces of milk. Girls average 34 ounces of soda a day
but only about 7 ounces of milk. That means youth are not getting the nutrients they
need. Soda single-handedly accounts for 15% or more of youth's calories. A 12-ounce can
of nondiet cola has about 10 teaspoons of sugar, 150 calories, and no other nutritive
value. Schools often promote soda consumption by entering into contracts to sell soft
drink products in their vending machines.

*Iron Deficiency Anemia*    **Iron deficiency anemia** is a consequence of poor eating habits among adolescents. Adolescent girls are at high risk for iron deficiency anemia because of inadequate intake of foods high in iron and vitamin C, which help the body absorb iron. Lacking sufficient iron, the young person's body has reduced ability to produce hemoglobin. Hemoglobin is needed to carry oxygen in the blood. Girls with iron deficiency anemia have difficulty paying attention and suffer from fatigue. They are also vulnerable to infections.

*Low Calcium Intake*    Adolescent females consume less **calcium** than is recommended by health experts. It is recommended that they consume at least 1,200 mg of calcium per day. To meet this recommendation, girls need to consume a minimum of three servings daily of milk or yogurt. A survey of 14- to 18-year-old girls showed that 90% of the girls consumed less than this amount. The study also found that girls' intakes of both milk and calcium have decreased since the 1980s and that calcium intake decreases among girls as they become teenagers.[2] Only 30% of school children consume the recommended milk group servings on any given day. Between 1989–1991 and 1994–1995, among children aged 2 to 17, the average consumption of milk and milk products dropped by 6%, while the average consumption of soft drinks rose by 41%.[3]

With almost half of an adult's bone mass being formed during the teen years, the inadequate calcium intakes among children and adolescents are a serious concern. Young females who consume inadequate amounts of dietary calcium are at increased risk for osteoporosis in later life. **Osteoporosis** is a decrease in the amount of bone so severe that the bones fracture easily. To reduce risk of osteoporosis, consuming enough calcium is particularly important during childhood, adolescence, and young adulthood. This helps bones to reach their maximum density. Regular participation in physical activity also can help prevent osteoporosis.

*Skipping Breakfast*    Many students start school with no breakfast or an inadequate breakfast. A study of Wisconsin students showed that 10% of elementary students, 25% of middle school students, and 30% of high school students started school without breakfast.[4] Many other students came to school without an adequate breakfast. Skipping breakfast is not limited to children who live in poverty. Many children who can afford breakfast come to school without eating breakfast. Those who skip breakfast do so for a variety of reasons. Some say that they don't have time to eat breakfast before leaving for school. Others say that they don't feel hungry when they wake up. Often, parents have left for work or are too busy to prepare breakfast. Even those who eat before leaving the house may become hungry way before lunch time. A long bus ride requires some children to leave home early, so their breakfast may wear off by midmorning.

Starting the school day off hungry puts students at a disadvantage. The physical symptoms of hunger include stomach pain, headache, muscle tension, muscle fatigue, and sleepiness. The emotional and psychological effects include anxiety, nervousness, anger, aggression, indecisiveness, and confusion. Teachers see the results of these symptoms. The hunger interferes with students' ability to learn and to perform academically. Often when children act out it is a behavioral response to being hungry. A study by Kleinman and colleagues found that elementary students who attended school hungry had significantly lower arithmetic scores, were more likely to repeat a grade, and more likely to have seen a psychologist and to have difficulty getting along with other children.[5] This study also found that secondary students who attended school hungry were more likely to have seen a psychologist, been suspended from school, and had difficulty getting along with other students.

The ideal option is for students to eat breakfast at home. However, when factors contribute to a child arriving at school hungry, schools can provide a nutritionally balanced breakfast before classes begin. Or, breakfast foods can be made available after classes have started, during recess or at a midmorning break. According to the U.S. Department of Agriculture, about 7 million students eat breakfast at school (compared with about 27 million eating school lunch), and 74,000 schools nationwide provide breakfast to students. About 85% of those eating breakfast receive their meals free or at reduced price.[6]

***Snacking***  Snacks are an important part of most adolescents' diets. Unfortunately, the snack foods typically consumed by adolescents tend to be high in fat, cholesterol, sugar, and sodium but lacking in real nutritive value. Snacks consisting of nonfat milk, raw vegetables, and fruits can be an important source of essential nutrients, and they do not contain the excessive fats, calories, sodium, sugar, or cholesterol of junk food.

***Undernutrition***  An estimated 4 million children experience prolonged food insufficiency and hunger each year. This represents 8% of children in the United States.[4] **Undernutrition** can have lasting effects on children's cognitive development and school performance. Chronically undernourished children attain lower scores on standardized achievement tests, especially tests of language ability. When children are hungry or undernourished, they:

❖ Have difficulty resisting infection and are therefore more likely than other children to become sick, to miss school, and to fall behind in class

❖ Are irritable and have difficulty concentrating, which can interfere with learning

❖ Have low energy, which can limit their physical activity

***Diet-Related Chronic Diseases***  Poor eating habits can contribute to the development of chronic diseases in adulthood. **Coronary heart disease, stroke, high blood pressure, diabetes,** osteoporosis, and **cancer** are some of the chronic diseases that are related to poor dietary habits. The eating practices that contribute to chronic disease are established early in life. Young people who have unhealthy eating habits tend to maintain these habits as they age. For this reason it is critical that healthy eating patterns are taught before poor habits become firmly established.

One diet-related chronic disease that can develop during childhood or adolescence is **type 2 diabetes**. Type 2 diabetes has been a disease that primarily affected adults. In fact, it used to be called *adult-onset diabetes* because it occurred mostly in men and women over age 50. But now it is showing up at an increasing rate among children, especially those who are obese and physically inactive. A decade ago, pediatricians would have been surprised to see a case of type 2 diabetes in a child. The rise in type 2 diabetes cases in young people has led experts to label the disease an emerging epidemic.

In type 2 diabetes the pancreas is usually producing enough insulin, but for unknown reasons the body cannot use the insulin effectively, a condition called **insulin resistance**. After several years, the insulin production decreases. Uncontrolled blood sugar can injure blood vessels, leading to serious health problems. If not treated, type 2 diabetes can cause serious and even life-threatening conditions, such as blindness, kidney disease, nerve damage, and heart disease. Children and adolescents diagnosed with type 2 diabetes have a longer time in which to develop these complications than individuals who develop the disease later in life. It appears that type 2 diabetes is a more aggressive disease when it occurs at a young age, increasing risk of complications.

Among children, cases have occurred in early childhood, but the peak age for diagnosis usually occurs after the onset of puberty. Changes in hormone levels during puberty can cause insulin resistance and decreased insulin action.

The symptoms of type 2 diabetes develop gradually. They are not as sudden in onset as in type 1 diabetes. Some people have no symptoms. Symptoms may include fatigue or nausea, frequent urination, unusual thirst, weight loss, blurred vision, frequent infections, and slow healing of wounds or sores.

Over the last decade, the prevalence of diabetes in the United States has escalated upward. Health experts attribute this increase to the fact that Americans have become heavier and that obesity is rising at an alarming rate. These experts are worried that the number of cases of diabetes in the United States could double in the next 50 years if the prevalence of obesity continues at the present rate.

## Availability of Junk Food in Schools

In the past, the primary source of foods for students at schools was school lunch. Today, school lunch represents a smaller part of the school food environment because many schools now provide increased food options:

foods are for sale in vending machines, school stores, and snack bars; and à la carte foods are for sale in the cafeteria. In addition, less nutritious options are now available to students at younger ages than ever before. The increased availability of low-nutritive foods at schools appears to be a major cause of poor eating habits in youth.[7]

With increasing financial pressures and limited resources, schools often put nutrition at the bottom of the priority list. School foodservice programs must often now be completely financially self-supporting because of declining allocations for operating budgets. As a result, many schools are compensating for the loss of funds from budget cuts by increasing the sale of à la carte foods and fast-food options. For many schools, entering into contracts with food or beverage marketers has become a source of additional income. A recent trend is for school districts to negotiate exclusive "pouring contracts" with soft drink companies. Many of these contracts have provisions to increase the percentage of profits schools receive when sales volume increases. This is a substantial incentive for schools to promote soft drink consumption by adding vending machines, increasing the times they are available, and marketing the products to students.[7]

## The Influence of Television and Media

Preschool and school-age children watch on average about 25 hours of television per week, 15% of which consists of advertisements. A high proportion of these advertisements are for food products. Many of the advertised food products are of low nutritional value and contain excessive amounts of sugar, fat, or sodium.

Preschoolers are perhaps the age group most vulnerable to this kind of advertising because they cannot differentiate the ads from the program and do not have the cognitive ability to understand why the advertised products are not good for them. Many commercials promote the false impression that consumption of certain foods will make children more like their heroes. As a result, preschoolers put heavy pressure on parents to buy the advertised foods and are genuinely confused and frustrated when parents do not comply.

Sedentary leisure activities, such as television watching, playing video games, and personal computing, have contributed to the increasing prevalence of overweight in the United States.[8] Television viewing and other sedentary activities are major contributors to physical inactivity in many school-age children. These sedentary activities take time away from participation in energy-expending physical activities. Studies have documented that the adolescents who are frequent viewers of television participate in physical activity less than their peers who watch less television.[9] Television viewing is also associated with snacking on high-energy, low-nutrient foods. As mentioned earlier, the average school-age youth spends approximately 25 hours per week watching television. In the United States, more than one-fourth of children watch four or more hours per day. Next to sleeping, television watching occupies the greatest amount of leisure time during childhood for most children. On average, youth spend more time watching television over the course of a year than they spend in school.

The media have a large influence in shaping attitudes about eating and physical activity. Because adolescence is a time of changing body image, young people are vulnerable to media messages that define one's sense of what is physically attractive. Adolescents are bombarded by magazines, television, and movies containing distorted images of what makes a person physically attractive and sexually desirable—excessively slim females and muscular males. In their attempt to approach these "ideals," adolescents often engage in poor nutritional habits and excessive exercise. Fad diets, diet pills, skipping meals (especially breakfast and lunch), and nonnutritious snacking put many adolescents at nutritional and psychological risk.

**Targeting Kids**  Food advertising often targets children and teenagers because they are so valuable to the food market industry. Children between the ages of 7 and 12 spend more than $2 billion of their own money on snacks and beverages each year, and teenagers spend more than $13 billion at fast-food restaurants. It is also estimated that children influence almost three-quarters of their families' food and beverage purchases. Is it any wonder then that the U.S. food industry spends $36 billion a year on advertising and is the second largest advertiser in the American economy? The most advertised products are convenience foods, confectionaries, snacks, and soft drinks; 95% of the 10,000 food commercials that children see each year are for foods high in sugar or fat or both. These advertisements frequently use cartoon and movie tie-ins to attract children to their products.*

Fast-food restaurants, such as McDonald's and Burger King, target children with on-site playgrounds, cartoon characters, and kids' meals that include toy giveaways. For example, McDonald's had a Happy Meal promotion that featured Mickey Mouse and several other Disney characters, and Burger King has promoted its food to kids with toys from movies such as *Ice Age* and others. During the 1990s, both Burger King and McDonald's offered toys from characters in the television show *Teletubbies*. *Teletubbies* is a show that is aimed at babies, and so this caused controversy over the marketing of fast food to 1- and 2-year-olds. Another controversial move by McDonald's is a TV advertisement in which a young father is playing with his infant child. In the background, a female voice says, "There will be a first step, a first word, and of course, a first french fry." This picture

---

* The statistics used in this paragraph are from Mediascope, "Children, Health and Advertising: Issue Briefs." Studio City, CA: Mediascope Press, 2000. Available at http://www.mediascope.org/pubs/ibriefs/cha.htm.

then fades to show the Golden Arches and a french fry curved into a smile. This ad ran numerous times during the television coverage of the 2002 Olympic Games. Another McDonald's ad shows a crying toddler who can be consoled only by Ronald McDonald waving at the child. These messages suggest that children can be started on fast foods (e.g., hamburgers, fries, shakes) at a very young age and seek to build brand loyalty in these children. These ploys certainly work, because every month more than 90% of children in the United States eat at McDonald's—and that's just one fast-food chain.

There can be no doubt that this constant and relentless promotion of high-calorie, high-fat food is contributing to the epidemic of childhood obesity. Advertisements targeting kids encourage preferences for junk food and contribute to the poor eating habits that we have discussed in this chapter.

***Advertising Thinness as the Ideal***    It is pretty hard not to be affected by the media's constant message that "Thin is in!" By the time a girl is 17, she is likely to have seen 250,000 commercials and advertisements through the media, many of which emphasize the importance of beauty and physical attractiveness and use thinness as a standard of beauty. However, the women portrayed in almost every ad are not typical of normal, healthy women. Fashion models weigh substantially less than the average women, and it has been estimated that a young woman in the United States has only a 1% chance of being as thin as a supermodel.

The apparent motive of advertisers in purposefully normalizing unrealistically thin bodies in ads is to create an unattainable desire that drives product purchase and consumption. In other words, when individuals realize that their own bodies are not in line with the desired or ideal body shape, they become anxious, frustrated, and disappointed. The overriding message is that we need to change something about ourselves in order to be accepted, loved, or successful. If we have thin, fit bodies, we are promised that our lives will be perfect. Yet, perhaps fewer than 5% of the population can in reality achieve the shapes and sizes the media portray as ideal. Still, the media hold this unrealistic ideal up to us and suggest that we try to reach it.

The dissatisfaction with body image that the media help to create leads to increased purchasing of products, but wreaks havoc on the psyches and well-being of many. No wonder so many men and women are struggling with body image dissatisfaction. Girls who spend their time reading women's magazines with lots of female-oriented advertisements are more likely to feel bad about their own appearance and to obsess over their physical appearance as a measure of their own worth than those who do not read these magazines. Is it any wonder then that three-quarters of normal-weight women think they are overweight and that 9 of 10 women overestimate their body size? Health experts are concerned that depicting thin models in ads may lead girls into unhealthy weight-control habits because the ideal they are seeking to emulate is unattainable for many and unhealthy for most. Girls who are dissatisfied with their bodies show more dieting, anxiety, and bulimic symptoms after exposure to fashion and advertising images in teen magazines. A study published in the March 1999 issue of *Pediatrics* showed that girls aged 10 to 18 who read women's fashion magazines are two to three times more likely to diet than girls who do not read these magazines.

The women featured in the media keep getting slimmer and slimmer. In 1999 *People* magazine ran an article about this trend entitled "How Thin Is Too Thin?" that depicted several famous actresses (Heather Locklear, Jennifer Aniston, Lara Flynn Boyle, Victoria Beckham, Calista Flockhart, Courtney Cox Arquette, Helen Hunt, Paula Devicq, Gwyneth Paltrow, Kelly Ripa, and others) before and after they had become excessively thin. The article noted the impact that these stars' appearances has on young people:

> "We're seeing quite an increase in inquiries [from parents and therapists] about girls 9, 10, and 11 years old trying to emulate their favorite stars," says Adrienne Ressler, body-image specialist at the Renfrew Center in Coconut Creek, Fla. "For adolescents, the ideal for the person they want to be when they grow up is either a movie star, TV actress or supermodel, and the emphasis is very much on external appearance. Our patients would die—and practically do—to look like Calista Flockhart. They say, 'I want to look like her. I want to *be* her.'"(pg. 120)[10]

## The Epidemic of Overweight and Obesity

Over the past 30 years, the prevalence of overweight and obesity among both children and adults has increased dramatically, prompting U.S. health organizations and officials to warn of an epidemic of obesity (see Figure 4-4). In December 2001, *The Surgeon General's Call to Action to Prevent and Decrease Overweight and Obesity* was released.[11] In the report, Surgeon General David Satcher said, "Overweight and obesity may not be infectious diseases, but they have reached epidemic proportions in the United States." He also said, "Left unabated, overweight and obesity may soon cause as much preventable disease and death as cigarette smoking."

The report paints a grim picture of the extent of overweight and obesity in the United States. Nearly two of every three adults (61%) in the United States are overweight or obese, according to the report. The surgeon general's report defines being **overweight** as having a **body mass index (BMI)** of 25 to 29.9, and being **obese** as having a BMI of 30 or higher. Body mass index is computed by multiplying a person's weight in pounds by 703 and then dividing that number by a person's height in inches squared. Nationwide, 13% of children aged 6 to 11 years and 14% of adolescents aged 12 to 19 years were overweight. This prevalence has nearly tripled for adolescents in the past two decades. A study reported in the *Journal of*

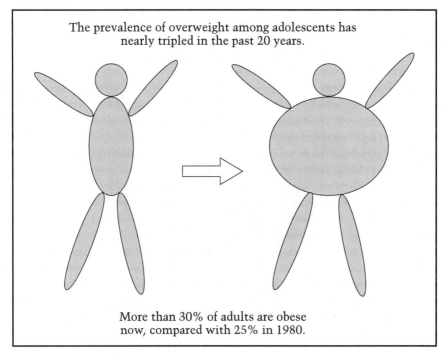

**FIGURE 4-4    Overweight youth**

*the American Medical Association* showed that among 4- to 12-year-olds, overweight is more of a problem for African-American and Hispanic children than for non-Hispanic white children.[12] Twenty-two percent of African-American and Hispanic children were overweight, compared with 12% of non-Hispanic children.

The surgeon general's report estimates that 300,000 people die each year of illness related to obesity or being overweight. This number of deaths is more than the number killed annually by pneumonia, motor vehicle accidents, and airline crashes combined. Overweight and obesity are associated with heart disease, high blood pressure, certain types of cancer, type 2 diabetes, stroke, arthritis, breathing problems, and psychological disorders such as depression. The economic cost of these problems is about $117 billion a year.

## Consequences of Overweight and Obesity in Children and Adolescents

The surgeon general's report points out several consequences of overweight and obesity in school-age youth (see Figure 4-5). Risk factors for heart disease, such as high cholesterol and high blood pressure, occur with increased frequency in overweight children and adolescents compared

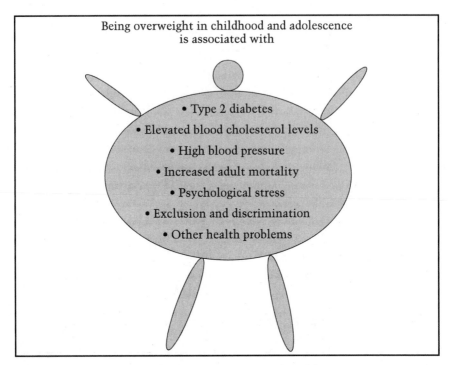

Being overweight in childhood and adolescence
is associated with

- Type 2 diabetes
- Elevated blood cholesterol levels
- High blood pressure
- Increased adult mortality
- Psychological stress
- Exclusion and discrimination
- Other health problems

**FIGURE 4-5   Problems associated with being overweight**

with children having a healthy weight. Type 2 diabetes, previously considered an adult disease, has increased dramatically in children and adolescents. Type 2 diabetes is closely linked to obesity and a sedentary lifestyle.

Fat children are very likely to grow into fat adults. Overweight adolescents have a 70% chance of becoming overweight or obese adults. This increases to 80% if one or more parent is overweight or obese. Overweight or obese adults are at risk for a number of health problems, including heart disease, type 2 diabetes, high blood pressure, and some forms of cancer.

The consequences of being overweight go beyond the physical health aspects. Children who are overweight or obese feel tremendous psychological pain as a result of their condition. They are likely to suffer from a poor self-image and feelings of inferiority and rejection. They are often teased, ridiculed, and left out of games, athletics, and other activities. The rejection and isolation that results from this treatment is a source of intense frustration and may cause a child to withdraw, act out, and overeat.

Substantial weight gain in very young girls can sometimes trigger premature puberty, as early as 8 or 9 in some girls. Puberty then triggers additional weight gain. About two years later a young girl begins menstruation and soon reaches full height. If extra weight gain triggers premature puberty, a young girl will often lose inches in height that she would otherwise have achieved, losing the opportunity for her height to catch up or "grow into" the added weight.

## Why Are Kids Getting Fatter?

Rising obesity rates in children and adults mean that more individuals are eating more and moving their bodies less. Children are sitting more, exercising less, and eating more than earlier generations. Today's children grow up in homes with televisions, VCRs, CD players, video game players, and computers, and they spend more time using these entertainment devices than they do in play or physical activity. Parents' worries about children's safety keep many children indoors instead of outdoors playing games or sports, walking, or biking.

Children don't get the amount of incidental physical activity that they used to obtain. In past generations, children were likely to run to the store on errands for a parent, walk to school, or bike to sports team practices. Forty years ago, half of all kids walked to school. Today's parents are not likely to have their children walk to school. Today only 10% do. Only one-third of children who live within a mile of school walk to school. Even among kids who live within a mile of school, fewer than one-third walk. One reason for this is that walking to school is not safe for many children. In many areas where children live, sidewalks, if they exist, usually end at the entrance to the subdivision or housing area. Modern suburban design often brings subdivision streets to connect to high-traffic roadways, which makes walking and biking dangerous. Many schools are located on busy highways or in areas that are dangerous for children to travel by foot or by bicycle.

Not only are many young people not active physically, but they are eating more calorie-dense foods, such as hamburgers, pizza, and chips, and drinking high-calorie, sugary drinks such as soda and other flavored drinks. The obesity epidemic developed concurrently with changes in the food supply such as increased consumption of fast foods and soft drinks, extraordinarily large serving sizes ("supersizing"), and a proliferation of food products. Businesses spend an estimated $13 billion a year marketing food and drinks to U.S. children and their parents—an increase of $5 billion from a decade ago.[13] About half of all advertisements aimed at kids are for food. And what's being marketed and consumed is primarily loaded with fat and sugar. Four of five food ads for children are for sugary cereal, soft drinks, fast food, or salty snacks. The food companies know that advertising works, so TV is full of food advertisements directed at kids. Only 2% of all advertising by food manufacturers is for fruits, vegetables, grains, or beans. Is it any surprise then that the average child gets about half of his or her calories from added fat and sugar? Very few children eat a diet that resembles the suggested food pyramid. Also, children have responded to the onslaught of ads for unhealthy foods by eating more and larger portions—often while watching TV or engaging in other sedentary activities.

## Pressure to Be Thin and Preoccupation with Weight

Young people, particularly girls and young women, feel tremendous pressure to be thin. For females in our society and culture, thinness has become synonymous with attractiveness. The current standard of beauty has been set so thin that females, almost without exception, consider themselves "overweight." The "weight problems" of many females would be defined out of existence if a health criterion were used to define obesity rather than the present societal standard.

The adolescent time period is characterized by intense preoccupation with appearance. Adolescents and children feel pressure to conform to a particular size, shape, or look. In order to achieve a desired look, weight reduction becomes a major focus for many young girls. Some rely upon extreme diet and exercise regimens in efforts to achieve their "ideal" body sizes. Fears of gaining weight abound in the minds of many young girls, and these fears propel efforts to either maintain or lose weight. The message has been delivered to our youth that "losing weight is good." Unfortunately, many are convinced that since losing weight is good, "the more weight I lose, the better I am." This drive for thinness plays a major role in the development of eating disorders in young people.

### Unsafe Weight-Loss Methods

Fear of weight gain and feeling pressure to be thin are desires that lead many young persons to practice unsafe weight-loss methods. **Unsafe weight-loss methods** include skipping meals, fasting for long periods of time, taking diet pills, using laxatives, and inducing vomiting after meals. Deliberately restricting food intake over long periods can lead to poor growth and delayed sexual development.

The 1999 Youth Risk Behavior Survey provides us with information about the frequency of unsafe weight-loss methods among high school students.[14] A substantially higher percentage of females (59.4%) than males (26.1%) report that they are currently trying to lose weight. More than half (56.1%) of the females and 25.0% of the males reported eating less food, fewer calories, or foods low in fat to lose weight or to keep from gaining weight during the past month. Taking laxatives or vomiting to lose or control weight in the past month was reported by 7.5% of females and 2.2% of males. Taking diet pills, powders, or liquids without a doctor's advice to lose weight or keep from gaining weight in the past month was reported by 10.9% of the females and 4.4% of the males.

Another unsafe means used by some young people to regulate weight is smoking cigarettes. Concern about weight gain is a major issue among young women smokers. Adolescents, and in particular adolescent girls, who diet or who are concerned about their weight have a higher rate of cigarette smoking than nondieters or girls having few weight concerns. Teens who smoke cigarettes are also more likely to report trying to lose weight through self-induced vomiting, taking diet pills, and using laxatives than nonsmoking teens.[15] Teachers need to inform children and adolescents that the health consequences of smoking outweigh any anticipated or realized effects of smoking on weight control. Because slenderness is highly prized, adolescents may be willing to overlook the very serious long-term consequences of smoking (e.g., emphysema, lung cancer) in order to achieve or maintain a desirable body weight.

## Eating Disorders

**Eating disorders** are food-related means by which individuals attempt to relieve emotional problems, such as low self-esteem, lack of social acceptance, fear of rejection, and the inability to express feelings in appropriate ways. Young girls are susceptible to eating disorders just before or just after puberty. The emergence of an eating disorder may be an unconscious effort to delay physical maturing. Stress also triggers eating disorders. Stressful life events that may trigger eating disorders include moving, parental divorce or death, a broken love relationship, or ridicule by others that the individual is fat or becoming fat.

It is common for young people with eating disorders to feel isolated, lonely, inadequate, and depressed. Despite low levels of self-esteem, those with eating disorders often do very well in school and other pursuits, such as athletics, music, drama, or other forms of art. This is confusing to parents, friends, and teachers because their achievements are so apparent. However, the drive to achieve comes not from the satisfaction of accomplishment but from an overwhelming fear of failure or rejection.

*Anorexia Nervosa*    **Anorexia nervosa** is a serious psychological disorder that affects many more females than males. This disorder is characterized by having a body weight at least 15% below normal weight for age and height, an intense fear of gaining weight or become fat, and body image distortion (e.g., claims of being fat even when emaciated, belief that one area of the body is too fat even when obviously underweight). Menstrual periods are also often absent in females with anorexia.

Anorexia nervosa is a very serious illness. It can be fatal. It is sometimes necessary to hospitalize severe cases to prevent death. The mortality rates for anorexia nervosa are among the highest for psychiatric disorders. Health experts estimate that between 15% and 20% of all anorexics die from the illness. Death is usually due to kidney failure or heart shrinkage.

Anorexia is misnamed, in that those with the condition do not lack appetite. (The term *anorexia* refers to a lack of appetite.) Anorexics refuse to eat, hungry or not.

The hallmark sign of anorexia nervosa is self-starvation and fanatical weight reduction. For anorexics, the idea of becoming fat creates intense fear and disgust even as they are becoming emaciated. As the self-starvation progresses, children and adolescents frequently experience behavioral and mood changes. Normal perception of what their bone and skin frames look like becomes distorted to the point of delusion. Even though they are emaciated, they typically feel too fat.

Anorexics often look and feel ill. They suffer fatigue and may be sensitive to cold. Their hair tends to thin and they experience numbing sensations in their hands and feet. Skin becomes dry and grayish. In advanced stages of the disease, a fine, downy covering of hair appears all over the body, which is the body's attempt to provide a thermal padding for lost fat layers. The reproductive organs may be permanently damaged by the self-starvation.

A central feature of anorexia nervosa in adolescents is the issue of control. Houck explains that by controlling one's weight through obsessive dieting, a young person is able to gain greater control over her or his life.[16]

> An anorexic tries to gain control of her life by controlling her weight, which by obsessive dieting and exercising, may drop by as much as 25 percent. She has little impact on the world, she believes, but has found that subduing her own body gives her that missing feeling of autonomy. As her illness develops, she often experiences, for the first time, power over her parents, as her family focuses its attention on her and joins her in becoming obsessed with her weight. Because self-inflicted starvation slows or reverses the onset of puberty by stopping menstruation and shrinking breasts, the anorexic—statistically most likely to be a girl between 10 and 18—may be avoiding womanhood, afraid of adult responsibilities and changes she doesn't feel up to handling. (pg. 138)

Many anorexics are from white, middle-to-upper socioeconomic families. They are frequently high achievers. However, it is common for grade point averages and other signs of high achievement to decline as the anorexia progresses. Anorexics have an overwhelming need to please their parents and teachers. Parents are often shocked at their child's starvation tactics because they are contrary to the usual good behavior and obedience that are characteristic of the child. Anorexic children usually conform to rules at home and outside of the home. This conforming is often to the point of losing self-esteem and the capacity for independent thought.

Feelings of self-doubt, ineffectiveness, and helplessness are characteristics of adolescents with anorexia nervosa, although they generally deny such feelings. Anorexics show decreased sexual feelings and drive, and at times fear contact with the opposite sex.

*Bulimia*  Bulimia is an eating disorder that consists of gorging on food, followed by self-induced vomiting or purging. This behavioral disorder may be part of anorexia nervosa or may constitute a distinct, separate disorder. As with anorexia nervosa, most persons with bulimic behaviors are female. Unlike anorexia nervosa, which typically emerges during early and middle adolescence, bulimia is most likely to occur during the late teenage years or early twenties.

Bulimic people are usually aware of their abnormal eating habits and fear not being able to control their eating. Food-binging episodes are followed by efforts to control weight through dieting, fasting, or purging. These efforts include vomiting, compulsive exercising, or the use of laxatives, diuretics, enemas, and weight-reducing drugs (e.g., amphetamines). Food binges are often responses to intense emotions such as depression, anger, loneliness, stress, or feelings of inadequacy. Binges serve to tranquilize or calm these negative feelings. Bulimics consume as many as 1,000 to 10,000 calories or more per binge. Binges sometimes continue for hours and stop only when all available food has been consumed, or the binger is exhausted or experiences abdominal pain or discomfort. Self-induced vomiting produces a sense of relief and often a feeling of euphoria. Vomiting episodes are often described by bulimic persons in sexual terms, ascribing to the vomiting an orgasmic quality. The resulting relief and euphoria are often associated with a sense of calmness, relaxation, and tiredness. These feelings, however, are short-lived and replaced by disgust, guilt, shame, and self-condemnation. A progression to more serious feelings of depression, hopelessness, and suicidal ideation is also common.

Muuss provides a case history of a bulimic's binge-purge behavior.[17] Notice the compulsive nature of the binging, the quantities and types of foods consumed, and the preoccupation with the binging.

The first vomiting period perpetuated itself into a five-year-long habit in which I had daily planned and unplanned binges and self-induced vomiting sessions up to four times daily. I frequently vomited each of the day's three meals as well as my afternoon "snack" of three or four hamburgers, four to five enormous bowls of ice cream, dozens of cookies, bags of various potato chips, packs of Swiss cheese, two large helpings of french fries, at least two milkshakes, and to top it off, an apple or banana followed by two or more pints of cold milk to help me vomit more easily.

During the night, I sneaked back into the dark so I would not risk awakening any family members by turning on a light. . . . Every night I wished that I could, like everyone else, eat one apple as a midnight snack and then stop. However, every night I failed, but continuously succeeded in consuming countless bowls of various cereals, ice cream sundaes, peanut butter and jelly sandwiches, bananas, potato chips, Triscuits, peanuts, Oreos, orange juice and chocolate chip cookies. Then I tiptoed to the bathroom to empty myself. Sometimes the food did not come up as quickly as I wanted; so, in panic, I rammed my fingers wildly down my throat, occasionally making it bleed from cutting it with my fingernails. Sometimes I would spend two hours in the bathroom trying to vomit, yet there were other nights when the food came up in less than three minutes. I always felt immensely relieved and temporarily peaceful after I had thrown up. There was a symbolic sense of emptying out the anxiety, loneliness, and depression inside of me, as well as a sense of rebellion to hurt my body, to throw up on the people who hurt me, so to speak. (pg. 261)

Mental health professionals look for the presence of certain character-istics when diagnosing bulimia. There must be recurrent episodes of binge eating and regular engagement in purging behaviors such as self-induced vomiting, use of laxatives or diuretics, strict dieting or fasting, or vigorous exercise to prevent weight gain. Bulimics will express that they lack con-trol over their eating behavior during the eating binges. Persistent overcon-cern with body shape is another sign of bulimia.

Although most bulimics maintain normal body weight, bulimia car-ries the risk of serious medical complications. Kidney impairment and heart irregularities may develop. In addition, the stomach or esophagus may rupture in response to binging or purging episodes. Chronic hoarse-ness, premature facial wrinkles, electrolyte disturbances, and hemorrhages in the conjunctiva of the eye are other complications. Tooth decay and ero-sion result from regurgitation of acidic gastric contents.

Syrup of ipecac, an over-the-counter drug used for inducing vomiting in poison victims, is sometimes abused by bulimics to purge after food binges. Repeated use of syrup of ipecac can cause irreversible heart dam-age. One famous victim of syrup of ipecac abuse was Karen Carpenter, a popular singer and performer during the 1970s.

## Physical Inactivity

Physical inactivity among young people is a serious cause for concern (see Figure 4-6.). A pattern of inactivity may persist throughout youth and

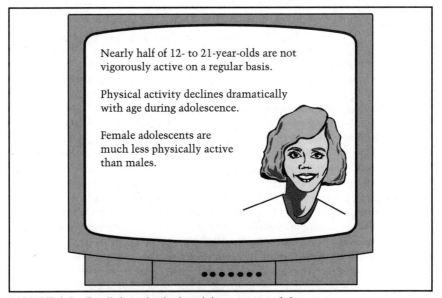

Nearly half of 12- to 21-year-olds are not vigorously active on a regular basis.

Physical activity declines dramatically with age during adolescence.

Female adolescents are much less physically active than males.

**FIGURE 4-6    Declining physical activity among adolescents**

into adulthood. Physically inactive individuals are likely to miss out on the many health benefits enjoyed by those who are physically fit. The first *Surgeon General's Report on Physical Activity and Health* outlined the benefits of physical activity on health.[18] These benefits include the following:

❖ Lowered death rates for adults

❖ Decreased risk of death from coronary heart disease

❖ Reduced blood pressure in people with high blood pressure

❖ Decreased risk of colon cancer

❖ Lowered risk of non-insulin-dependent diabetes mellitus

❖ Maintenance of normal muscle strength and joint function later in life

❖ Decreased risk of osteoporosis

❖ Maintenance of a healthy body weight

❖ Relief of symptoms of depression and anxiety

❖ Improved mood

The surgeon general's report made clear that the health benefits of physical activity are not limited to adults. Regular participation in physical activity in childhood and adolescence:

❖ Helps build and maintain healthy bones, muscles, and joints

❖ Helps control weight, build lean muscle, and reduce fat

❖ Prevents or delays the development of high blood pressure and helps reduce blood pressure in some adolescents with hypertension

❖ Reduces feelings of depression and anxiety

The surgeon general's report also concluded that only about one-half of young people in the United States (ages 12 to 21 years) regularly participate in vigorous physical activity. One-fourth report no vigorous physical activity. Young males are more likely than females to participate in vigorous physical activity, strengthening activities, and walking or bicycling. Participation in all types of activity declines strikingly as age or grade level increases.

The report also paints a bleak picture of the physical activity patterns of adults. One-fourth of adults are completely sedentary, reporting no physical activity at all in their leisure time. Only 15% of adults in the United States engage regularly (three times a week for at least 20 minutes) in vigorous physical activity during leisure time.

Physical inactivity affects more than the physical dimension of health. Emotional health is improved through participation in physical activity. The President's Council on Physical Fitness and Sports states that physical activity reduces anxiety, reduces depression, improves self-esteem, and increases the ability to respond to stress.[19] Physical activity among adolescents is associated with higher self-esteem and self-concept and lower anxiety and stress. A study by Page and Tucker found that adolescents who participate infrequently in physical activity experience more loneliness, shyness, and hopelessness than their more active peers.[20] Another study by Page and colleagues showed that elementary children who are lonely are less physically fit than children who are not lonely.[21]

Students who participate in interscholastic sports are less likely to be regular or heavy smokers or to use drugs and are more likely to stay in school and have good conduct and high academic achievement than non-participants. Sports and physical activity programs can introduce young people to skills such as teamwork, self-discipline, sportsmanship, leadership, and socialization. Lack of recreational activity, on the other hand, may contribute to making young people more vulnerable to gangs, drugs, and violence.

One of the major benefits of physical activity is that it helps young people improve their physical fitness. Physical fitness is a state of well-being that allows individuals to perform daily activities with vigor, participate in a variety of physical activities, and reduce their risks for health problems. Five basic components of fitness are important for good health: cardiorespiratory endurance, muscular strength, muscular endurance, flexibility, and body composition (percentage of body fat). A second set of attributes, referred to as sport- or skill-related physical fitness attributes, includes power, speed, agility, balance, and reaction time. Although skill-related fitness attributes are not essential for maintaining physical health, they are important for athletic performance or physically demanding jobs such as military service and emergency and rescue service.

# Guidelines

Educators need to be aware of the guidelines for healthy eating and physical activity. These guidelines are designed by health experts to promote good health and development.

## The 2000 Dietary Guidelines for Americans

The **Dietary Guidelines for Americans** are recommendations for diet choices among healthy Americans who are aged 2 years or more. In addition to recommendations for healthy eating, these guidelines emphasize the importance of being physically active each day and of

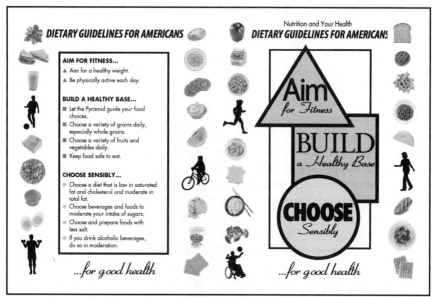

Source: http://www.health.gov/dietaryguidelines/dga2000/10guidelines.pdf. Accessed 9/18/02.

**FIGURE 4-7    Dietary guidelines for Americans**

observing food safety. The guidelines are organized under three basic messages for health: Aim for Fitness, Build a Healthy Base, and Choose Sensibly (see Figure 4-7).

## Food Guide Pyramid

The **Food Guide Pyramid** (see Figure 4-8) is a blueprint for what to eat each day to ensure a healthy diet. The pyramid encourages eating from five major food groups and provides a guide for how many servings to eat from each group. Following the Food Guide Pyramid helps a person to meet the Dietary Guidelines for Americans, getting the nutrients he or she needs while avoiding too many calories or too much fat, saturated fat, cholesterol, sugar, sodium, or alcohol. Because most American diets are too high in fat, the pyramid focuses on reducing fat consumption. A diet low in fat helps a person maintain a healthy weight and reduces the chance of getting certain diseases associated with a high-fat diet. The pyramid also calls for eating a variety of foods each day. See Table 4-1 for what constitutes a serving size and how many servings are needed each day.

## Physical Activity Guidelines for Young People

The National Association for Sport and Physical Education established a guideline recommending that elementary school children be physically

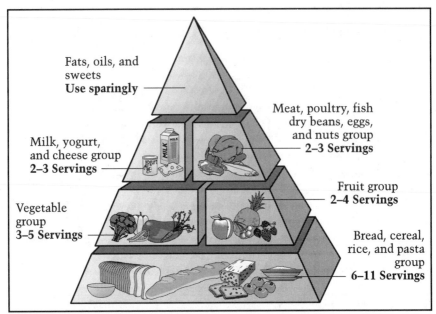

Source: U.S. Department of Agriculture and U.S. Department of Health and Human Services.

**FIGURE 4-8    Food Guide Pyramid**

active a total of at least 60 minutes a day and up to several hours per day.[22,23] Elementary school children should engage in a variety of physical activities of various levels of intensity. It is advised that physical activity occur intermittently in periods lasting 10 to 15 minutes or more, and include moderate to vigorous activity. There should be brief periods of rest and recovery between periods of activity. Extended periods of inactivity are not appropriate for normal, healthy children.

This recommendation is based on the physical developmental needs of children. Participating in physical activity helps children develop skills and increases the likelihood that physical activity will become a regular part of their lifestyle. Adequate time in physical activity is required before these skills are acquired. Those who are physically active in childhood are more likely to be physically active as adolescents and adults.

The International Consensus Conference on Physical Activity Guidelines for Adolescents recommends that healthy adolescents be physically active daily or nearly every day.[24] Physical activity should be part of play, games, sports, work, transportation, recreation, physical education, or planned exercise in the context of family, school, and community activities. It is recommended that adolescents engage in three or more activity sessions per week that last 20 minutes or more and that require moderate to vigorous levels of exertion.

**TABLE 4-1    Serving sizes**

| What Constitutes a Serving Size? |
| --- |

One serving of breads, cereals, rice, and pasta equals
   1 slice of bread
   ½ cup of coked rice or pasta
   ½ cup of cooked cereal
   1 ounce of ready-to-eat cereal

One serving of vegetables equals
   ½ cup of chopped raw or cooked vegetables
   1 cup of leafy raw vegetables

One serving of fruit equals
   1 piece of fruit or melon wedge
   ¾ cup of juice
   ½ cup of canned fruit
   ¼ cup of dried fruit

One serving of milk, yogurt, or cheese equals
   1 cup of milk or yogurt
   1½ to 2 ounces of cheese

One serving of meat, poultry, fish, dry beans, eggs, and nuts equals
   2½ to 3 ounces of cooked lean meat, poultry, or fish

The following are equivalent to 1 ounce of lean meat
   ½ cup cooked beans
   2 eggs
   2 tablespoons of peanut butter

| How Many Servings Do You Need Each Day? | | |
| --- | --- | --- |
|  | *Children and Teenage Girls* | *Teenage Boys* |
| Calories | about 2,200 | about 2,800 |
| Bread group | 9 | 11 |
| Vegetable group | 4 | 5 |
| Fruit group | 3 | 4 |
| Milk group | 3 | 3 |
| Meat group | 2, for a total of 6 ounces | 3, for a total of 7 ounces |

Source: Adapted from the U.S. Department of Agriculture and U.S. Department of Health and Human Services.

# Promoting Healthy Eating in Schools*

Schools are ideal settings for promoting healthy eating for several reasons:

❖ Schools can reach almost all children and adolescents.

❖ Schools provide opportunities to practice healthy eating. More than one-half of youths in the United States eat one of their three major

---

* This section of the chapter is adapted from Centers for Disease Control and Prevention, "Guidelines for School Health Programs to Promote Lifelong Healthy Eating," *Morbidity and Mortality Weekly Report*, 45(RR-9), 1996.

meals in school, and 1 in 10 children and adolescents eats two of his or her three main meals in school.

❖ Schools can teach students how to resist social pressures. Eating is a socially learned behavior that is influenced by social pressures. School-based programs can directly address peer pressure that discourages healthy eating and can harness the power of peer pressure to reinforce healthy eating habits.

❖ Skilled personnel are available. After appropriate training, teachers can use their instructional skills and foodservice personnel can contribute their expertise to nutrition education programs.

❖ Evaluations suggest that school-based nutrition education can improve the eating behaviors of young persons.

## Nutrition Education

Nutrition education should be part of a comprehensive health education curriculum that focuses on understanding the relationship between personal behavior and health. This curriculum should give students the knowledge and skills they need to be "health literate." The comprehensive health education approach is important to nutrition education for these reasons:

❖ Unhealthy eating behaviors may be interrelated with other health risk factors (e.g., cigarette smoking, sedentary lifestyle).

❖ Nutrition education shares many of the key goals of other health education content areas (e.g., raising the value placed on health, taking responsibility for one's health, increasing confidence in one's ability to make health-enhancing behavioral changes).

❖ State-of-the-art nutrition education uses many of the social learning behavioral change techniques used in other health education domains.

Therefore, nutrition education activities can reinforce, and be reinforced by, activities that address other health education topics as well as health in general.

Linking nutrition and physical activity is particularly important because of the rising proportion of overweight youths in the United States. Nutrition education lessons should stress the importance of combining regular physical activity with sound nutrition as part of an overall healthy lifestyle. Physical education classes, in turn, should include guidance in food selection.

***Sequential Lessons and Adequate Time***    Students who receive more lessons on nutrition have more positive behavioral changes than students who have fewer lessons. To achieve stable, positive changes in students' eating behaviors, adequate time should be allocated for nutrition education lessons. The curriculum should be sequential from preschool through secondary school; attention should be paid to scope and sequence. When designing a curriculum, schools should assess and address their students' needs and concerns. A curriculum targeted to a limited number of behaviors might make the most effective use of the scarce instructional time available for nutrition education.

*Integration into Other Subject Areas*    To maximize classroom time, nutrition education can be integrated into the lesson plans of other school subjects; for example, math lessons could analyze nutrient intake, or reading lessons could feature texts on nutrition. Integration into other courses can complement, but should not replace, sequential nutrition education.

*Focusing on Promoting Healthy Eating Behaviors*    The primary goal of nutrition education should be to help young persons adopt eating behaviors that will promote health and reduce risk for disease (see Box 4-1). Behaviorally based education encourages specific healthy eating behaviors (e.g., eating less fat and sodium and eating more fruits and vegetables).

*Developmentally Appropriate and Culturally Relevant Activities*    Different educational strategies should be used for young persons at different stages of cognitive development. Nutrition education for young children should focus on concrete experiences (e.g., increasing exposure to many healthy foods and building skills in choosing healthy foods). More abstract associations between nutrition and health become appropriate as children approach middle school. By this age, children can understand and act on the connection between eating behaviors and health. Nutrition education for middle and high school students should focus on helping students assess their own eating behaviors and set goals for improving their food selection. Lessons for older children should emphasize personal responsibility, decision-making skills, and resisting negative social pressures.

Nutrition education presents opportunities for young persons to learn about and experience cultural diversity related to food and eating. Students from different cultural groups have different health concerns, eating patterns, food preferences, and food-related habits and attitudes. These differences need to be considered when designing lesson plans or discussing food choices. Nutrition education can succeed only when students believe it is relevant to their lives.

*Active Learning and Emphasis on Fun*    Students are more likely to adopt healthy eating behaviors when:

❖ They learn about these behaviors through fun, participatory activities rather than through lectures

❖ Lessons emphasize the positive, appealing aspects of healthy eating patterns rather than the negative consequences of unhealthy eating patterns

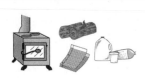
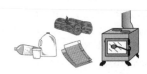

IN THE
CLASSROOM
*4-1*

## Crash Dieting

At any given time nearly half of the girls and over 10% of the boys in a school may be dieting. Young people often begin dieting while in elementary school. These youth are particularly vulnerable to using unsafe weight-loss methods and developing poor eating habits. Part of promoting healthy eating in schools is teaching students why crash dieting doesn't work. Teachers can do so using the following facts and analogy:

1. We burn calories in our muscles. Think of our muscles as wood-burning stoves. They can burn three kinds of fuel:
   Fat—think of it as big logs
   Glucose—think of it as paper (long paper chains are carbohydrates)
   Protein—think of it as plastic explosives
2. Paper and plastic explosives easily burn by themselves, but a log needs some kindling to burn. Fat, acting like a log, will not burn without glucose, which acts like kindling.
3. When the body doesn't have any glucose to burn (and thus can't burn fat), it burns protein.
   - We don't want to burn protein. Our muscles are made out of protein. If we lose muscle mass while dieting, we diminish the number of "stoves" we have to burn calories.
   - When you go on a crash diet, you quickly use up what glucose there is and your body begins to burn protein (muscle) for fuel.
   - You lose weight, but most of it is from dehydration, empty intestines, and lost muscle (not the fat you wanted to get rid of). Once you begin eating again your body quickly regains some weight as it replaces lost water and as your intestines refill.
   - You might continue to gain more weight because you do not have as many muscle cells (wood-burning stoves) as you once did. With fewer "stoves" you don't burn as many calories during a day and can gain weight more easily than before. This often happens to people who go on lots of diets when they are young.
4. The healthy way to lose weight is to eat foods high in nutrition and low in fats and sugars, while getting lots of physical activity.
   - Only reduce the number of calories you eat per day by about 30%. Consume these calories throughout the day rather than all in one meal.
   - Eat complex carbohydrates. Your body will slowly break down these large chains of sugar into glucose, providing you with a steady source of this fuel. If you eat simple sugars (pop, candy, cookies) your bloodstream will get a large surge of glucose all at once, which will be burned quickly.
   - Burn more calories by being more physically active.

❖ The benefits of healthy eating behaviors are presented in the context of what is already important to the students

❖ The students have repeated opportunities to taste foods that are low in fat, sodium, and added sugars, and high in vitamins, minerals, and fiber

Computer-based lessons on nutrition can also be effective, especially when teacher time is limited or when student self-assessment is appropriate. Interactive, highly entertaining, and well-designed computer programs are now available to help young persons learn healthy food-selection skills and assess their own diets. Computer-based lessons allow students to move at their own pace and can capture their attention.

*Social Learning Techniques*    Most of the nutrition education programs that result in behavioral change use teaching strategies based on social learning theory. In such lessons, increasing student knowledge is only one of the many objectives. Social learning instruction also emphasizes the following:

❖ Raising the value students place on good health and nutrition and identifying the benefits of adopting healthy eating patterns, including short-term benefits that are important to young persons (e.g., physical appearance, sense of personal control and independence, capacity for physical activities)

❖ Giving students repeated opportunities to taste healthy foods, including foods that they have not yet tasted

❖ Working with parents, school personnel, public health professionals, and others to overcome barriers to healthy eating

❖ Using influential role models, including peers, to demonstrate healthy eating practices

❖ Providing incentives (e.g., verbal praise, small prizes) to reinforce messages

❖ Helping students develop practical skills for, and self-confidence in, planning meals, preparing foods, reading food labels, and making healthy food choices through observation and hands-on practice

❖ Enabling students to critically analyze sociocultural influences— including advertising—on food selection, to resist negative social pressures, and to develop social support for healthy eating

❖ Helping students analyze their own eating patterns, set realistic goals for changes in their eating behaviors, monitor their progress in reaching those goals, and reward themselves for achieving their goals

*Integration of School Foodservice*    The school cafeteria provides a place for students to practice healthy eating. This experience should be coordinated with classroom lessons to allow students to apply critical thinking skills taught in the classroom. School foodservice personnel can do the following:

- ❖ Visit classrooms and explain how they ensure that meals meet the standards of the Dietary Guidelines for Americans

- ❖ Invite classes to visit the cafeteria kitchen and learn how to prepare healthy foods

- ❖ Involve students in planning the school menu and preparing recipes

- ❖ Offer foods that reinforce classroom lessons (e.g., whole-wheat rolls to reinforce a lesson on dietary fiber)

- ❖ Post nutrition posters and fliers in the cafeteria

- ❖ Display nutrition information about available foods and give students opportunities to practice the food analysis and selection skills learned in the classroom

**Family and Community Involvement**    The attitudes and behaviors of parents and caretakers directly influence children's and adolescents' choice of foods. Parents control most of the food choices available at home, so changing parents' eating behaviors may be one of the most effective ways to change the eating behaviors of their children. Although parental involvement can enhance the effects of nutrition education programs at the elementary school level, it is not known whether involving parents at the secondary school level helps improve the students' eating behaviors. For older youths, self-assessment and peer educators might be more influential than parental involvement.

Parents are usually more receptive to activities that can be done at home than to those that require their attendance at school. To involve parents and other family members in nutrition education, schools can do the following:

- ❖ Send nutrition education materials and cafeteria menus home with students

- ❖ Ask parents to send healthy snacks to school

- ❖ Invite parents and other family members to periodically eat with their children in the cafeteria

- ❖ Invite families to attend exhibitions of student nutrition projects or health fairs

- ❖ Offer nutrition education workshops and screening services

- ❖ Assign nutrition education homework that students can do with their families (e.g., reading and interpreting food labels, reading nutrition-related newsletters, preparing healthy recipes)

Through school health advisory councils or through direct contact with community organizations, schools can engage community resources and services to respond to the nutritional needs of students. Schools can also participate in community-based nutrition education campaigns sponsored by public health agencies or voluntary organizations. Students are most likely to adopt healthy eating behaviors if they receive consistent messages through multiple channels (e.g., home, school, community, the media) and from multiple sources (e.g., parents, peers, teachers, health professionals, the media).

## Supportive School Environment

A supportive school environment reinforces the promotion of lifelong healthy eating for its students. In addition to providing adequate time for nutrition education, a supportive school environment involves a commitment to serving healthy and appealing foods at school, food-use guidelines for teachers, supporting healthy school meals, and establishing links with nutrition service providers.

*Junk Food Reduction*    Healthy and appealing foods should be available in meals, à la carte items in the cafeteria, snack bars, and vending machines, as classroom snacks, and at special events, athletic competitions, staff meetings, and parents' association meetings. In addition, schools should discourage the sale of foods high in fat, sodium, and added sugars (e.g., candy, fried chips, soda) on school grounds and as part of fundraising activities. Although selling low-nutritive foods may provide additional revenue for school programs, such sales tell students that it is acceptable to compromise health for financial reasons. The school thereby risks contradicting the messages on healthy eating given in class. If schools contract with food-service management companies to supply meals, the contractors should be required to serve appealing, low-fat, low-sodium meals that comply with the standards of the Dietary Guidelines for Americans.

*Food-Use Guidelines for Teachers*    Schools should discourage teachers from using food for disciplining or rewarding students. Some teachers give students low-nutritive foods, such as candy, as a reward for good behavior, and punish misbehaving students by denying a low-nutritive treat. These practices reinforce students' preferences for low-nutritive foods and contradict what is taught during nutrition education. Schools should recommend that both teachers and parents serve healthy party snacks and treats. When foods are served in the classroom, teachers must use hygienic food-handling practices and consider possible food allergies and religious prohibitions.

*Support for Healthy School Meals*    Schools are required to serve meals that comply with the standards of the Dietary Guidelines for Americans. To encourage students to participate in school meal programs and to make healthy choices in cafeterias, schools can use marketing-style incentives and promotions; use healthy school meals as examples in class; educate parents about the value of healthy school meals; involve students and parents in planning meals; and have teachers, administrators, and parents eat in the cafeteria and speak favorably about the healthy meals available there. Students should also be given adequate time and space to eat meals in a pleasant and safe environment.

***Links with Nutrition Service Providers***    Schools should establish links with qualified public health and nutrition professionals who can provide screening, referral, and counseling for nutritional problems; inform families about supplemental nutrition services available in the community, such as WIC, food stamps, local food pantries, the Summer Food Service Program, and the Child and Adult Care Food Program; and implement nutrition education and health promotion activities for school faculty, other staff, school board members, and parents. These links can help prevent and resolve nutritional problems that can impair a student's capacity to learn, demonstrate the value placed on good nutrition for the entire school community, and help adults serve as role models for school-age youths.

## Promoting Physical Activity Among Young People in Schools*

Schools are an efficient vehicle for providing physical activity instruction and programs because they reach most children and adolescents. Schools have the potential to improve the health of young people by providing instruction, programs, and services that promote enjoyable, lifelong physical activity.

### Health Education

Health education can effectively promote the health-related knowledge, attitudes, and behaviors of students. The major contribution of health education in promoting physical activity among students should be to help them develop the knowledge, attitudes, and behavioral skills they need to establish and maintain a physically active lifestyle.

Health education curricula should provide information about physical activity concepts. These concepts should include the physical, social, and mental health benefits of physical activity; the components of health-related fitness; principles of exercise; injury prevention and first aid; precautions for preventing the spread of bloodborne pathogens; nutrition; physical activity and weight management; social influences on physical

---

* This section is adapted from Centers for Disease Control and Prevention, "Guidelines for School and Community Programs to Promote Lifelong Physical Activity Among Young People," *Morbidity and Mortality Weekly Report*, 46(RR-6), 1997.

activity; and the development of safe and effective individualized physical activity programs.

Health instruction should also generate positive attitudes toward healthy behaviors. These positive attitudes include perceptions that it is important and fun to participate in physical activity. Ways to foster positive attitudes include emphasizing the multiple benefits of physical activity, supporting children and adolescents who are physically active, and using active learning strategies.

*Behavioral Skills*    Children and adolescents should develop behavioral skills that may enable them to adopt healthy behaviors. Certain skills (e.g., self-assessment, self-monitoring, decision making, goal setting, identifying and managing barriers, self-regulation, reinforcement, communication, advocacy) may help students adopt and maintain a healthy lifestyle that includes regular physical activity. Active learning strategies give students opportunities to practice, master, and develop confidence in these skills.

*Active Learning Strategies*    Health education instruction should include use of active learning strategies. Such strategies may encourage students' active involvement in learning and help them develop the concepts, attitudes, and behavioral skills they need to engage in physical activity. Additionally, health education should encourage students to adopt healthy behaviors (e.g., physical activity) in the school, community, and home.

*Teacher Collaboration*    Collaboration allows coordinated physical activity instruction and should enable teachers to provide a range and depth of physical activity-related content and skills. For example, health education and physical education teachers can collaborate to reinforce the link between sound dietary practices and regular physical activity for weight management. Collaboration also allows teachers to highlight the influence of other behaviors on the capacity to engage in physical activity (e.g., using alcohol or other drugs) or behaviors that interact with physical activity to reduce the risk of developing chronic diseases (e.g., not using tobacco).

## Physical Education

Most states and school districts require some physical education. Physical education curricula and instruction are vital parts of a comprehensive school health program. One of the main goals of these curricula should be to help students develop an active lifestyle that will persist into and throughout adulthood. Curricula should emphasize knowledge about the benefits of physical activity and the recommended amounts and types of physical activity. Physical education should help students develop the attitudes, motor skills, behavioral skills, and confidence they need to engage in lifelong physical activity. Physical education should emphasize skills for lifetime physical activities (e.g., dance, strength training, jogging, swimming, bicycling, cross-country skiing, walking, hiking).

Knowledge of physical activity is viewed as an essential component of physical education curricula. Related concepts include the physical, social, and mental health benefits of physical activity; the components of health-related fitness; principles of exercise; injury prevention; precautions for preventing the spread of bloodborne pathogens; nutrition and weight management; social influences on physical activity; and the development of safe and effective individualized physical activity programs. For both young persons and adults, knowledge about how to be physically active may be a more important influence on physical activity than is knowledge about why to be active.

Positive attitudes toward physical activity may affect young people's involvement in physical activity. Positive attitudes include perceptions that physical activity is important and fun. Ways to generate positive attitudes include providing students with enjoyable physical education experiences that meet their needs and interests, emphasizing the benefits of physical activity, supporting students who are physically active, and using active learning strategies.

For physical education to make a meaningful and consistent contribution to the recommended amount of young people's physical activity, students at every grade level should take daily physical education classes in which they are physically active for a large percentage of class time. National health objectives call for students to be physically active for at least 50% of physical education class time, but many schools do not meet this objective. In addition, the percentage of time students spend in moderate or vigorous physical activity during physical education classes has decreased over the past few years (see Figure 4-9.)

## Supportive School Environment

The physical and social environments of children and adolescents should encourage and enable their participation in safe and enjoyable physical activities. School environments encourage safe and enjoyable physical activity by providing access to safe spaces and facilities for physical activity, establishing and enforcing measures to prevent physical activity-related injuries and illness, providing time within the school day for unstructured physical activity, discouraging the use or withholding of physical activity as punishment, providing health promotion programs for school faculty and staff, and involving parents in physical activity programs.

***Access to Safe Spaces and Facilities for Physical Activity***   School spaces and facilities should be available to young people before, during, and after the school day, on weekends, and during summer and other vacations. These spaces should also be readily available to community agencies and organizations offering physical activity programs.

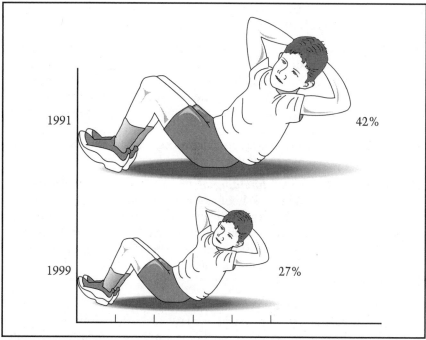

1991    42%

1999    27%

**FIGURE 4-9    Percentage of students enrolled in daily physical education classes**
The number of students enrolled in daily physical education classes and the percentage of
time students spend in moderate or vigorous physical activity during physical education
classes have decreased over the past few years.

Schools should ensure that spaces and facilities meet or exceed recommended safety standards for design, installation, and maintenance. For example, playgrounds should have cool water and adequate shade for play and rest. Young people also need places that are free from violence and free from exposure to environmental hazards (e.g., fumes from incinerators or motor vehicles). Spaces and facilities for physical activity should be regularly inspected, and hazardous conditions should be immediately corrected.

***Prevention of Physical Activity-Related Injuries and Illnesses***    Minimizing physical activity-related injuries and illnesses among young people is the joint responsibility of teachers, administrators, coaches, athletic trainers, other school and community personnel, parents, and young people. Preventing injuries and illness includes having appropriate adult supervision, ensuring compliance with safety rules and the use of protective clothing and equipment, and avoiding the effects of extreme weather conditions. Explicit safety rules should be taught to, and followed by, young people in physical education, health education, extracurricular physical activity programs, and community sports and recreation programs. Adult supervisors should consistently reinforce safety rules.

***Provide Time for Unstructured Physical Activity***     During the school day, opportunities for physical activity exist within physical education classes, during recess, and immediately before and after school. For example, students in grades 1 to 4 have an average recess period of 30 minutes. School personnel should encourage students to be physically active during these times. The use of time during the school day for unstructured physical activity should complement, rather than substitute for, the physical activity and instruction children receive in physical education classes.

***Discourage the Use or Withholding of Physical Activity as Punishment***     Teachers, coaches, and other school and community personnel should not force participation in, or withhold opportunities for, physical activity as punishment. Using physical activity as a punishment can create negative associations with physical activity in the minds of young people. Withholding physical activity deprives students of health benefits important to their well-being.

***Health Promotion Programs for School Faculty and Staff***     Enabling school personnel to participate in physical activity and other healthy behaviors should help them serve as role models for students. School-based health promotion programs have been effective in improving teacher participation in vigorous exercise, which in turn has improved their physical fitness, body composition, blood pressure, general well-being, and ability to handle job stress. In addition, participants in school-based health promotion programs may be less likely than nonparticipants to be absent from work.

***Parental Involvement***     Parental involvement in children's physical activity is key to the development of an environment that promotes physical activity among young people. Involvement in these programs provides parents the opportunity to be partners in developing their children's physical activity-related knowledge, motor skills, behavioral skills, confidence, and behavior. Thus, teachers, coaches, and other school personnel should encourage and enable parental involvement. For example, teachers can assign homework to students that must be done with their parents and can provide flyers designed for parents that contain information and strategies for promoting physical activity within the family. Parents can also join school health-advisory councils, booster clubs, and parent-teacher organizations. Parents who have been trained by professionals can also serve as volunteer coaches or leaders of extracurricular physical activity programs and community sports and recreation programs. Parents may be able to influence the quality and quantity of physical activity available to their children by advocating for comprehensive, daily physical education in schools and for school and community physical activity programs that promote lifelong physical activity among young people. Parents should also be advocates for safe spaces and facilities that provide their children the opportunities to engage in a range of physical activities.

### Extracurricular Physical Activities

Extracurricular activities are activities offered by schools outside of formal classes. Interscholastic athletics, intramural sports, and sports and recreation clubs are believed to contribute to the physical and social development of young people. These activities can help provide students with opportunities to engage in physical activity and to develop the knowledge, attitudes, motor skills, behavioral skills, and confidence needed to adopt and maintain physically active lifestyles.

Interscholastic athletic programs are typically limited to the secondary school level and usually consist of a few highly competitive team sports. Intramural sports programs are not uncommon, but, where they are offered, usually emphasize competitive team sports. Such programs usually underserve students who are less skilled, less physically fit, or not attracted to competitive sports. One reason that participation in sports declines steadily during childhood and adolescence is that undue emphasis is placed on competition.

After the needs and interests of all students are assessed, interscholastic, intramural, and club programs should be modified and expanded to offer a range of competitive and noncompetitive activities. For example, noncompetitive lifetime physical activities include walking, running, swimming, and bicycling.

Frequently, schools have the facilities but lack the personnel to deliver extracurricular physical activity programs. Community resources can expand existing school programs by providing intramural and club activities on school grounds. For example, community agencies and organizations can use school facilities for after-school physical fitness programs for children and adolescents, weight management programs for overweight or obese young people, and sports and recreation programs for young people with disabilities or chronic health problems.

## Key Terms

essential nutrients   123
calories   123
carbohydrate   123
fat   123
protein   123
iron deficiency anemia   126
calcium   126
osteoporosis   126
undernutrition   127
coronary heart disease   127

stroke   127
high blood pressure   127
diabetes   127
cancer   127
type 2 diabetes   128
insulin resistance   128
overweight   132
body mass index (BMI)   132
obese   132
unsafe weight-loss methods   136

## Review Questions

1. Identify the poor dietary habits often displayed by adolescents. Explain why girls are at higher risk than boys for failing to meet nutritional requirements.
2. Explain the problems associated with iron deficiency anemia, low calcium intake, and undernutrition. What dietary practices are placing young people at risk for these problems?
3. What chronic diseases are diet related?
4. Explain the influence of television and media on eating habits, physical activity levels, and body image of young people.
5. Discuss why junk food is so readily available in schools.
6. How do today's rates of being overweight and obese compare with rates in the past? Why do you think these changes have taken place? What do you predict will be the trend in the future?
7. Why do young people, particularly girls, feel pressure to be thin? Identify several unsafe weight-loss methods being used today.
8. Explain why crash diets don't work and how to more safely lose weight.
9. Describe who is at risk for anorexia nervosa (consider personality and family characteristics as well as antecedents). Identify symptoms of anorexia and explain why anorexics starve themselves.
10. What is bulimia? Why do individuals engage in bulimic behaviors? What are the risks associated with it?
11. Identify the benefits of physical activity for health and explain why our society is so physically inactive.
12. Identify the new Dietary Guidelines for Americans. Explain why they are important.
13. Make a Food Guide Pyramid indicating each food group and the recommended servings. Identify what constitutes a serving size for each group and how many servings children, teenage girls, and teenage boys need.
14. What are the physical activity guidelines for young people?
15. Identify and briefly explain the eight elements identified in the chapter that should be part of nutrition education.
16. Explain why crash dieting doesn't work, using the analogy of a wood-burning stove.
17. Identify what the goals and objectives should be of physical education.
18. Identify elements of a supportive school environment and explain how extracurricular physical activities can benefit students.

# References

1. Centers for Disease Control and Prevention (1997). "Guidelines for School and Community Programs to Promote Lifelong Physical Activity Among Young People." *Morbidity and Mortality Weekly Report*, 46(RR-6).

2. National Dairy Council (1998). "Teenage Girls Need to Drink More Milk." *Nutrition News*, 61(1): 1.

3. Gleason, P., and C. Suitor (2001). *Changes in Children's Diets: 1989–1991 to 1994–1996* (Report No. CN-01-CD2). Alexandria, VA: U.S. Department of Agriculture, Food and Nutrition Service.

4. Allington, J. (2001, March). "Eating for Health and Academic Achievement." *Wisconsin School News*. Available at http://www.dpi.state.wi.us/dpi/dltcl/bbfcsp/doc/tnarticle.doc.

5. Kleinman, R. E., J. M. Murphy, M. Little, M. Pagano, C. A. Wehler, K. Regal, and M. S. Jellinek (1998). "Hunger in Children in the United States: Potential Behavioral and Emotional Correlates." *Pediatrics*, 101(1): E3.

6. U.S. Department of Agriculture, School Breakfast Program. "Facts—Healthy Eating Helps You Make the Grade!" Available at http://www.fns.usda.gov/cnd/Breakfast/SchoolBfastCampaign/Facts.htm.

7. U.S. Department of Agriculture (2001). "Foods Sold in Competition with USDA School Meal Programs: A Report to Congress." Available at http://www.fns.usda.gov/cnd/Lunch/CompetitiveFoods/competitive.foods.report.to.congress.htm.

8. Andersen, R. E., C. J. Crespo, S. J. Bartlett, L. J. Cheskin, and M. Pratt (1998). "Relationship of Physical Activity and Television Watching with Body Weight and Level of Fatness Among Children: Results from the Third National Health and Nutrition Examination Survey." *Journal of the American Medical Association*, 279(12): 938–942.

9. Page, R., J. Hammermeister, A. Scanlan, and O. Allen (1996). "Psychosocial and Health-Related Characteristics of Adolescent Television Viewers." *Child Study Journal*, 26(4): 319–331.

10. Schindehette, S. (1999, October 18). "How Thin Is Too Thin?" *People*, 112–119.

11. Office of the Surgeon General (2001). *The Surgeon General's Call to Action to Prevent and Decrease Overweight and Obesity*. Rockville, MD: U.S. Department of Health and Human Services, Public Health Service. Available at http://www.surgeongeneral.gov/topics/obesity/calltoaction/toc.htm.

12. Strauss, R. S., and H. A. Pollock (2001). "Epidemic Increase in Childhood Overweight, 1986–1998." *Journal of the American Medical Association*, 286(22): 2845–2848.

13. Nestle, M. (2002). *Food Politics: How the Food Industry Influences Nutrition and Health*. Berkeley, CA: University of California Press.

14. Centers for Disease Control and Prevention (2000). "Youth Risk Behavior Surveillance—United States, 1999." *Morbidity and Mortality Weekly Report*, 49(SS-05).

15. Page, R. M., O. Allen, L. Moore, and C. Hewitt (1993). "Weight-Related Concerns and Practices of Male and Female Adolescent Cigarette Smokers and Nonsmokers." *Journal for Health Education*, 24(6): 339–346.

16. Houck, C. (1986, September). "Eating Disorders." *New Woman*, 138–151.

17. Muuss, R. E. (1986). "Adolescent Eating Disorder: Bulimia." *Adolescence*, 21: 257–267.

18. U.S. Department of Health and Human Services (1996). *Physical Activity and Health: A Report of the Surgeon General*. Atlanta, GA: Centers for Disease Control and Prevention.

19. President's Council on Physical Fitness and Sports (1997). "The Influence of Exercise on Mental Health." *Research Digest*, 2(12): 2.

20. Page, R. M., and L. A. Tucker (1994). "Psychosocial Discomfort and Exercise Frequency: An Epidemiological Study of Adolescents." *Adolescence*, 29(113): 183–191.

21. Page, R. M., J. Fray, R. Talbert, and C. Falk (1992). "Children's Feelings of Loneliness and Social Dissatisfaction: Relationship to Measures of Physical Fitness and Activity." *Journal of Teaching and Physical Education,* 11(3): 211–219.

22. Colorado Alliance for Health, Physical Education, Recreation and Dance (1998). "NASPE Physical Education Guidelines." Available at http://mscd.edu/~quatrocj/ position_state/NASPEGuide.html.

23. Finholm, V. (1998, August 23). "Taking the Couch Potato Battle to School." *Hartford Courant.* Available at http://www.bergen.com/physkids199808231.hml.

24. Sallis, J. F., and K. Patrick (1994). "Physical Activity Guidelines for Adolescents: Consensus Statement." *Pediatric Exercise Science,* 6: 302–314.

# 5

## SEXUAL ACTIVITY

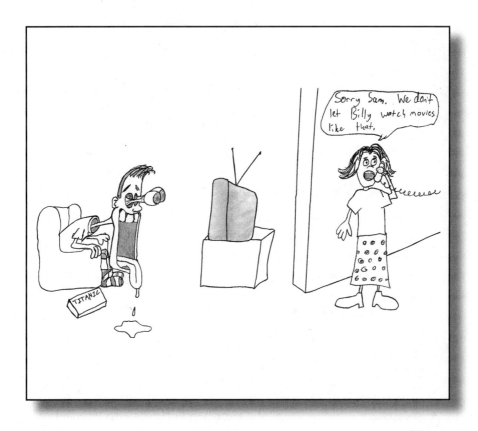

## *In Your Opinion*

*The following are polled answers to the question: Should condoms be made available on high school campuses?*

*Yolanda Jackson, high school student* Sure. Almost everyone I know is sexually active. What's the big deal? Having condoms available won't make kids do it more, but might help them be more responsible. AIDS is scary, but pregnancy is the real problem. Four of my friends have already had babies.

*Edith Rollings, teacher* No. I'm all for responsible sex education, which, in my opinion, should be abstinence education. Giving out condoms in high schools is going too far. It's like telling kids to not drink and drive and then giving them a beer.

*Earl Richardson, teacher* No. Sex is more prevalent and more dangerous than when I was a kid, but the problem isn't obtaining condoms. We could easily get them back then and so can kids now. Kids have trouble remembering to use condoms, not get them. They don't need a free handout at school.

*Tie Owyang, high school student* No. I think the real answer is in having TV condom advertisements. I guess some people are scared of erotic commercials, but what's the difference between that and movie previews or MTV?

*Susan Nelson, mother and PTA member* Yes. Let's face it, TV is this nation's biggest sex educator. I know some parents who are dead set against sex education in the schools, but don't monitor the TV shows or movies their kids watch. Kids need help, especially now that sex is so dangerous. Few kids find that help at home, so let the schools do it.

*Gary Sorenson, principal* I know school districts in Seattle, New York City, Chicago, Baltimore, and Los Angeles are distributing condoms in their high schools. I don't think that we are ready for that here, but then this is a question for the school board to answer.

A dolescence is a developmental time period that is largely about forging a personal identity. During adolescence, youth undergo the process of puberty and attain physiological sexual maturation. Most adolescents are extremely sensitive about their physical appearance and many are confused about issues of sexual activity. Adolescents feel newly developed biological sexual urges and impulses. There is much in society to arouse these feelings. Sex is pervasive in advertising, on television shows, in movies and videos, and in other forms of media. Parents and schools encourage abstinence from sexual activity at the same time that the mass media glamorize sex. Peer pressure about sexual activity can be either negative or positive. For example, it is common for youth to report feeling pressure from peers to experiment and engage in early sexual activity. Yet, on the other hand, some youth say that they feel support for sexual abstinence from peers. Religious and cultural beliefs also exert strong influence on decisions about sexual activity. Young people observe that the issues surrounding youth sexual activity are emotionally charged and evoke a wide range of opinions and reactions from teens, parents, and educators.

In the midst of such confusion, young people must make decisions about their involvement in sexual activity. Young people face developmental challenges in making decisions. Teens and preteens often lack the maturity, experience, and range of options that adults have when making decisions about sexual activity. There is a tendency to engage in short-range thinking, focusing more upon present desires than on long-term consequences of decisions. Also, it is common for young people to feel a strong sense of personal invulnerability. As a result, they do not perceive the need to avoid risks. These factors help explain why a high percentage of young people engage in sexual behaviors that place them at great risk for unintended pregnancy and acquiring sexually transmitted diseases (STDs), including HIV (human immunodeficiency virus) infection.

## Sexual Activity of Teenagers

Results from the 1999 **Youth Risk Behavior Survey** show that sexual activity begins early for many teens.[1] The percentage of high school students who initiated sexual intercourse before 13 years of age was 8.3% (12.2% of males and 4.4% of females). Almost 39% have had intercourse by the ninth grade, and 64.9% have had intercourse by twelfth grade. More than one-third (36.3%) of students in grades 9 through 12 reported having had sexual intercourse within the past three months. Half (50.6%) of twelfth graders reported having sexual intercourse in the past three months. The percentage of high school students who reported having four or more sex partners during their lifetime was 16.2% (19.3% of males and 13.1% of females).

The Youth Risk Behavior Survey was conducted in 1991, 1993, 1995, 1997, and 1999 (see Table 5-1). This makes it possible to determine trends in teen sexual activity and behaviors. The percentage of students reporting having ever had sexual intercourse, having had sexual intercourse in the past three months, and having had four or more sexual partners decreased from 1991 to 1997, but increased from 1997 to 1999. The percentage of students using a condom at last sexual intercourse improved at each survey through the 1990s, while the percentage of sexually active students using birth control pills at last sexual intercourse declined at each survey. Nine in 10 high school students report having been taught about HIV/AIDS in school.

**TABLE 5.1    Sexual behaviors of teenagers**

|  | 1991 | 1993 | 1995 | 1997 | 1999 |
|---|---|---|---|---|---|
| Ever had sexual intercourse | 54.1 | 53.0 | 53.1 | 48.4 | 49.9 |
| Had sexual intercourse in the past three months | 37.5 | 37.5 | 37.9 | 34.8 | 36.3 |
| Had four or more sexual partners | 18.7 | 18.7 | 17.8 | 16.0 | 16.2 |
| Used a condom at last sexual intercourse | 46.2 | 52.8 | 54.8 | 56.8 | 58.0 |
| Used birth control pills at last sexual intercourse (among those who have had sexual intercourse in the past three months) | 20.8 | 18.4 | 17.4 | 16.6 | 16.2 |
| Had been taught about HIV/AIDS in school | 83.3 | 86.1 | 86.3 | 91.5 | 90.6 |

Source: Centers for Disease Control and Prevention, *Fact Sheet: Youth Risk Behavior Trends*. Available at http://www.cdc.gov/nccdphp/dash/yrbs/trend.htm.

## Pervasiveness of Sex in the Media

American media, both programming and advertising, are highly sexualized in their content. The American Psychological Association estimates that the average young viewer is exposed to 14,000 sexual references and innuendos per year on television alone. This number does not come close to the many other sexual messages conveyed through exposure to other media, including movies, music, magazines, billboards, radio, and the World Wide Web. Television, movies, and music videos now routinely air images that were taboo not too many years ago.

The amount of sexual material, including sexually violent material, has increased over the past decade. Studies by the Kaiser Family Foundation show that 75% of television programs include sexual content and that there are on average 5.8 scenes per hour containing sexual talk and/or behavior.[2] Further, there are eight sexual incidents per hour during the "family hour" on television (8 to 9 P.M. in Eastern and Pacific time zones, 7 to 8 P.M. in Western and Central time zones), which is a fourfold increase since the mid-1970s. Network sitcoms were the most frequent offenders, and only 3% of their scenes contained information related to risks and responsibilities.

The followings facts and statistics about the increasing presence of sex in the media were compiled by Mediascope:[3]

❖ During a 10-year span, implicit references to sex in popular music decreased approximately 20%, while sexually explicit language increased by 15%. This shows that the amount of sexual references did not increase, but the language used to describe the sexual behavior became more graphic and explicit.

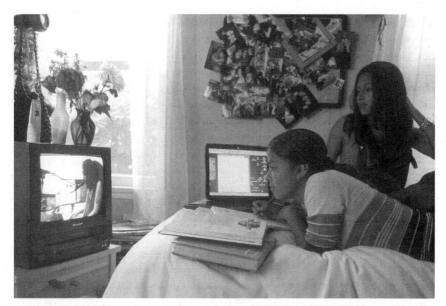

Nearly two-thirds of teenagers have television sets in their bedrooms. This is concerning in light of the amount and type of sexual content portrayed during nighttime programming.

- ❖ Six of 10 music videos show sexual behavior, and music videos contain more sex per minute than any competing media genre.

- ❖ Many print magazine editorials and advertisements feature seductive models; 40% of female models in the 1990s were considered "provocatively" dressed, compared with 28% in the 1980s. That was true for 18% of male models in the 1990s, compared with 11% in the 1980s.

- ❖ One in four young people aged 10 to 17 has inadvertently encountered sexual content on the World Wide Web, and one in five has been exposed to unwanted sexual solicitation while online in the past year.

Advertisers are increasingly using sexual titillation to attract the attention of potential customers, with much of the sexual imagery and depiction bordering on what would have been considered pornography a decade or two ago. Sexual images and themes are used in an attempt to grab the consumer's attention. Sexy bodies used to sell products are seen almost everywhere in our environment:

> The corner store is plastered with posters of busty models in wet T-shirts, hawking Budweiser. On a billboard that hovers over a busy intersection, a young woman in a clingy bathing suit arches her back in apparent sexual ecstasy beside an enlarged bottle of Wild Irish Rose. In an ad for Bugle Boy clothes, the camera moves in on the pelvis of a model in panties, pans out to show barely clothed beauties at the beach, and so on, ad nauseam.

The use of women's bodies in ads is essentially a cheap trick that marketers use instead of making more thoughtful arguments on behalf of their products. The mechanism used in these ads is quite simple: Attractive bodies are employed to grab attention and stimulate desire, which advertisers hope will then be transferred to the product. Buy the beer, get the girl. In this way, women's bodies are equated with commodities, presented as the rewards of consumption. (pg. 82)[4]

Given the heavy dose of sexual messages that young people receive through media sources, the entertainment industry is our nation's primary source of sex education. This is a scary fact when you consider what might be portrayed during a typical week of network TV fare. In 1993, *USA Today* analyzed a week's worth of programming on ABC, CBS, NBC, and Fox.[5] They found that of the 45 sex scenes on the shows, only 4 were between married heterosexuals; singles or cheaters had sex 39 times. That was 1993, and television has since become increasingly sexualized. Also, there has been a proliferation of cable TV channels and movie channels into the homes of many families—bringing more seductiveness to young people. The inappropriateness of much of what is on the popular media is even more disconcerting in light of the fact that young teens (ages 13 to 15) rank entertainment media as their top source of information about sexuality and sexual health.[3]

We no longer question the negative consequences of viewing violent material in the media and its impact on young people. Scientists have repeatedly confirmed that watching acts of violence leads to increased aggression and violent acting out. Isn't it plausible and probable that the heavy dose of sexual material that children are being exposed to is also harming them? Educators, legislators, and parents need to join together in telling the entertainment media to become more responsible in the messages they produce for our consumption. The inappropriate material they produce is irresponsible and certainly harms us all—children and adults alike. It is interesting to note that while many of our school-based sex education programs promote abstinence to avert problems such as unintended pregnancy and sexually transmitted diseases, our media mock abstinence as a choice.

## Understanding Adolescence and Sexual Development*

Adolescence is often portrayed as the "difficult" life stage. Understanding why young people behave the way they do provides us with ideas for how to effectively work with and support young people through this life stage.

---

* This section on understanding adolescence is adapted from National Clearinghouse on Families and Youth, "Preventing Adolescent Pregnancy: A Youth Development Approach," 1998. Available at http://www.ncfy.com/prevpreg.htm.

Adolescence is a time for young people to define their place in the family, their peer groups, and the larger community. During this stage of their lives, youth struggle with the transition from childhood to adulthood. During childhood, they depended mainly on their parents for economic and emotional support and direction. In adulthood, however, they will be expected to achieve independence and make choices about school, work, and personal relationships that will affect every aspect of their futures.

During this period, young people must contend with physical changes, pressure to conform to current social trends and peer behaviors, and increased expectations from family members, teachers, and other adults. Adolescents also must deal with sometimes conflicting messages from parents, peers, or the media. They struggle with an increasing need to feel as if they "belong."

During adolescence, young people begin to take risks and experiment. They do so because they are moving from a family-centered world to the larger community within which they will begin to define their own identities. They may choose friends of whom their parents do not approve or try alcohol or other drugs. They may wear clothing that is trendy and generational, begin comparing their families' lifestyles with those of other families, or break rules imposed by their parents or the larger community.

Adolescence is also a time of great cognitive and physical change. During this life stage, young people develop the ability to think about more than facts. They begin formulating possibilities and making connections between thoughts. Concurrent with this cognitive development are increasingly pronounced physical changes, including sexual maturation. Sexual maturation is as inevitable a part of the lifespan as growing old. Although young people have some capacity to make choices about whether or not to smoke or take drugs, they have little control over their physiological sexual development. Moreover, while society may be interested in preventing young people from ever becoming involved with drugs or violence, sexual activity is something to be guided or delayed until adulthood or marriage, not stopped entirely.

Today, adolescents are maturing at an earlier age than did previous generations (see Figure 5-1). This increases the likelihood that they will not have been exposed to sexual education before they experience changes caused by their own sexual development. It also increases the period of sexual exploration between puberty and marriage. Moreover, youth 10 to 12 years of age may be physically mature, but their still-limited cognitive reasoning abilities make providing information about, or discussing, sexuality issues all the more challenging. Moreover, their emotional or social development may not be keeping pace with their new physical maturity.

By the time most youth reach the age of 13 or 14, they have some sense of their body image and have developed a general sense of their self-worth, for better or for worse. At that age, most of that sense of self is related to how their parents, teachers, other significant adults, and peers

---

**Teens Before Their Time**

- Signs of sexual development in girls appear at younger ages today than in the past.
- One in seven white girls starts to develop breasts or pubic hair by age 8.
- Nearly one of every two African-American girls shows these signs by the age of 8.
- Early sexual maturation causes pressures that young girls are not prepared to handle—pressure to act like teenagers or even adults.
- Early maturing girls have to cope with pressures from boys who are interested in them sexually.
- Scientists haven't figured out what's causing early sexual maturation with certainty.
- Some scientists believe it may be due in part to the increase in obesity—overweight girls tend to mature earlier, and very thin girls, such as those with anorexia nervosa, tend to mature later than normal.
- Some scientists believe that seeing sexualized messages in the media and elsewhere might trigger brain chemicals that "jumpstart" sexual development.

---

Source: M. Lemonick, "Teens Before Their Time," *Time*, 156(18), October 30, 2000. Available at http://www.time.com/time/magazine/archives.

**FIGURE 5-1    Teens before their time**

have treated them. Clearly, young people do not grow up in isolation. They do so in families, schools, and communities. The culture of each affects young people's self-perception, their decision making, their behavior, and their view of the future.

Youth also are socialized regarding their sexual development through a range of cultural images and messages from their parents, their religious advisors, the media, and their peers. Yet, this socialization is more random than that which occurs in most other areas. Consider the example of teaching young people to brush their teeth, a dissimilar activity but relevant in terms of the discipline necessary to maintain a healthy lifestyle. Parents teach their children about brushing their teeth at a relatively early age and then spend considerable time coaching youngsters to develop the habit of brushing at least twice a day.

In the area of sexuality, almost the reverse happens. The cultural norms regarding sexuality tend to limit open discussion. Even in close families, parents often do not display physical affection, and most do not talk with their children about relationships or intimacy. Young people, therefore, have few role models with regard to relationships and little exposure to appropriate sexual behavior. When introduced to sexuality education and concepts such as reserving sexual activity for a loving relationship later in life, young people can grasp these ideas intellectually, but often they do not have an experiential or real-life frame of reference.

## Surgeon General's *Call to Action*

In 2001, Surgeon General David Satcher released *The Surgeon General's Call to Action to Promote Sexual Health and Responsible Sexual Behavior.*[6] The *Call to Action* was developed through a collaborative process by a work group formed by Surgeon General Satcher with the charge to find ways to move forward on promoting sexual health and responsible sexual behaviors. In releasing the report, he said, "We face a serious public health challenge regarding the sexual health of our nation. Doing nothing is unacceptable. If we are to meet this challenge, we must find common ground and reach consensus on the nature of these problems and their possible solutions, consistent with the best available science."

The *Call to Action* notes that strategies geared toward increasing awareness must include a recognition that parents are the child's primary educators and should guide a child's sexuality education in a way that is consistent with their values and beliefs. Strategies for doing so must also recognize that families differ in their levels of knowledge and comfort in discussing such issues, making school education a vital component in providing equity of access to information. The report also notes that churches and other community settings can play a role in providing such education.

Such information should be thorough and wide-ranging, begin early, and continue throughout the lifespan. Education should recognize the special place that sexuality has in everyday life; stress the value and benefits of remaining abstinent until involved in a committed, enduring, and mutually monogamous relationship; and ensure awareness of optimal protection from sexually transmitted diseases and unintended pregnancy, while also stressing that there are no infallible methods of contraception aside from abstinence, and that condoms cannot protect against some forms of STDs. Strategies for promoting sexual health and responsible sexual behavior must be based on sound scientific evidence and research.

## Helping Young People Make Responsible Decisions About Sexual Activity

All young people need careful guidance about making decisions about sexual activity. They need the skills necessary to successfully avoid dangerous or risky behavior. It is critical for young people to recognize the dangers they may encounter and to be taught negotiation and decision-making skills. Then, adequate time must be given to young people and their peers to practice those skills. In addition, young people need to develop a sense of personal responsibility to protect both themselves and others from risky behavior. They need to know that they are valued and have worth as individuals so that they will feel important enough to protect themselves.

The most appropriate and effective place for this guidance is from loving parents. The role of parents is vital to the successful development of children and adolescents. It is a difficult job that requires support and assistance from educational institutions and community agencies. Unfortunately, many young people do not have adults in their lives who can effectively provide the nurturing and guidance that they need. Some of these young people are particularly vulnerable to involvement in sexual activity that places them at risk of unintended pregnancy and infection with sexually transmitted diseases. For this reason, schools must play an active and vital role in teaching young people how to make responsible decisions about sexual activity.

## Sex Education

Due to increased concerns about issues such as AIDS, sexually transmitted diseases, teenage pregnancy, and child sexual abuse, schools are being called upon to offer human sexuality education curricula that help young people make thoughtful and informed choices about sexual behavior. Sexuality education, when done properly, reflects the needs of the community. **Sex education** programs need to be locally determined and consistent with parental and community values. Therefore, those who teach sex education must not only be familiar with the subject matter, but must also be sensitive to the attitudes of their students, the parents of students, community groups, and school administrators. They must examine their own personal attitudes toward sensitive and controversial topics and be prepared for how students, parents, and administrators might react to these issues. They must be thoroughly familiar with state and district policies regarding the teaching of sex education.

A major obstacle facing sex education is the perception of a lack of support for it. Some sex education teachers encounter negative reactions from parents or community groups opposing certain sex education topics. However, when parents are provided the opportunity to visit the school to learn what will be addressed through the sex education curriculum (and how it will be taught), most parents welcome support in helping their children develop healthy relationships that are based on information, choice, respect, and responsibility. Most parents support the teaching of sex education in schools.

Most states have policies supporting sex education. Many of these policies emphasize human reproduction and family life education. In response to the HIV epidemic, most states have adopted policies requiring or supporting HIV prevention education.

Effective sex education is much more than teaching about pregnancy and sexually transmitted diseases. It requires going beyond just providing accurate information. In order to help young people, sex education must assist them in their decision-making process. It must also offer life skills training (e.g., communication skills, negotiation skills, refusal skills, relationship skills) that helps young people avert adverse consequences from sexual activity and fosters healthy development. To do this, educational programs must present both the risks of involvement in sexual activity and the specific actions young people can take to avoid these risks. Particular emphasis must be given to helping youth build relationship skills, because relationships are the context in which sexual activity occurs. Learning activities should also address media influences on sexual behavior because the media are a strong and pervasive influence on youth. See Box 5-1 for suggested activities.

Effective sexual education programs also help young people to examine the risks of becoming sexually active within the context of planning for their future. Sex education programs take into account the cognitive developmental level of students and the various capacities of students at each particular grade level. Sufficient time must be devoted to building student trust because the issues addressed in sex education programs are more complex and personal than in any other area of the curricula. Specialized support and/or immediate referral to such support must be in place for youth who, as a result, disclose sexual abuse or other serious problems.

Teaching sex education is also challenging due to the breadth and range of topics. Some of these topics include the following:

- ❖ Reproductive anatomy and physiology (e.g., male and female reproductive systems, menstruation, nocturnal emissions)

- ❖ Sexual development (e.g., physiological development [puberty], psychological development, cultural and societal influences, sex roles)

- ❖ Human reproduction (e.g., fertilization and conception, prenatal development, pregnancy, childbirth)

- ❖ Family life issues (e.g., parent-child relationships, parenting skills, marriage, divorce, single parenting)

- ❖ Relationships and interpersonal skills, including decision making, assertiveness, and peer refusal skills

- ❖ Responsibility regarding sexual activity, including addressing abstinence and how to resist pressures to become prematurely involved in sexual activity

- ❖ Contraception and/or birth control

- ❖ HIV infection and other sexually transmitted diseases

IN THE
CLASSROOM
*5-1*

# Sex Education Teaching Activities

## *Counterfeits of Love*

Use the following chart to help you discuss the differences between lust, infatuation, and love with your students. Discuss how literature and the media often portray lust and infatuation as love. Talk about the many relationship problems that develop from believing the love myths perpetuated by fictional characters in books and on the screen. (I, J, H)

| Lust | Infatuation | Love |
| --- | --- | --- |
| Visceral. | Cupid's arrow—fall into and out of it. No control over it. | Takes time, develops, not discovered. Is something you do, not something that happens to you. |
| Self-centered, predatory. Uses other person as an object. | Self-gratifying—someone you want to be seen with, or fear of being left behind or missing out (everyone else is paired up). | Deep concern for the welfare of the loved one. True love gives. |
| Can consume thoughts, comments, and activities. Focuses on "stimuli," not person. | Feelings based on illusions and idealizations; exaggerations of other's good points. | Feelings based on reality— mature love sees more, not less, but because it sees more, it is willing to see less. |
| Varying states of physical arousal. | Loss of appetite; hard to concentrate. Can be short-tempered and irritable. | Eat, study, excel because you want to be your best for the other. |
| No desire for relationship other than for physical gratification. | Insecure; in love with being loved; jealousy. | Happy because you are sure and secure. |
| Tells lies in order to get sex. | Disagree easily. Focused on love feeling rather than on coming to deeply know and understand the other. | Readiness to listen to and understand others' perspective. |

*continued*

| Lacks self-control or restraint. | Feel like must have sex or marry to cement relationship. | Recognize sex is a natural part of love, but have sexual restraint to prevent consequences for self and loved one and don't want sex to get in the way of developing the relationship. Marriage and sex can wait till the right time. |

## TV Analysis

Assign various students to watch different TV channels for specific blocks of time during one week. (Use wisdom and care in making these assignments.) Have the students record the number and types of sexual material presented on the programming and commercials. Combine all the student's reports into a graph format for an analysis of one week. Discuss the amount and appropriateness of the sexual material presented in light of the time of day and probable audience; the messages "taught" or "caught" from such material, the misconceptions and myths perpetuated, the demographics of those involved in sexual behaviors in contrast to real life (married vs. single, etc.), and the relative number of negative consequences of sexual behaviors depicted. Have students write letters of concern to the advertisers of programs they found troubling, or to the companies whose advertising was found distasteful. (J, H)

## Wheel of Misfortune

Divide the class into groups. Have each group design a "Wheel of Misfortune" game based on the TV program *Wheel of Fortune*. Instruct students to design their wheels so that they contain physical and emotional problems associated with premature sexual involvement. (I, J, H)

## Great Comebacks

Ask the class to identify and list on the board 10 or more examples of sexual pressure (e.g., "Don't worry, I'll take care of everything," "Nobody will know but us," "If you love me ..."). Divide the class into pairs. Have each pair come up with a great comeback for each of the listed pressures (e.g., "If you love me ..."—"If *you* loved me you wouldn't pressure me!"). Have class members share their comebacks. Write the best comebacks next to their corresponding pressures on the board. (I, J, H)

*continued*

*continued*

### *Life Line*

Give each student seven small pieces of paper (three-by-five inch). Have students write at the top of each of their papers their name, a future age (e.g., 18, 23, 28, 35, 45, 55, 65) and what they want to be doing or have accomplished by the indicated age. Have the students clip their "age papers" to a life line made by stringing a clothesline or similar cord from one end of the classroom to the other. Encourage students to read one another's papers as they are clipping theirs up. Discuss how decisions made in their adolescence can affect the rest of their lives. (I, J, H)

### *Drawing the Line*

Create a sexual continuum on the board ranging from holding hands to intercourse. Ask the students to mentally draw a line on the continuum that they do not want to cross at this point in their lives. Tell the following two stories to impress upon students the importance of "drawing the line" early, way before the point they don't want to cross. After telling the stories, discuss safety rules for "flying well above the trees" and staying far away from "dangerous cliffs." Such rules might include "date in groups" and "avoid being alone with the other person." (J, H)

**Story 1.** In World War II some pilots participated in "tree topping" to impress others with their flying skills. They would fly close enough to break off the very tips of trees. This practice became prohibited because of the number of planes that ended up in the trees. A new safety rule was set in place so that the minimum altitude at which a pilot could fly was well above the trees.

**Story 2.** A company was interviewing truck drivers for hauling precious cargo across a mountain pass. When asked about a particularly hazardous curve on a steep cliff, one applicant said, "I could take that corner going 60 miles an hour while driving on the outside shoulder." A second applicant said, "I would gear down, and drive slowly and as close as possible to the hill side of the road." Which of the two applicants would you hire to drive your precious cargo?

### *Everybody's Not Doing It*

(Read "Normative Education" on page 203.) Poll students to determine what percentage of their peers they believe are sexually active. Discuss how and why youth often overestimate the number of adolescents who are sexually active. Discuss the true figures. (National figures can be found in this chapter. Your school district might have access to local or regional data. You might want to conduct a survey of your school with principal and school board approval.) Discuss how everyone is *not* doing it—that many youth choose to be or become sexually inactive. (J, H)

❖ Sexual abuse and assault (e.g., date rape, incest, child sexual abuse, sexual harassment)

❖ Controversial issues (e.g., abortion, homosexuality, pornography)

A study published in *Family Planning Perspectives* compares the findings of a nationally representative sample of nearly 4,000 seventh- through twelfth-grade public school teachers responsible for teaching subjects (biology, health education, family or consumer science, physical education) that typically include sexuality education with a comparable national survey conducted in 1988.[7] School nurses were also included in the study. In 1999, 93% of all respondents reported that sexuality education was taught in their school at some point in grades 7 to 12; sexuality education covered a broad number of topics, including sexually transmitted diseases, abstinence, birth control, abortion, and sexual orientation. Some topics—how HIV is transmitted, STDs, abstinence, how to resist peer pressure to have intercourse, and the correct way to use a condom—were taught at lower grades in 1999 than in 1988. In 1999, 23% of secondary school sexuality education teachers taught abstinence as the only way of preventing pregnancy and STDs, compared with 2% who did so in 1988. Teachers surveyed in 1999 were more likely than those in 1988 to cite abstinence as the most important message they wished to convey (41% vs. 25%). In addition, steep declines occurred between 1988 and 1999, overall and across grade levels, in the percentage of teachers who supported teaching about birth control, abortion, sexual orientation, and STD services, as well as in the percentage actually covering those topics. However, 39% of the respondents in 1999 who presented abstinence as the only option also told students that both birth control and condoms can be effective.

Most states have adopted laws governing sex education. A review of states' laws and policies by the Alan Guttmacher Institute found that 39 states require that some sex education be provided throughout the state.[8] Twenty-one states require that both sexuality and STD education be provided. Seventeen states require provision of STD information specifically, but not sexuality education. Only one state (Maine) requires sexuality education but not STD education, and 11 states leave the decision to teach sexuality education entirely to local school districts.

Local school districts are given wide latitude in determining the content of their sexuality education programs. According to a survey conducted by the Alan Guttmacher Institute, about two-thirds of public school districts have a policy mandating sexuality education.[9] This survey of school districts also showed that:

❖ Eighty-six percent of school districts with a sexuality policy require promotion of abstinence

❖ Fifty-one percent require that abstinence be taught as the preferred option but also permit discussion of contraception as an effective

means of protecting against unintended pregnancy and sexually transmitted infections

❖ Thirty-five percent require abstinence to be taught as the only option
for unmarried people, while either prohibiting discussion of contraception altogether or limiting discussion to contraceptive failure rates

❖ Fourteen percent of school districts currently have policies that are
truly comprehensive and teach both contraception and abstinence

## Abstinence Education

It is important that young people make healthy and safe choices about
sex. Abstinence from sex is often stressed in school-based sex education
programs because it is the most effective way to prevent unintended
pregnancy and sexually transmitted diseases, including HIV. Also, engaging in early sexual activity can delay emotional and personal development and limit opportunities for young people to build a strong future.
For this reason, **abstinence education** is emphasized in most school-based
sex education programs. However, there is considerable debate and lack
of agreement about how to carry out abstinence education. Some sex
education programs are broadly classified as "abstinence-only," while
others are categorized as "abstinence-plus." **Abstinence-only education**
generally teaches abstinence from all sexual activity as the only appropriate option for unmarried people. These programs often do not teach
about contraception or condom use or, if discussed, do not provide
detailed information. **Abstinence-plus education** emphasizes the benefits of abstinence while also teaching about contraception and disease-
prevention methods, including condom and contraceptive use. Abstinence-
plus programs are also sometimes referred to as **comprehensive sex
education**.[10]

Since the early 1980s, the U.S. Congress has allocated large sums of
federal funding toward abstinence-only education. In 1981, Congress
passed the Adolescent Family Life Act (AFLA), which provided federal
funding "to promote self-discipline and other prudent approaches to the
problem of adolescent premarital sexual relations, including adolescent
pregnancy." Funding for abstinence-only education has increased steeply
since 1996 as a result of a provision attached to the welfare reform legislation, which creates an automatic annual appropriation for abstinence-only
education as part of the Social Security Act. Funds for this appropriation
are only provided to programs that meet the legislation's strict definition
of abstinence education.

Educators can reinforce abstinence as a healthy choice by emphasizing
the concerns and skills addressed in this section.

***Health Concerns*** Because of concerns about sexually transmitted diseases and HIV, as well as teenage pregnancy, educators are choosing to

emphasize abstinence from sexual intercourse to lower the health risks and prevent disease.

*Emotional Concerns*   Choosing to abstain from sexual activity gives youth the time and freedom to discover who they are and make long-range goals for the future, rather than becoming caught up in defining themselves in terms of a dating game. Abstinence gives youth time to learn how to develop quality relationships, rather than superficial ones based primarily on physical drives. Abstinence also helps youth develop social skills, discover healthful ways of expressing emotions and needs, gives them time to focus on developmental tasks, and helps them develop character as they learn self-control, delayed gratification, respect for self and others, and responsibility for their own actions. Abstinence also protects them from the emotional baggage that can come with promiscuity.

*Parent-Child Communication*   Communication between parents and their children is an important factor in deterring sexual activity among teenagers. Many school, community, and religious groups are offering parent-child sexuality classes. These classes help parents articulate the value they put on abstinence and help them to define, with their teens, exactly what they want them to abstain from and why. It is interesting that many parents who have resisted sexuality education for their children often support classes that include them. Such programs provide activities that increase parent-child communication about sexuality and give opportunities for parents to share expectations and values with their children. (You will find additional information on communication skills in Chapter 2.)

*Refusal Skills*   Teenagers report that the pressures to engage in sexual activity are strong. Many curricula provide **refusal skills** activities to teach young people to resist this pressure. Many of these skills are also useful in resisting pressures to engage in other health-risky behaviors (e.g., substance use). Resisting the pressure to engage in sexual activity with someone a young person cares for is much more difficult than refusing sex from a "creep." Young people should be taught that pressure may also come from someone they like and/or find attractive. This requires stronger commitment and adherence to personal values. (Refusal skills are also discussed in Chapter 6.)

*Decision-Making Skills*   Youth need to understand that they are responsible for their own behavior and that it carries consequences, both favorable and unfavorable. Unfortunately, many young people do not see this link between personal behavior and behavioral consequences for their life goals. Providing opportunities for youth to grapple with decision making often leads to the determination that delaying sexual activity is best for their futures. (Specific guidelines and teaching activities regarding decision-making skills can be found in Chapter 2.)

*Goal-Setting Skills*  As young people mature, they develop the cognitive ability to begin analyzing their feelings and developing their own sense of self. They begin to understand what is in their best interest, not only for today but for the future. When young people receive guidance in setting and working toward goals that will ensure a bright future, they understand that an adverse consequence from engaging in sexual activity (e.g., unintended pregnancy, HIV infection) could prevent them from achieving those goals. This focus on the future is central to effective prevention education and should be at the core of all related activities. Discussions of how engaging in sexual activity can damage future opportunities are central to promoting abstinence as a healthful choice. (Chapter 2 provides additional information on goal setting.)

## HIV Prevention Education

A major focus of HIV prevention should be on school-based sex education, with emphasis on increased responsibility of sexual decision making. Schools are a highly effective and appropriate place to teach young people HIV prevention skills before they begin the behaviors that put them at risk for HIV infection. Young people are best equipped to protect themselves from HIV when they are provided accurate information and given opportunities to develop the skills needed to avoid HIV infection.

Most states mandate HIV prevention education in schools. Health experts urge that education about HIV should start in early elementary school and at home so that children can grow up knowing how to protect themselves against HIV infection. They further emphasize that HIV prevention education should be offered in the context of a comprehensive school health education program (grades K–12). In addition to simply providing information about HIV transmission, students should be provided with opportunities to develop skills for decision making and resisting personal and social pressures. Building self-esteem is also an important HIV prevention tool.

School-based programs are critical for reaching youth before behaviors are established. Because risk behaviors do not exist independently, topics such as HIV, STDs, unintended pregnancy, tobacco, nutrition, and physical activity should be integrated and ongoing for all students in kindergarten through high school. The specific scope and content of these school health programs should be locally determined and consistent with parental and community values. Research has clearly shown that the most effective programs are comprehensive ones that include a focus on delaying sexual behavior and provide information on how sexually active young people can protect themselves.[11]

*Kindergarten Through Third Grade*  Kindergarten through third grade is the time for educators to establish a foundation for a more detailed

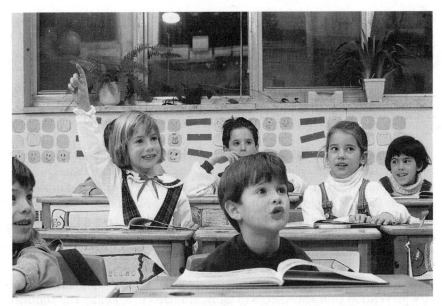

What do our children know about AIDS? Education about AIDS should start in elementary school, providing information about HIV transmission and developing skills for making decisions and resisting pressure.

discussion of sexuality in later grades. Children should be encouraged to feel positive about their bodies. It is also important for them to know about their body parts and the differences between girls and boys. The primary goal during the early elementary years should be to dispel the fear of AIDS. To do this teachers can tell students that young children rarely get AIDS. Teachers should also communicate that there is no need to worry about playing with children who have family members with AIDS or have AIDS themselves. They cannot get the disease from playing with these children. Because children at this age are interested in germs and how disease is spread, discuss HIV as one of many diseases. Questions about AIDS should be answered directly and simply; responses can be limited to questions asked by students. Children should be warned not to play with hypodermic needles that they may find in neighborhoods or elsewhere. They should also be taught to avoid contact with other people's blood and the importance of cleaning up bodily fluids in a safe manner. Educators can also discuss having compassion for those living with AIDS.

*Upper Elementary Grades*    Children in upper elementary grades should be provided with basic information about human sexuality. They will need help understanding puberty and the associated changes in their bodies. Part of this understanding is affirming that their bodies will have natural sexual feelings. Children should be urged to examine and affirm their own family values about sexuality. Upper elementary level children need to have answers to their questions about AIDS and HIV prevention. It is appropriate at this age level to begin discussing the ways HIV is transmitted (e.g., sexual intercourse, sharing needles). Students should also recognize that alcohol and other drugs can increase the risk of infection by lowering a person's ability to act responsibly.

*Secondary Level*   At the secondary level, the major emphasis of HIV prevention education should be to teach students to protect themselves and others from infection with HIV. Information about HIV prevention should focus on healthy behaviors rather than on the medical aspects of the disease. Students should clearly understand that they have a right to abstain from sexual intercourse and to postpone becoming sexually active. Adolescents should be taught that abstaining from sexual activity is the best way to prevent HIV infection. It should be stressed to secondary students that alcohol and other drugs influence individuals to make very poor choices. HIV prevention education needs to allow students to examine and confirm their own values. Decisions can be reinforced by providing adequate opportunities to rehearse resisting peer and social pressure to engage in risky behaviors. Questions about HIV must always be answered honestly and factually.

It should not be assumed that all students will choose to abstain from sexual activity and/or substance use. For these students, proper information concerning risk reduction (e.g., using condoms, avoiding injecting drugs) should be provided. Still, these behaviors must never be condoned by school personnel. It is important to stress that young people do not have to continue their risky behavior. High-risk youth should be offered assistance in changing their risky behavior patterns.

Effective HIV prevention must take place over the course of many years and be developmentally appropriate. Teachers should strive to provide information about HIV prevention clearly and in sufficient detail for each grade level. Students should also be encouraged to ask questions and be given the opportunity to ask questions anonymously. HIV prevention education should also include discussion of critical social issues associated with HIV infection (e.g., civil liberties, protection of public health, health care costs, compassionate care of HIV-infected people) and be taught skills that will enable them to continue to evaluate HIV-related issues.

The importance of HIV prevention is too great to be left to health educators alone. All teachers and school personnel who work with young people should receive HIV prevention information as part of inservice and preservice training. In this way all school personnel can effectively and sensitively assist in HIV prevention efforts.

## Contraceptives

Young people who are sexually active need to make decisions about the use of **contraceptives.** Talking about contraceptives in schools raises many concerns and points of view. Many argue that teaching about contraceptives is necessary because many unmarried adolescents are already sexually active. However, many teachers feel uncomfortable discussing sexual matters in the classroom, and many concerned parents, community groups, and religious organizations promote the idea that it is immoral or irresponsible to suggest the use of contraceptives to young people. Further, it is difficult to get sexually active adolescents to regularly and properly use contraception because all methods require planning. It should be pointed out that school programs that promote contraceptives do not lead to an increase in sexual activity.

Successful contraception for sexually active teens requires the performance and foreplanning of a complex sequence of behaviors. First, there must be an admission that one is sexually active. An advance decision about contraception is needed in anticipation of further sexual activity. The teen must learn relevant information about conception and contraception. Contraceptive methods must be evaluated in terms of personal advantages and disadvantages as well as the barriers to obtaining needed contraceptives. A difficult task for most young people is engaging in presex discussions and negotiation of contraception with a partner. A teen using contraception will need to acquire the contraceptive method. This usually requires a public acquisition, such as purchasing condoms at a store or a visit to a health department or health clinic. Once contraceptives have been obtained, the adolescent must consistently and correctly use the chosen contraceptive. Often, this requires action prior to each instance of sexual intercourse.

Anticipating sexual activity, consistently practicing contraception, acquiring contraceptives, and persuading partners to behave in a certain way are difficult tasks for adults, let alone teens. The complexity of such behavioral tasks is difficult considering the cognitive inability of many adolescents to consider and plan for future outcomes. Educators should consider using simulations to teach young people these skills. Simulations should allow students to make decisions about sex, social life, relationships, school, and work and then "live" with the consequences of their choices in all areas of their life. Perhaps such exercises will succeed in extending the time orientation of adolescents to a point where outcomes of choices can be envisioned and decisions more thoughtfully weighed.

Some areas of the country now offer contraceptive services through school-based clinics. The presence of school-based clinics in schools does not appear to increase the rates of sexual activity among students attending the schools.

## Peer-Led Prevention Programs

Peer education is a highly effective prevention strategy with youth. **Peer education** uses young people as credible prevention messengers to promote healthy lifestyles among other young people. Peer educators can present material about the risks of sexual activity in ways that are highly relevant to young people. Adolescents often find prevention messages more believable when they are delivered by their peers. Peer-led prevention efforts are popular at many schools. However, many more such efforts utilizing peer educators are needed. An example of an innovative peer-led prevention effort is the Sex Can Wait program. High school students are trained to work with middle school students. They teach self-respect and give concrete reasons for remaining abstinent. Instead of just telling the middle school students why they shouldn't have sex, the older teens also tell them how to say no. They perform skits emphasizing this message and assist the younger students in practicing ways of saying no to sexual activity. The program also has benefits for the peer educators. It teaches leadership and reinforces the skills that can keep them from falling to peer pressure to have sex. Making a public commitment to not have sex reinforces the decision to remain abstinent.

## Teen Parenthood Programs

Teens who have been sexually active, become pregnant, and choose to bear their babies need a considerable amount of support and help with making decisions. Comprehensive efforts need to be made to assist pregnant teens in ensuring adequate prenatal, obstetric, and pediatric care in order to prevent the adverse consequences associated with pregnancy and childbirth. Young teens with children usually need training in parenting skills, and programs to help keep them in school, so that they can finish their high school degree and meet other educational and career goals. These young people need to learn skills to prevent subsequent unintended pregnancies as well. Many of these needs are shared by both the adolescent mother and adolescent father.

## Programs for Out-of-School Youth

School-based programs do not reach all youths at risk. Those adolescents not in school—because they have graduated or dropped out—will need to be reached with the same kind of basic information that schools provide to all others. Many youth at very high risk for STDs, HIV infection, and unintended pregnancy, such as homeless or runaway youth, juvenile offenders, or school dropouts, can only be reached through intensive community-based programs. Integrating prevention programs with ongoing community efforts to provide shelter, medical care, or other services to out-of-school youth is essential. Schools can play an important role in supporting these programs and referring students who drop out to these programs and services.

# Problems Associated with Youth Sexual Activity

## Emotional Consequences

Even if promiscuous youth escape the harsh consequences of sexual activity—pregnancy, HIV infection, or an STD—they can experience negative emotional consequences. This is evidenced by the numerous young adults who state they wish they would have waited longer before becoming sexually active. It can take years for individuals to overcome the emotional baggage of early-age sexual activity. Some never completely overcome lingering emotional effects. Thomas Lickona identifies the following 10 emotional dangers of premature sexual involvement.[12]

1. *Worry about pregnancy and STDs.* Sexually active young people can experience a great deal of stress over the possibility of being pregnant or having contracted an STD. Receiving a negative pregnancy or STD screening test can relieve their fears, but the stress reemerges upon their next sexual encounter. Many youth don't get screened but remain sexually active, turning this stress into a chronic condition.

2. *Regret and self-recrimination.* Young women often report feeling used, stupid, and cheap after sexual encounters. Girls are especially vulnerable to this because they are more likely to think of sex as a way of "showing they care." They may become physically intimate in an effort to try to "keep the guy," but become ignored or "dumped." Giving one's self for nothing can be emotionally devastating. Youth can also regret losing their virginity as they realize sex isn't exactly what it is hyped to be.

3. *Guilt.* Many people report having a guilty conscience about having sex. This can come from not living up to religious expectations or from seeing the pain they have caused in others. Guilt can also come from knowing that their parents would be upset if they knew they were having sex. Parents can be crippled by guilt regarding their own early sexual activity. Their reluctance to be hypocritical can keep them from advising their children about the dangers of premature sexual involvement.

4. *Loss of self-respect and self-esteem.* Discovering that one is pregnant or has contracted an STD can have a monumental impact on one's sense of confidence and worth. Casual sex can also lower self-esteem. An oppressive cycle can develop of casual sex leading to lowered self-esteem leading to more casual sex. When we treat people as objects we not only hurt them but also lose respect for ourselves. Getting drunk and having sex with someone you can't remember or having sex for a sexual conquest results in a loss of self-respect for both parties.

5. *Corruption of character and the debasement of sex.* People corrupt their characters and debase their sexuality when they treat others as

sexual objects and exploit them for their own pleasure. The breakdown of the character traits of self-control and delayed gratification are major factors in many of the sex-related problems plaguing our society: pornography, sexual harassment, sexual abuse, infidelity in marriage, and rape. Character is also corrupted when people tell lies in order to get sex. Lies can range from "I love you" to "I've never had a sexually transmitted disease."

The debasement of sex is too often seen on school campuses. In school hallways students can be heard using "profane language." Teenage boy clubs have been reported to exist in which members compete to see how many girls they can sleep with. Elementary school children have been found playing sexual contact games in which points are earned by touching another's private parts. And sadly, many young people have stated that forced sex is permissible if a man and woman have been dating for six months or more.

6. *Shaken trust and fear of commitment.* Individuals who feel betrayed or used after breaking up from a sexual relationship can experience difficulty in future relationships. Girls can see guys as interested in just one thing and wonder if anyone will ever love and accept them without demanding sex to earn that love. Boys can also feel a loss of trust and a fear of commitment. Some young men report engaging in one-night stands because they are afraid of falling in love.

7. *Rage over betrayal.* Sex can create an emotional bond that hurts terribly when broken. Rage and violence can result when an individual feels betrayed. News networks often report on the violent acts of former lovers.

8. *Depression and suicide.* The emotional pain caused by a terminated sexual relationship can be enormous, especially if it was thought to be "the real thing." Sometimes the emotional turmoil of a broken relationship can lead to deep depression. Depression in turn can lead to suicide. Rage turned inward has also resulted in suicide.

9. *Ruined relationships.* Sex can turn a good relationship bad. It can quickly become the focal point, block other means of communicating love, and stunt the balanced growth of a relationship.

10. *Stunting personal development.* Some young people have used sex, like alcohol and drugs, ineffectively to try to cope with life's pressures. Teens caught up in intense sexual relationships thwart their individual growth and sense of identity. They are focusing on one thing when they need to be forming friendships with others, developing skills and interests, and taking on larger social responsibilities. Promiscuous youth can have trouble expressing and meeting their own needs and

the needs of others. They can also have trouble setting long-range goals and creating a plan for their lives.

## Unintended Teen Pregnancy

In the United States, teen pregnancy rates rose in the 1970s and early 1980s. After remaining at a steady level through the 1980s, teen pregnancy rates declined through the 1990s. The teen pregnancy rate in 1993 was 117 pregnancies per 1,000 girls aged 15 to 19; the rate by 1997 fell to 93 per 1,000 girls of the same age.[13] This was a decline of 19% in the teen pregnancy rate. Still, 4 of 10 girls get pregnant at least once before age 20 (see Figure 5-2). There are nearly one million teen pregnancies each year and about half as many teen births.[14] Most teen pregnancies are unplanned and occur outside of marriage. Among unmarried teens, almost 8 of 10 pregnancies are unintended. The United States has one of the highest rates of teenage pregnancy in the developed world (see Figure 5-3). This discrepancy exists despite evidence that teens in the United States are no more sexually active than teens in other developed nations.

Why has the teen pregnancy rate declined? Researchers at the Alan Guttmacher Institute conclude that approximately one-fourth of the decline is due to increased abstinence from sex, and the other three-quarters is the result of changes in contraceptive use. It appears that while teens' overall contraceptive use increased only slightly, there was a significant change to

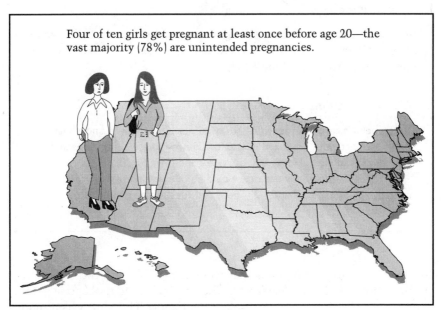

Four of ten girls get pregnant at least once before age 20—the vast majority (78%) are unintended pregnancies.

**FIGURE 5-2    Teen pregnancy in the United States**

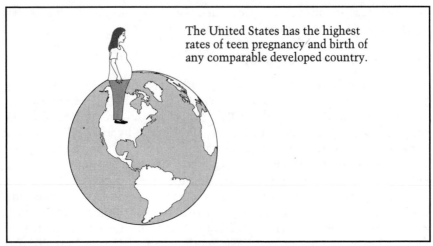

The United States has the highest rates of teen pregnancy and birth of any comparable developed country.

**FIGURE 5-3**    Teen pregnancy, a U.S. problem

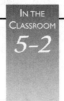

IN THE
CLASSROOM

*5-2*

### Virginity Pledges

As part of a larger sex ed program, give students the opportunity to pledge "I won't" until swearing "I do." These can be written documents that students sign on the dotted line. (I, J, H)

### Good Clean Fun

Youth need alternative activities to avoid sexual pressures and situations. Many such activities are listed in Box 6-1. Review these suggestions and ask students for additional ideas that provide good clean fun. (I, J, H)

Many additional activities that would be relevant in a sex education program can be found in Chapter 2. These activities can be altered to meet specific needs.

long-acting hormonal methods that were introduced into the U.S. market in the early 1990s—in particular the injectable contraceptive (Depo-Provera) and the contraceptive implant (Norplant). This shift was responsible for helping sexually active teens become more successful at avoiding pregnancy.[13]

In addition to becoming sexually active, lack of contraceptive use is a major cause of teenage pregnancy. Among the reasons that sexually active adolescents are reluctant to use contraceptives are that they:

❖ Do not believe they could conceive

❖ Do not expect to have intercourse

❖ Want to keep their sexual activity private

❖ Are embarrassed to discuss sexual matters with others (partners, friends, parents, counselors, physicians, health care providers)

❖ Believe using condoms takes all the pleasure out of intercourse

❖ Believe that birth control decisions are female decisions

❖ Believe myths such as the following:
   You can't get pregnant the first time you have intercourse.
   You can't get pregnant if you are standing during intercourse.
   You can't get pregnant if a girl is still having her period.
   You can't get pregnant if a boy withdraws in time.
   You can't get pregnant if you douche afterward.
   You can't get pregnant if you use foam afterward.
   You can't get pregnant if you take a birth control pill afterward.

There are other reasons that teens become pregnant besides failure to use contraception. Some desire to have a baby as a sign of maturity or even as a type of status symbol. Some teens view motherhood as a way of achieving love or feeling needed by someone else. Others use pregnancy as a means of escaping an unhappy or abusive family situation. Teen mothers can obtain federal and state aid to support their babies through such programs as Medicaid, AFDC (Aid to Families with Dependent Children), and food stamps.

There are serious consequences associated with teenage pregnancy. Babies carried by teenage mothers are at high risk for complications of pregnancy, birth, and infant development. The pregnancy outcomes of teenagers who receive good prenatal care are no different from those of older women. The problem is that pregnant adolescents, and particularly young adolescents, are much less likely to receive that care. As a result, pregnant adolescents are more likely to give birth to premature and low-birthweight infants. The babies born to adolescents are at risk for decreased rates of growth and intellectual development, and are susceptible to infections, injuries, and violence. Teens who become mothers are often poor and dependent on public assistance for their economic support.

The consequences for a teen mother or father often include the following:

❖ Early dropout from school

❖ Poor academic performance and achievement

❖ Increased economic needs due to the presence of a baby

❖ Decreased ability to earn and provide due to lack of education

❖ Increased likelihood of teenage girl being a single parent and staying a single parent

❖ Increased likelihood of repeat pregnancies

❖ Limited life options for teen parents and children reared by teen parents

Teen girls who have babies are likely to become pregnant again in the short-term future. According to Campaign for Our Children, 50% of the adolescents who have a baby become pregnant again within two years of the baby's birth, and 25% have a second baby within two years of the first baby's birth.[15] More than 20% of all births to teens are repeat births (i.e., a second birth or higher). Children of teen mothers are also at increased risk for being teen parents themselves. These children are at increased risk for dropping out of school as adolescents.

Approximately 55% of teen pregnancies end up in birth; 14% end up in a miscarriage, and 31% in abortion. In most states, teens who give birth can legally place their child for adoption without parental consent and involvement, but only a small percentage of these babies are placed in adoptive homes.

## HIV Infection

One-quarter of new HIV infections in the United States are believed to occur among teenagers.[16] Infection with **HIV (human immunodeficiency virus)** is the most frightening potential consequence of youth sexual activity. HIV is the cause of AIDS (acquired immunodeficiency syndrome). This virus attacks the cells of the immune system so that the body loses its ability to fight infection and certain cancers. As a result, people with AIDS are susceptible to life-threatening diseases, called **opportunistic diseases,** that are caused by pathogens that do not cause illness in healthy people.

The most common means of transmitting HIV from person to person is through sexual contact with an infected partner. During sexual contact, HIV can enter the body through the lining of the vagina, vulva, penis, rectum, or mouth. Another common means of transmitting HIV is the sharing of needles or syringes used to inject drugs. Transmission occurs when needles or syringes are contaminated with minute quantities of blood from someone infected with HIV.

The proportion of HIV infections due to heterosexual transmission is increasing. The potential for the sexual transmission to or among adolescents or children is real and of grave concern. Young people are at greatest risk of HIV infection if they have unprotected sex outside of a mutually monogamous relationship between two HIV-negative individuals, use

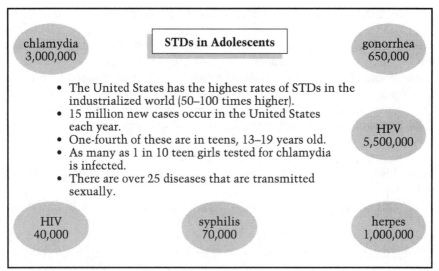

FIGURE 5-4     STDs in adolescents

injection drugs, or use alcohol or other drugs that impair their decision-making abilities. Those who have many different sex partners and who inject illicit drugs into their bloodstream are at even greater risk. Individuals with other sexually transmitted diseases (e.g., chlamydia, herpes) are at increased susceptibility of acquiring HIV infection during sex with an infected partner.

HIV-infected females can pass the virus to their fetuses during pregnancy or birth. About one-fourth of HIV-infected females who do not receive treatment pass the infection to their babies. The virus can also be passed to the baby through breast milk after delivery. The chances of passing HIV to a baby are greatly reduced if the pregnant female is given the drug AZT during pregnancy.

Concerns that HIV can be transmitted through casual contact are unfounded. The virus is not spread through the sharing of food utensils, towels and bedding, swimming pools, telephones, or toilet seats. Closed-mouth kissing does not carry risk of HIV transmission. However, health authorities advise against open-mouthed kissing ("French" kissing) with an infected person because of the possibility of contact with blood. HIV is also not spread by biting insects such as mosquitoes or bedbugs.

### Sexually Transmitted Diseases

According to the CDC, about 15 million cases of **sexually transmitted diseases (STDs)** are reported in the United States each year (see Figure 5-4). One-fourth of these cases of STDs are among teenagers.[17] Many of these young people will suffer long-term health consequences as a result.

The high rate of sexual activity among young people increases their likelihood of being exposed, infected, or transmitting a host of infectious diseases. There are now more than 25 known sexually transmitted diseases. Many of these diseases are passed from one person to another unknowingly because the carrier may not feel ill or may come to feel ill after he or she has already passed the disease to unknowing victims. Some diseases regarded as STDs can be transmitted through other means (e.g., from a mother to an unborn or newborn child, through blood transfusions, by sharing contaminated needles).

The primary means of transmission of these diseases, however, is through sexual contact. Therefore, the most effective means of prevention is to avoid sexual contact.

Young people who are sexually active put themselves at high risk of acquiring a sexually transmitted disease. The greater the number of partners with whom an individual has sexual contact, the greater the risk of developing an STD. *Safe sex* refers to sexual practices that are important in preventing the spread of STDs. One safe-sex practice is the use of a condom during sexual activity. This reduces but does not eliminate the risk of STD transmission from one partner to another. Use of nonoxynol-9, a common ingredient in spermicidal jellies and foams, in combination with a condom reduces the risk of spreading an STD from one person to another during sexual intercourse. Avoiding other practices, such as oral-genital and anal-genital contact, also reduces the risk of contracting an STD.

Young people who are sexually active should seriously consider the risks of developing an STD and consider postponing sexual contact. They should also know the potential signs and symptoms of STDs. If any of the following are present, early medical advice and treatment should be sought:

❖ Any unusual discharges from the genitals

❖ Pain in the genital area

❖ Burning sensation in or around the genitals (especially during urination)

❖ Sores on or near the genitals

❖ Frequent urination

❖ Lower abdominal pain

❖ Itching around the genital or anal area

❖ Growths or warts in the genital area

***Common STDs Among Teens***  Teens are at high risk for acquiring most STDs. Teenagers and young adults are more likely than any other age groups to have multiple sex partners and to engage in unprotected sex. Also, young females are likely to choose sexual partners older than themselves.

Chlamydia and gonorrhea are the most common curable STDs among teens. **Chlamydia** is the result of a bacterial infection and is the most common sexually transmitted disease in the United States today. Forty percent of all chlamydia cases are reported among 15- to 19-year-old adolescents.[17] **Gonorrhea**, also a bacterial infection, is one of the oldest and most widespread sexually transmitted diseases. Chlamydia and gonorrhea produce similar symptoms, and most females with these infections are asymptomatic and unaware that they are infected. These bacterial infections can easily be treated with antibiotics if detected early enough. However, if these diseases remain undetected and untreated, they can result in severe health consequences later in life, including pelvic inflammatory disease (PID), a major infection of the entire female reproductive tract that can lead to permanent sterility or even death. Babies born to females with chlamydial or gonorrheal infections can acquire serious eye infections that lead to blindness.

An increasing number of individuals acquire genital herpes or genital warts, both viral STDs, during the teenage years. **Genital herpes** is a viral infection caused by a herpes simplex virus that cannot be cured. These viruses are very contagious, and their resulting infection is characterized by recurrent and unpredictable outbreaks. Herpes infection results in painful, blisterlike sores that may appear on the sex organs, the mouth, or the face. Although the sores go away, the herpes virus remains in the body, so the sores reappear periodically throughout the person's lifetime. The herpes virus can be spread from a mother to her baby during vaginal delivery and can be fatal to the baby. **Genital warts** are the result of infection with the human papilloma virus (HPV). They cause considerable discomfort and embarrassment for an infected person. They are highly contagious and can easily spread to a sexual partner and to a baby during delivery. Females with genital herpes and genital warts are at higher risk for having cervical cancer in their lifetimes than those who have not been infected.

Syphilis, hepatitis B, and chancroid are STDs that are declining among teens and other age groups. **Syphilis** is a bacterial infection that when detected early can be treated effectively with antibiotic drugs. However, untreated syphilis can cause destructive effects in the body and even birth defects in a developing baby if a pregnant female carries the infection. Infection with **hepatitis B virus** can cause serious viral infection of the liver. Hepatitis B is preventable through vaccination. **Chancroid** is a highly infectious sexually transmitted disease caused by a bacterium that can cause ulcers in the genitals or painful swelling in the groin area, or both. Chancroid can be effectively treated with antibiotics.

Other STDs that teens may acquire include trichomoniasis, candidiasis, and pubic lice. **Trichomoniasis** is a common STD caused by a protozoal organism. This organism can be also spread by towels, sheets, and other objects because the protozoan can remain alive on external objects for up to 1.5 hours. **Candidiasis** is caused by *Candida albicans*, a yeastlike fungus that creates intense vaginal itching and burning sensations. **Pubic lice**, known as "crabs," are parasites that are spread by sexual contact. These lice attach to the pubic hair and feed on the blood of a host.

## Key Terms

Youth Risk Behavior Survey   163
sex education   170
abstinence education   176
abstinence-only education   176
abstinence-plus education   176
comprehensive sex
   education   176
refusal skills   177
contraceptives   181
peer education   182
human immunodeficiency
   virus (HIV)   188
opportunistic diseases   188

sexually transmitted diseases
   (STDs)   189
chlamydia   191
gonorrhea   191
genital herpes   191
genital warts   191
syphilis   191
hepatitis B virus   191
chancroid   191
trichomoniasis   191
candidiasis   191
pubic lice   192

## Review Questions

1. Describe the sexual activity patterns of teenagers today and any increasing or decreasing trends.
2. Discuss the pervasiveness of sex in the media, why this should be alarming, and what educators can do to try to change the current trend.
3. Explain why adolescence is often a difficult life stage. Include in your answer the pressures from family, peers, and society; physical, mental, and social changes; risk-taking behaviors; and problems associated with early physical maturation.
4. What indications are there that sexual development occurs at a younger age today? What are associated pressures and possible causes?
5. What are the major points of the *Surgeon General's Call to Action to Promote Sexual Heath and Responsible Sexual Behavior*.
6. Discuss state laws governing sex education.
7. Identify the wide range of topics often included in sex education. Explain why decision making and other life skills must be a part of sex education.
8. Discuss the differences between abstinence-only and comprehensive sex education. Explain why abstinence education is emphasized in most school-based programs. Identify and discuss the six components in the chapter that are highlighted in abstinence programs.

9. Why do most states mandate HIV prevention education in schools? Identify what should be taught regarding HIV in kindergarten through third grade, upper elementary grades, and secondary level.

10. Explain why teaching about contraceptives in school is controversial. Cite some arguments found for and against it.

11. Describe peer-led prevention programs, teen parenthood programs, and programs for out-of-school youth.

12. Identify the negative emotional consequences associated with premature sexual involvement.

13. Cite some statistics concerning teenage pregnancy in the United States. How do these compare with other countries?

14. Explain the causes of teenage pregnancy and the consequences associated with it.

15. How many HIV infections in the United States are among teenagers? Who is at greatest risk of HIV infection? About how many HIV-infected females pass the infection to their babies? How can this occur? How can the HIV virus be spread other than intercourse? How can it not be spread?

16. What percentage of STDs occur among teenagers? Identify the potential signs and symptoms of STDs.

# References

1. Centers for Disease Control and Prevention (2000). "Youth Risk Behavior Surveillance—United States, 1999." *Morbidity and Mortality Weekly Report*, 49(SS-05).

2. Kunkel, D. C., K. M. Cope, W. M. Farinola, R. Biely, E. Rollin, and E. Donnerstein (1999). *Sex on TV: A Biennial Report to the Kaiser Family Foundation* (No. 1457). Washington, DC: The Henry J. Kaiser Family Foundation.

3. Mediascope (2001). "Teens, Sex, and the Media: Issue Briefs." Studio City, CA: Mediascope Press. Available at http://www.mediascope.org/pubs/ibriefs/tsm.htm.

4. Jacobsen, M. F., and Mazur, L. A. (1995). "Sexism and Sexuality in Advertising." In M. F. Jacobsen and L. A. Mazur (Eds.), *Marketing Madness: A Survival Guide for a Consumer Society*, (pp. 74–87). Boulder, Co: Westview Press.

5. Hansen, B., and C. Knopes (1993, July 6). "TV vs. Reality: Prime Time Tuning Out Varied Culture." *USA Today*, 1A–2A.

6. Office of the Surgeon General (2001). *The Surgeon General's Call to Action to Promote Sexual Health and Responsible Sexual Behavior*. Washington, DC: U.S. Department of Health and Human Services. Available at http://www.surgeongeneral.gov/library/sexualhealth/call.htm.

7. Darroch, J. E., D. J. Landry, and S. Singh (2000). "Changing Emphases on Sexuality Education in U.S. Public Secondary Schools, 1988–1999." *Family Planning Perspectives*, 32(5): 204–211, 265.

8. Gold, R. B., and E. Nash (2001, August). "State-Level Policies on Sexuality, STD Education." *The Guttmacher Report on Public Policy*, 4(4). Available at http://www.guttmacher.org/pubs/journals/gr040404.html.

9. Dailard, C. (2001, February). "Sex Education: Politicians, Parents, Teachers and Teens." *The Guttmacher Report on Public Policy*, 4(1). Available at http://www.guttmacher.org/pubs/journals/gr040109.html.

10. Collins, C., P. Alagiri, and T. Summers (2002). *Abstinence Only vs. Comprehensive Sex Education: What Are the Arguments? What Is the Evidence?* (Policy Monograph Series). San Francisco: AIDS Research Institute, University of California.

11. Centers for Disease Control and Prevention (2002). "Young People at Risk: HIV/AIDS Among America's Youth." Available at http://wsww.cdc.gov/hiv/pubs/facts/youth.htm.

12. Lickona, T. (1994, Summer). "The Neglected Heart: The Emotional Dangers of Premature Sexual Involvement." *American Educator*, 34–39.

13. Boonstra, H. (2002). "Teen Pregnancy: Trends and Lessons Learned." *The Guttmacher Report on Public Policy*, 5(1). Available at http://www.guttmacher.org/pubs/journals/gr050107.html.

14. The National Campaign to Prevent Teen Pregnancy (2002, February). *Recent Trends in Teen Pregnancy and Birth, Sexual Activity, and Contraceptive Use* [Brochure]. Washington, DC: The National Campaign to Prevent Teen Pregnancy.

15. Campaign for Our Children (2002). "Fact Sheet on Adolescents Who Have Babies." Available at http://www.cfoc.org/5_educator/5_facts.cfm?Fact_ID=125&FactCat_ID=2.

16. AIDS Action (2001). *What Works in HIV Prevention for Youth* [Brochure]. Washington, DC: AIDS Action.

17. Centers for Disease Prevention and Control (2000). "Tracking the Hidden Epidemics 2000: Trends in STDs in the United States." Available at http://www.cdc.gov/nchstp/od/news/RevBrochure1pdftoc.htm.

# 6

# Substance Use and Abuse

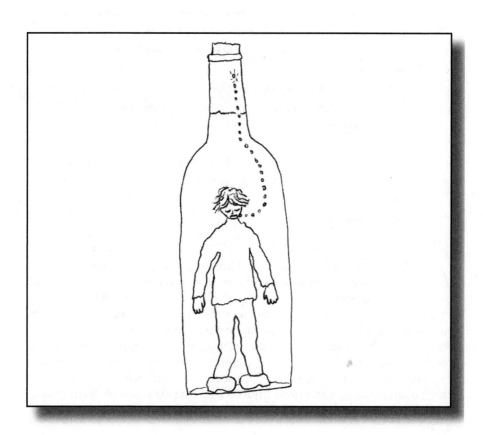

The following was turned in by a university student in a personal health class. The assignment was to write a short story about a family suffering from alcoholism.

## Once Upon a Time . . . My Story

*Once upon a time there lived a family of six—a mom, an alcoholic (Dad), and four children. The mother was kind of crazy trying to keep up with her alcoholic husband. She loved him, so in her eyes she had to drink along with him to prove her love to him.*

*Out of the four kids there was only one family hero. She was 16 at the time, but she had to grow up a lot faster than she ever expected. She took care of the two younger children and covered up the alcoholic's mistakes constantly. She took care of everything because she had to become the mother and father and still keep up with her own life.*

*The other two girls in the family were labeled between a scapegoat and the family mascot or clown. They were the reason the alcoholic dad lost four jobs and was drinking his life away. Yet, at times they brought relief to the family due to their humor.*

*The youngest child was the lost child of the family. He fit all the classic characteristics of a lost child. He died at age 15 due to someone choosing a life in the bottle over his family.*

*This is a true story. It's my story.*

Alcohol and other drugs are facts of life in most communities. The use of psychoactive substances by children and adolescents is a national problem that demands the attention of all professionals who work with young people. Substance use poses many problems for young people. Youthful substance users are vulnerable to life-threatening accidents and injuries. Substance abuse is the major cause for most of the premature life lost and morbidity seen in adolescents in the United States and many other nations as well. The Centers for Disease Control and Prevention (CDC) reports that three-quarters of unintentional injuries (the leading cause of death in adolescents) among adolescents are directly or indirectly related to substance abuse.

Substance users are often impulsive and engage in risk-taking behavior and illegal activity that increases risk of injury and serious medical consequences. Young people who use drugs often expose themselves to sexually transmitted diseases, including HIV infection. The effects of psychoactive drugs erode emotional, social, and cognitive development in youth, making it difficult to face developmental challenges during adolescence and in later stages of life. Involvement with substances interferes with school achievement and contributes to school dropout and truancy. School systems are adversely affected by substance use. Students under the influence of psychoactive substances cannot learn, and teachers cannot teach such students. Substance-using students alter the learning environment for everyone in a school.

Compared with non-substance-using youth, teenage substance users:

❖ Have a greater chance of getting into trouble with parents, friends, and teachers

❖ Have a greater chance of engaging in problematic behavior, such as truancy, vandalism, petty theft, and property damage

❖ Have a greater chance of not learning many of the emotional and social skills necessary for a safe and productive life

❖ Have a greater chance of causing an accident or injury to themselves or others

❖ Have a greater chance of engaging in sexual behavior that can put them at risk of unintended pregnancy and sexually transmitted diseases

❖ Have a greater chance of progressing to heavy use and drug dependency

## Substance Use Trends

The Monitoring the Future study is an annual survey funded by the National Institute on Drug Abuse that measures the extent of drug use among high school seniors, tenth graders, and eighth graders.[1] The 2001 survey showed that the primary drug showing an increase in 2001 was Ecstasy (MDMA), whose use had been rising sharply since 1998. Despite the continuing increase in Ecstasy use among secondary students, the rate of increase was not as high as in 1999 or 2000. This may be due to a sharp increase in the proportion of students seeing Ecstasy use as dangerous. However, the proportion of schools in 2001 having at least one student who has ever used Ecstasy increased in 2001. This indicates that Ecstasy use is diffusing to new communities. The reported availability of Ecstasy continued to rise quite dramatically. The use of anabolic steroids increased among high school seniors in 2001, but decreased among younger students.

A number of other drugs showed evidence of some decline in 2001. One of these drugs was heroin, which had been at or near peak levels in recent years. In the 1990s heroin use increased in popularity in large part because young people were using heroin without a needle. Because of the availability of high-purity heroin, users were able to smoke or snort heroin. The Monitoring the Future study also showed continuing declines in use for LSD, inhalants, and cocaine (crack and powdered cocaine).

The use of marijuana appears to be holding steady or slightly below the peak rates reached in 1997 among tenth and twelfth graders. Eighth graders, who had shown a steady decline in marijuana use after their recent peak in 1996, also showed no further improvement in 2001. Other drugs that showed no significant changes in use in 2001 included hallucinogens other than LSD, narcotics other than heroin with a needle, amphetamines, barbiturates, and three of the so-called club drugs—Rohypnol, GHB, and ketamine. It is important to point out that the use of most illicit drugs increased among secondary students during the 1990s until about 1997. Hopefully, these trends showing declining use of substances will continue. The Monitoring the Future study also shows that there has been a modest decrease in the prevalence of alcohol use (in the past 30 days) among students at all three grade levels since the peaks reached in 1996 or 1997. Reports of being drunk also decreased in 2001 among students in eighth and tenth grades.

Cigarette smoking by adolescents in all three grades continued to decline sharply in 2001. This decline began after 1996 (among eighth and tenth graders) or 1997 (among twelfth graders). The use of smokeless tobacco (chewing tobacco and snuff), which had declined considerably in recent years, did not decline any further in 2001.

When children advance from elementary school to middle school or junior high, they often face social challenges, such as learning to get along with a wider group of peers. It is at this stage, early adolescence, that children are likely to encounter drug use for the first time. Children most often begin to use drugs at about age 12 or 13, and many researchers have observed young teens moving from the illicit use of legal substances (such as tobacco, alcohol, and inhalants) to the use of illegal drugs (marijuana is usually the first). The sequence from tobacco and alcohol use to marijuana use and then, as children get older, to other drugs has been found in almost all long-term studies of drug use. The order of drug use in this progression is largely consistent with social attitudes and norms and the availability of drugs. But it cannot be said that smoking and drinking at young ages are the cause of later drug use.

## Media Promotion of Alcohol and Tobacco Use

Alcohol and tobacco companies spend billions of dollars each year promoting their products through advertisements and other means. These industries proclaim that they do not target children and adolescents and that they are not in the business of recruiting new users. In your mind, do the following facts refute or support this claim?

❖ Beer companies use cute and alluring animals and cartoon characters in TV ads and other promotions (e.g., billboards, magazine ads, T-shirts), such as the Budweiser frogs and lizards, Spuds MacKenzie, and Whassup space-alien dogs.

❖ Children consistently name Budweiser commercials as among their favorites.

❖ Alcohol companies are continually bringing new products to the market that have special appeal to kids and heavily advertising them. Several "alcopops" have recently appeared on the market. **Alcopops** include hard lemonades (e.g., Two Dogs, Hootch, Mike's Hard Lemonade) and other fruit-flavored alcoholic beverages that resemble soft drinks in taste and looks.

❖ Liquor-branded malt beverages, such as Smirnoff Ice, are increasingly being advertised on TV at times when young people are viewing.

❖ A survey of elementary students in Washington, D.C., found that children could name more brands of beer than they could U.S. presidents.[2]

❖ Beer companies air their ads on cable television during the times and on shows where the audience is made up of primarily underage viewers.

❖ Beer companies frequently air commercials during TV coverage of popular sporting events that are viewed by large numbers of youth, such as the Super Bowl, NBA championships, the World Series, and the Olympic Games. During the Super Bowl, 20% to 25% of the large audience is younger than 21. This game is used annually to showcase several trend-setting, youth-oriented beer ads. You can't watch a football game on TV without seeing 10 to 20 beer commercials.

❖ Beer and liquor companies deliberately target young people through sponsoring "extreme" sporting events such as snowboarding, mountain biking, and inline skating that especially appeal to youth and in which many of the contestants are teenagers. These companies also sell related sports paraphernalia with beer company brand logos. In a recent snowboarding competition, contestants wore Captain Morgan bibs until a parent complained.[3]

❖ Alcohol and tobacco companies design Internet websites that are particularly attractive to underage audiences, featuring popular music, games, contests, animations, and downloads.

❖ Makers of distilled beverages, in an effort to compete favorably with the beer industry, are increasingly using images in liquor ads designed to catch the attention of young people.

❖ The Marlboro Man is considered by advertising experts as the top advertising icon of the century and accounts for Marlboro's phenomenal success in growing to become the top-selling cigarette in the world. Marlboros are the most popular brand among teen smokers.

❖ The Joe Camel ad campaign was wildly successful in increasing sales of Camel cigarettes among teens. The R.J. Reynolds company did not give up using Joe Camel as an advertising icon out of concern for the welfare of children but because they were under pressure from consumer groups and the threat of expensive litigation.

❖ Children are able to recognize Joe Camel as much as Mickey Mouse and other popular childhood icons. Children as young as 3 years link him with cigarettes.

❖ Nearly 90% of teen smokers smoke one of the three most heavily advertised brands of cigarettes: Marlboros, Camels, and Newports.

❖ Cigarette ads regularly appear in magazines with a large underage readership, such as *Sports Illustrated, Glamour, People,* and *Rolling Stone.*

❖ The three largest tobacco companies increased the amount of cigarette advertising in magazines with high youth readership after the November 1998 Master Settlement Agreement, in which the tobacco companies agreed not to market to kids. Also, after tobacco billboards were banned in the Master Settlement Agreement, cigarette companies increased their advertising and promotions in retail outlets such as convenience stores.

❖ Beer and tobacco companies would suffer enormous financial losses if underage drinking and tobacco use stopped because of all the revenue they receive from the huge amounts consumed by teenagers.

❖ Tobacco companies have developed and marketed "starter products" that have special appeal to youth, such as smokeless tobacco products with cherry flavoring.

❖ One-third of teenagers own tobacco-brand promotional items sporting tobacco company logos, such as T-shirts, backpacks, hats, and CD players.

❖ Numerous internal tobacco industry documents, revealed in various recent tobacco lawsuits, show that the tobacco companies have perceived kids as young as 13 years as a key market, studied the smoking habits of kids, and developed products and marketing campaigns aimed at them.[4]

The list of facts that you have just read attests to the fact that the alcohol and tobacco industries do target kids and use the media as a major tool to do so.

The Philip Morris Company, maker of Marlboro cigarettes, has launched its own "youth smoking prevention" media campaign, which uses the slogan "Think. Don't Smoke." This campaign shows a variety of teens in different settings explaining that cigarettes make you uncool and that young people should stay away from cigarettes. A recent study in the *American Journal of Public Health* concluded that youth exposed to the "Think. Don't Smoke" advertisements were more likely to be open to the idea of smoking.[5] They were less likely to deny that cigarettes cause harmful diseases and to say that they want cigarette companies to go out of business in the future. They were more likely to say that they would smoke in the future. This same study looked at the effects of exposure to the American Legacy "truth" ad campaign, which included media images of young people placing 1,200 body bags at the door of a cigarette company office building and cowboys leading horses with body bags over the saddle. Teenagers exposed to the "truth" countermarketing ads showed an increase in anti-tobacco attitudes and beliefs.

It is not surprising that the American Legacy ads are more effective tobacco prevention tools than the Philip Morris campaign. The "Think. Don't Smoke" ads are very careful not to make the connection between cigarettes and death or to point out the devious tactics of the cigarette companies in marketing a lethal, deadly product to young people. It appears that this campaign is not designed to prevent young people from smoking but rather is merely a public relations tool to build respectability for the company. On the other hand, the media can be an effective tool for smoking prevention by airing hard-hitting, truthful messages such as the "truth" ad campaign.

Advertisements for addictive products (alcohol and tobacco) influence people so deeply because they create associations between the product and powerful emotions about relationships, sex, good times, lifestyle, and self-esteem:

> What Madison Avenue has done is to take every desirable aspect of life that you can imagine and tie it to beer. Close and loving relationships, bonding with your friends and buddies, great sex, having attractive girl-friends and boyfriends, glamorous lifestyle, good health, rugged outdoor life, sports and athletics, cool cars—you name it—if it is something desirable in life—something that we all want for ourselves—then it has been tied to beer. The liquor industry spends well over a billion dollars a year to rope in young viewers.[6]

Another media vehicle for promoting alcohol and tobacco is movies. Many popular movies show likeable and charismatic characters using and enjoying tobacco and alcohol products. Movie scenes showing stars using alcohol, cigarettes, or cigars are in many ways an advertisement for one of these addictive products. Young people are susceptible to this influence. Recent studies show that kids who see stars smoking in films are more likely to start smoking and have higher receptivity to the idea of smoking.[7,8] This is particularly concerning given the fact that adolescents are three times more likely to go to the movies than adults.

During the 1990s there was a marked increase in smoking in movies. Cigarette smoking has become so pervasive in movies that the vast majority of popular films in the last decade showed people smoking. According to the Smoke Free Movies website (www.SmokeFreeMovies.ucsf.edu), of America's 25 top grossing movies each year, 9 in 10 dramatize use of tobacco. More than 1 in 4 depicts a particular brand of cigarettes. Eighty percent of the time, the featured brands are the same ones most heavily advertised in other media (e.g., billboards, magazines). Marlboro cigarettes have been featured in at least 28 of Hollywood's top-grossing movies in the past decade.

Smokers are frequently lead characters in movies and are usually likeable, rebellious, attractive, and successful. Women are often displayed smoking to convey sex appeal, power, emotional control, and body-image control. Males smoke to portray masculinity, power, prestige, authority, and male bonding.[9] Some examples of youth-appealing movies in which leading characters were portrayed as smokers are *Charlie's Angels*, *Erin Brockovich*, *There's Something About Mary*, *Thelma and Louise*, *What Women Want*, *Titanic*, *Independence Day*, *My Best Friend's Wedding*, *Bridget Jones's Diary*, *Good Will Hunting*, *Men in Black*, *Reality Bites*, *Romeo and Juliet*, *Jerry Maguire*, *Payback*, *Escape from LA*, *Lethal Weapon*, *Kate and Leopold*, *Vanilla Sky*, and *Proof of Life*.

Television is another medium that routinely portrays the use of alcohol and tobacco in the programs shown. Seven of 10 prime-time TV programs have scenes of alcohol use, averaging 3.5 scenes an hour, and the music videos most popular with teens show 4.2 drinking episodes per hour.[10] Television shows also frequently feature smoking at high levels. And, of course, most movies eventually show up on cable and network television so that young people view thousands of media depictions of alcohol and tobacco use in their own homes and, increasingly, on their own bedroom TV sets.

## Substance Abuse Prevention Education

Next to the family, schools are the primary societal institution serving young people, and so it is vital that schools assume some responsibility for substance abuse prevention. Substance abuse interferes with school goals by disrupting the educational process. Schools employ personnel who have the necessary skills to plan and implement programs to prevent substance abuse. Schools also provide important access to youth.

Substance abuse is a family and community problem; therefore, it is unrealistic to expect the schools alone to solve drug abuse problems. The responsibility for the well-being of children and for assisting in substance abuse prevention is shared by all individuals and institutions affected by substance abuse: parents, students, school staff, communities, professional organizations, colleges, businesses, policy makers, the media, social services, health care professionals, and mental health agencies. Effective prevention programs evolve only with the collaboration of these groups in developing coordinated and comprehensive efforts.

## Information-Based Strategies

Most substance abuse education programs in the 1960s and 1970s relied solely on information about the legal and medical consequences of drug use as a prevention strategy. These programs often used scare tactics in an effort to change attitudes and behavior regarding substance use and abuse. It was common for drug prevention programs to invite into the classroom local police to tell stories about drug abusers and the troubles that drug abuse made in their lives. Police officers would place emphasis upon showing young people what drugs looked like and maybe even demonstrating what burning marijuana smelled like. The rationale was that children would then know what to avoid. Another common strategy for schools was to invite former addicts to explain to children how easy it is to get hooked on drugs and the horrible life that results from addiction. Scary antidrug films were also shown to young people in order to scare them away from using drugs.

This approach to preventing substance use and abuse assumed that if students understood that drugs are harmful, they would avoid experimentation and drug use. Information-only approaches are considered ineffective because information is only one of the many factors that govern an individual's decision to use or not use substances. However, sound information about drugs and their effects and consequences is fundamental to substance abuse prevention efforts. Information provides the foundation for effective substance prevention programs.

Information about how specific substances produce immediate effects (e.g., yellow stains on teeth and bad breath from cigarette smoking) may be more effective than information about the possible long-term consequences (e.g., lung cancer or emphysema). Regardless of the focus or strategy of a program any information presented in a substance abuse prevention program must be accurate.

## Normative Education

It is typical for young people to overestimate the prevalence of tobacco, alcohol, and other drug use among their peers. Consequently, a critical component of a substance abuse prevention program should be clearing up misconceptions about the perception that "everybody is drinking, smoking, or doing drugs." This approach is sometimes referred to as **normative education.** Students gain more accurate perceptions when they are provided with information concerning drug use prevalence rates among their peers from national and local surveys. This information is then compared with their own estimates of drug use. Misconceptions can also be cleared up when students organize and conduct surveys of drug use in their school and community. Research shows that normative education, which posits that drug use is not the norm, is an effective strategy in lowering substance abuse behavior.[11] This research also showed refusal skills and enhancing competence in personal and social skills to be effective strategies in reducing drug use among youth.

## Resistance Strategies

Peer group acceptance and identification are major concerns of young people. Peer pressure to use various substances or engage in other health-risky behavior can be great for many young people. Therefore, teaching upper-elementary, middle-school, and high-school-specific skills to resist peer pressure may be effective in deterring substance use and abuse. A typical refusal skills technique includes a film or video depicting the various social pressures students are likely to encounter from peers, media, and others. After "inoculation," or exposure to these anticipated pressures ("germs"), students brainstorm and discuss possible refusals to the pressures. Role-play is then used to practice and rehearse these skills. These skills can assist young people to not only refuse pressure from peers and others, but also to resist the persuasive influence of advertising. Students are then better able to recognize the appeals in ads and formulate counter-arguments to them.

## Personal and Social Skills Training and Enhancement Approaches

Educators must realize that youth do not begin to use substances simply because they lack knowledge about drugs and their consequences. Rather, there are several cognitive, affective, and environmental factors that influence substance use and abuse. In addition to peer and media pressure, factors such as poor self-concept, anxiety, low social confidence, external locus of control, impulsivity, and low assertiveness increase the risk of substance use. The recognition that problem behaviors, including substance abuse, result from an interplay of these personal and social factors has led to the development of effective prevention programs such as the Life Skills Training program. The program deals directly with the interpersonal and social factors that promote drug use by teaching general self-management and social competence skills. The Life Skills Training program includes teaching the following:[12]

❖ General problem-solving and decision-making skills

❖ Critical thinking skills for resisting peer and media influences

❖ Skills for increasing self-control and self-esteem (e.g., self-appraisal, goal setting, self-monitoring, self-reinforcement)

❖ Adaptive coping strategies for relieving stress and anxiety through the use of cognitive coping skills or behavioral relaxation techniques

❖ Skills for communicating effectively (e.g., how to avoid misunderstandings by being specific, paraphrasing, asking clarifying questions)

❖ Skills for overcoming shyness

❖ Skills for meeting new people and developing healthy friendships

❖ Conversational skills

❖ Complimenting skills

❖ General assertiveness skills

Skills training requires instruction, demonstration, feedback, and reinforcement. Adequate classroom time is devoted for practicing the skills (behavioral rehearsal) as well as for extended practice outside of class through behavioral homework assignments. The Life Skills Training program has been shown to effectively reduce drug use behavior, particularly when the training is followed by booster sessions to reinforce retention of personal and social skills.

## Peer Approaches

Many youth substance abuse prevention programs utilize peer leaders. The rationale for using peer leaders is that they often have higher credibility with young people than do teachers or other adults. Peer leaders may lead discussions in classroom or group settings or serve as facilitators of skills training by demonstrating skills taught in prevention programs (e.g., refusal skills). Peer leaders also serve as role models who do not use drugs. Peer leaders can be about the same age as prevention program participants or may be older students who work with younger students. **Peer tutors** are usually older students who teach younger students about drugs and how to resist pressures to use them.

**Peer counselors** are students who have received specific training in how to listen, avoid making judgments, maintain confidentiality, and be supportive of others. Peer counselors make themselves available to their peers who need to discuss problems and then refer students with serious problems to an appropriate professional or school staff member.

Some advocate peer-led programs as being more effective in preventing and reducing high-risk behavior than teacher-led programs. This may be explained by the fact that peers have more social information than teachers and other adults. Further, modeling appropriate behaviors outside of school, where youth use substances, may explain the effectiveness of peer-led programs. To ensure successful implementation of peer approaches, it is imperative that school administrators and personnel provide extensive support, guidance, and training.

## Drug-Free Activities and Alternatives to Drugs

It may be assumed that some children and adolescents take drugs in order to achieve an altered state of consciousness. As a result, some substance abuse prevention programs teach and/or provide youth with opportunities to achieve "natural highs" or altered states of consciousness through drug-free activities. Stimulating, relaxing, creative, or growth-enhancing activities such as meditation, exercise, sports, or performing arts are used as alternatives to drugs (see Box 6-1). Service projects in which youth volunteer to assist people in need also serve as alternatives to substance abuse activities.

---

IN THE
CLASSROOM

### 6-1

## Good Clean Fun

Here are some great ideas for having fun without getting drunk, high, or "in bed." Have your students add some ideas of their own.

### Quick and Easy

Buy a cheap model at the store and put it together.

Eat cornflakes by candlelight.

Watch TV without the sound on. Figure out the plot and supply your own dialogue.

Teach boys how to make bread or other baked items.

### Outdoor Activities

Create a treasure hunt for teams or each other.

Make and fly kites.

Create sidewalk chalk drawings.

Go ice blocking—ride down a grassy slope on a block of ice.

*continued*

---

Go hay sledding—ride down a mowed hay hill on cardboard.

Go gravestone rubbing—pace a blank piece of paper on an illegible grave and rub chalk over the paper. You can then read it.

Play frisbee golf.

Organize a frisbee football game.

Play water-balloon volleyball or baseball.

Climb trees at the park.

## Service Ideas

Plan a date for other couples and then be their chauffeurs, chefs, waiters, and so forth.

Have a candlelit dinner ready for someone at a park, hill top, or elsewhere.

Bake cookies for someone who could use a tender touch—a crabby neighbor, a shut-in, someone feeling low.

Read stories to children in the hospital or elsewhere.

Take flowers or goodies to new mothers at the hospital.

Baby-sit for a young married couple so that they can go out on a date.

## Get a Little "Crazy"

Have dinner on the roof.

Have a Christmas party in July.

Have a marathon dinner.

Have a three-armed dinner. Each couple ties one pair of their arms together and then is in charge of making some part of the dinner—dessert, salad, main course, or other.

As teams, visit travel agencies and pretend you are planning a trip. Compete to see who can come up with the best vacation for a predetermined time and budget. Get together over treats to determine who won.

As teams, pretend to be engaged and go shopping for a wedding ring. Return to treats and to share stories.

Give each couple 99 cents and see how many items they can purchase with it. Each item must be different.

Pretend to be tourists and do local sight-seeing. Take pictures or videos.

*continued*

*continued*

Have a hairdo party where the boys do the girls' hair. Have an awards ceremony and don't forget to videotape!

Play hide-and-seek at the mall.

Build sand castles. (Get sand at a cement company and put it into wading pools.)

Take lawn chairs to the side of the road. Hold up cards with numbers 1–10 to rate the cars going by.

Go on a "sound" scavenger hunt, using a point system like the following.

| Sounds | Points |
|---|---|
| 1. Cow mooing | 8 |
| 2. Someone singing in the shower | 10 |
| 3. Someone speaking over a store's public address system | 7 |
| 4. Ask for water at a fast-food restaurant | 5 |
| 5. Squealing car brakes | 7 |
| 6. Toilet flushing | 4 |
| 7. Baby crying | 7 |
| 8. Police siren | 6 |

## Student Assistance Programs

These programs, modeled after employee assistance programs in business and industry, provide professional counseling to students at risk for substance abuse or other problems. In addition, these programs can provide intervention for students already abusing substances and can refer students and their families to outside agencies and professionals. Student assistance programs are partnerships among people inside and outside of schools (e.g., substance abuse and mental health treatment professionals, businesses, law enforcement personnel) and can serve communities in the following ways:

❖ Provide substance abuse education to teachers, students, and parents

❖ Help identify youth with problems

❖ Accept self-referral of students and referral by teachers, parents, and peers of youth needing evaluation and/or services

❖ Help students and families find and use community resources

❖ Conduct discussion groups to allow youth troubled by substance abuse (or other problems) to talk about their concerns

❖ Conduct reentry groups for students returning to school after receiving treatment for substance abuse

## Parent Approaches

A variety of parent approaches have been used in substance abuse prevention programs. Information programs strive to give parents basic information about drugs and the impact they have on health and society. Programs on parenting skills assist parents in learning and developing personal and interpersonal skills that may serve to prevent drug abuse in the family. For example, parents refine skills in communicating with children, decision making, setting goals and limits, and even how and when to say no to their children. These important skills can improve weak family relationships and poor family communication, which are often found in families where youth use drugs.

Parent support groups help parents to cope with drug problems in their homes and neighborhoods. Parents meet to gain mutual support by discussing problem solving, communication skills, parenting and child-management skills/strategies, and ways to take action against drug problems. These groups often provide supervision for young people's activities that are free of alcohol and other drugs.

Some of the most promising drug prevention programs are those in which parents, students, schools, and communities join together to send a firm, clear message that the use of alcohol and other drugs will not be tolerated. Parents should be encouraged to visit their children's school and learn how substance abuse education is being taught. Parents can evaluate substance abuse education programs by asking questions. Are the faculty members trained to teach about alcohol and other drug use? Is drug education a regular part of the curriculum or limited to a special week? Is it taught through the health class, or do all teachers incorporate drug education into their subject area? Do children in every grade receive drug education, or is it limited to selected grades? Is there a component for parents? Do drug education materials contain a clear message that alcohol and other drug use is wrong and harmful? Is the information accurate and up-to-date? Does the school have referral sources for students who need special help?

Parents can help their children to remain drug-free by supporting community efforts to give young people healthy alternatives. Alcohol- and drug-free proms and other school-based celebrations are growing in popularity around the country. Parents can help to organize such events, solicit contributions, and serve as chaperones.

## Principles of Effective Substance Abuse Prevention

Principles of effective substance abuse prevention are outlined in the National Institute on Drug Abuse publication *Preventing Drug Use Among Children and Adolescents: A Research-Based Guide.*[13] These principles are as follows:

1. Prevention programs should be designed to enhance protective factors and move toward reversing or reducing known risk factors.

2. Prevention programs should target all forms of drug abuse, including the use of tobacco, alcohol, marijuana, and inhalants.

3. Prevention programs should include skills to resist drugs when offered, strengthen personal commitments against drug use, and increase social competency (e.g., in communications, peer relationships, self-efficacy, assertiveness), in conjunction with reinforcement of attitudes against drug use.

4. Prevention programs for adolescents should include interactive methods, such as peer discussion groups, rather than didactic teaching techniques alone.

5. Prevention programs should include a component for parents or caregivers that reinforces what the children are learning—such as facts about drugs and their harmful effects—and that opens opportunities for family discussions about use of legal and illegal substances and family policies about their use.

6. Prevention programs should be long-term, over the school career, with repeat interventions to reinforce the original prevention goals. For example, school-based efforts directed at elementary and middle school students should include booster sessions to help with critical transitions from middle to high school.

7. Family-focused prevention efforts have a greater impact than strategies that focus on parents only or children only.

8. Community programs that include media campaigns and policy changes, such as new regulations that restrict access to alcohol, tobacco, or other drugs, are more effective when they are accompanied by school and family interventions.

9. Community programs need to strengthen norms against drug use in all drug abuse prevention settings, including the family, the school, and the community.

10. Schools offer opportunities to reach all populations and also serve as important settings for specific subpopulations at risk for drug abuse, such as children with behavior problems or learning disabilities, and those who are potential dropouts.

11. Prevention programming should be adapted to address the specific nature of the drug abuse problem in the local community. The higher the level of risk of the target population, the more intensive the prevention effort must be and the earlier it must begin.

12. Prevention programs should be age-specific, developmentally appropriate, and culturally sensitive.

## School-Based Programs That Work

The drug education that students receive in schools varies considerably from school district to school district. Drug education is sometimes delivered as early as kindergarten; in other districts, it may not be delivered until late elementary, middle school, or junior high. Sometimes drug education is designed to stand alone as a course, whereas sometimes it is integrated into a health education, family life, or life skills course. It may be taught by a school's own teachers or may be taught by outside personnel (e.g., police officers). Some school districts purchase drug education curricula from commercial vendors. Others develop their own curricula and materials.

The most widely used drug education program is DARE (Drug Abuse Resistance Education). DARE began in 1983 in Los Angeles and is found today in more than three-quarters of all school districts in the United States. The program is taught by police officers to students mainly in fifth or sixth grade. The effectiveness of this program was challenged by a study in the *Journal of Consulting and Clinical Psychology* showing that DARE not only did not affect adolescents' rate of experimentation with drugs, but may also have actually lowered their self-esteem.[14] The authors of this study suggested that one reason DARE may not be effective is because it emphasizes the role of peer pressure in drug use. Many young people may be motivated to use drugs by other factors, such as curiosity or thrill-seeking. Also, DARE may teach children drug resistance skills years before they need them. DARE has been criticized for asserting that drug abuse is more prevalent or normal than it is in reality. As a result of studies showing the ineffectiveness of DARE, cities such as Salt Lake, Seattle, Houston, and others have dropped the program. Also, changes have been made to the DARE curriculum to reach not only youth in the fifth grade but in seventh and ninth grade as well. There is also less reliance on lecturing to students and more emphasis on discussion groups. Further, the message is presented that not everyone uses drugs.

Only a handful of school drug prevention programs have been subjected to rigorous scientific evaluation and meet high standards for determining effectiveness. These programs are highlighted and described on the World Wide Web (http://www.preventionnet.com). The following are some of the programs highlighted on the website.

❖ *Project STAR (Students Taught Awareness & Resistance)*. This program consists of five components that are introduced in sequence to communities over a three- to five-year time period: school, parent, community organization, health policy, and mass media. These components focus on helping adolescents develop drug use resistance and counteraction skills, helping parents and other adults serve as role models for adolescents, and helping schools and communities promote and support social norms and expectations of nondrug use.

❖ *Adolescent Alcohol Prevention Trial (AAPT).* This classroom program is designed for fifth-grade students and is supported by booster sessions conducted in the seventh grade. Resistance skills training gives children the social and behavioral skills they need to refuse explicit drug offers. Normative education counteracts the influences of passive social pressures and social modeling effects. It corrects erroneous perceptions about the prevalence and acceptability of substance use and establishes conservative group norms.

❖ *Preparing for the Drug Free Years (PDFY).* This program helps reduce drug use and other delinquent behaviors by helping parents of children aged 9 to 13 years to create meaningful ways to interact with their families, strengthen family bonds, set clear expectations for their children's behavior, teach their children skills to resist peer pressure, reduce family conflict and control emotions, and practice consistent family management. The program is facilitated by two leaders, one of whom is a parent.

❖ *Life Skills Training.* This program was discussed earlier in this chapter. It focuses on the major social and psychological factors promoting substance use and abuse. It consists of 15 classes that can be implemented in the first year of middle school (usually the sixth grade) or the first year of junior high (usually the seventh grade). Life Skills Training is designed to provide students with the necessary skills to resist social (peer) pressures to smoke or drink; help them develop greater self-esteem, self-mastery, and self-confidence; enable children to effectively cope with social anxiety; and increase their knowledge of the immediate consequences of substance use. The program also includes a booster curriculum in the second and third years of middle or junior high. A new version of this program has been developed that can be taught to upper elementary school students.

## Substance Abuse Prevention Curricula

Substance abuse curricula must present a clear and consistent message that the use of alcohol, tobacco, and other illicit drugs is unhealthy and harmful. Curricula should be designed to promote healthy, safe, and responsible attitudes and behavior. It is critical that curricula be sensitive to the specific needs of the local school and community in terms of cultural appropriateness and local substance abuse problems. Developmental considerations should also be carefully taken into account when designing and organizing substance abuse curricula. Efforts to infuse prevention education into other curricular subjects can increase the amount of drug prevention education delivered to students. Box 6-2 provides some suggestions.

# Substance Abuse Prevention Activities

## Smoking Machine

Make a simple smoking machine as shown in the diagram. Place cotton balls in the jar to collect the tars. Have students take turns squeezing the ball to simulate taking a "drag" from a cigarette. Discuss the accumulation of tars in the body. Take care not to let tobacco smoke accumulate in the classroom or school; open windows or use fans when possible.    (P, I, J, H)

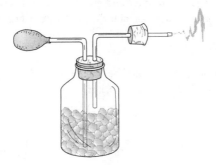

## Money up in Smoke

◆ Have students calculate the cost of smoking one pack of cigarettes every day for one year. Compare the cost to a stereo system or other items students would enjoy owning. Multiply the yearly cost of smoking by 5, 10, 15, and 20 years and determine what could be purchased with the same amounts of money.    (I, J, H)

◆ Calculate the additional cost smokers pay for car and home insurance, medical care, laundry, and home cleaning.    (I, J, H)

◆ Discuss the costs of smoking to all Americans in terms of medical care, lost work productivity, and loss of lives.    (I, J, H)

## Government and Tobacco

◆ Have students research and report on U.S. legislation and aid to support the tobacco industry.    (J, H)

◆ Have students check on passive smoking laws. Assign students to interview employees in public buildings and other work environments affected by the legislation.    (J, H)

*continued*

*continued*

◆ Have students research and report on the results of state lawsuits against tobacco companies in the past decade.

### Clean Up

Initiate a school clean-up campaign and log the effects of smoking on the property and facilities.　(J, H)

### Reward

Design awards, badges, or plaques and give them to tobacco users (students and adults) who have reduced or quit their tobacco habits.　(P, I, J, H)

### White Line

Have students walk a white chalk line and discuss, "Would you want to ride with a driver who couldn't do it?"　(I, J, H)

### Guest Speakers

◆ Have a representative from MADD, Mothers Against Drunk Driving, speak to your class about the organization and the problem of drinking and driving.　(J, H)
◆ Have a representative from a detoxification unit speak about available services and experiences in treating alcoholics.　(H)
◆ Have a highway patrol officer talk to your class about the effect of alcohol on drivers and others.　(J, H)

### SADD

Have students organize their own chapter of Students Against Drunk Driving.　(H)

### TV Observation

Assign students to count the number of alcoholic beverages consumed by television characters during a certain time period.　(P, I, J, H)

### Math

Have students calculate how many drinks it would take individuals of various weights to become legally drunk. Discuss the role of food in the stomach, alcoholic content of beverages, and other factors in blood alcohol levels.　(I, J, H)

*continued*

## Meetings

Have students attend and report on Alcoholics Anonymous, Al-Anon, or Alateen meetings. (H)

## Warning Labels

Have students design warning labels about fetal alcohol syndrome to place on all alcoholic beverages. (I, J, H)

## Recipes

Have students collect recipes for nonalcoholic beverages. Prepare and try some of the recipes in class. (I, J, H)

## Skit

Write a skit in which each student plays the part of a different body organ and expresses how tobacco, alcohol, or other drugs affects it. (I, J, H)

## Posters

Have students design and make antitobacco, antidrug, or antidrinking-and-driving posters. Encourage parental involvement. Hang the posters around the school and have students vote on the top three. Award the creators of the top three posters. (P, I, J, H)

## Bulletin Boards

◆ Create or have students create a bulletin board illustrating the short-term and long-term effects associated with tobacco, alcohol, or other drug use. (P, I, J, H)
◆ Create or have students create a bulletin board illustrating how drug abuse (tobacco, alcohol, and others) affects family life, social life, school-work, and the economy. (P, I, J, H)
◆ Illustrate alcohol's cost to society in terms of fatalities, medical costs, job absenteeism, job loss, decreased productivity, and family life. (I, J, H)
◆ Illustrate the short- and long-term effects of alcohol on the body. (P, I, J, H)

*continued*

*continued*

## Commercials

Review common advertising appeals and have students use these strategies to write commercials against tobacco, alcohol, and other drug use.   (P, I, J, H)

## Ad Deconstruction

Have students deconstruct tobacco and alcohol ads they view on TV, in magazines, or on billboards. For each ad, have students identify:

1.  Who the target audience is
2.  What the "hooks" are (techniques used to get attention and create appeal
3.  What emotional associations are made (happiness, maturity, sex, body image, success, security, independence, power, adventure, escape, romance, love and belonging, etc.)
4.  What messages are conveyed overtly and subtly
5.  The types of models or actors used and why they were selected
6.  The behaviors the ad tries to create or shape
7.  Important facts that were omitted
8.  The estimated number of people the ad reached and an estimate of the average number of exposures per person (frequency)
9.  Minute details that were choreographed into the ad showing that a great deal of time and money went into the ad's construction

## PSA

Have students write and record a Public Service Announcement for radio about the dangers of drinking and driving. Have them submit announcements to local radio stations.   (I, J, H)

## Bumper Stickers

Have students create bumper stickers with strong messages against tobacco, alcohol, or other drug use.   (I, J, H)

## Letters

Have students write a letter to a hypothetical friend to persuade him or her to stop smoking or obtain help in overcoming a drug abuse problem.   (I, J, H)

## Demonstration

Display three white mixtures (e.g., laundry detergents, salt, sugars, rat poisons, baking powder, soda) and ask the students which they want. Discuss how drugs are cut and that a person buying drugs on the street doesn't know what he or she is getting.   (I, J, H)

## Developmental Considerations

*Grades K–3*   The knowledge gained in grades K–3 should be the foundation for all future substance abuse prevention education. Much of the early health education experience for children should emphasize wellness. **Wellness** is an approach that stresses the positive physical, social, and emotional benefits of being healthy and acting safely. Wellness is a key concept in developing young children's determination to avoid drugs. At this age children should also begin to develop a sense of responsibility toward themselves and others, including the responsibility to tell adults if something is wrong.

Substance abuse prevention education for this age group should discuss alcohol, tobacco, marijuana, cocaine, Ecstasy, and methamphetamine. Children should also be introduced to the dangers of inhalants because inhalant abuse may be one of the first forms of drug abuse with which children experiment. A special effort should be made to counter the myths that marijuana and other substances are not harmful. K–3 students should learn how to identify a responsible adult through homework assignments involving parents and through classroom presentations by police officers, school nurses, doctors, clergy, and human service professionals. Parents can participate in homework assignments by identifying family rules for behavior, conducting safety checks, and helping with class assignments. Having parents sign homework assignments is a good way to involve them and keep them informed of what is going on in class.

At the early elementary level, instruction may include both formal curricula and other types of classroom activity, including songs and skits and the use of character props such as puppets, cartoon characters, and clowns. These are particularly useful for relaying messages about safety, personal health, and dangerous substances. Skits enable children to practice resistance skills by acting out scenarios in which they encounter dangerous substances or situations. Songs encapsulate important information in an easily remembered form. Some packaged curricula incorporate standardized songs and skits; teachers often enjoy creating their own.

*Grades 4–6*   In grades 4–6, peer influences continue to grow. Because of an expanding world of friends and experiences, older elementary school children have a particular need to deal with increased pressures. Some in this age group may experiment with tobacco, alcohol, and other drugs. Therefore, they need more information, more analysis of why people use drugs, stronger motivation to avoid drugs, and specific skills for avoiding drug use. In particular, children in the upper elementary grades need specific strategies for resisting pressures.

Curricula at these grade levels should emphasize personal safety. Children in grades 4–6 have more freedom than younger children, may travel alone to and from school and other local destinations, and may be left alone part of the day. Personal safety lessons can include using the "buddy" system of always traveling in groups or at least in pairs, why to avoid certain routes, how to get help (such as through the local emergency telephone number), and how to answer the telephone or door.

It is important to help children understand rules and laws at this age level. They should learn about society's interest in protecting people from dangerous substances and behavior. They need to understand that they have certain rights—the right to be safe, to learn, and to say no. Along with these rights come duties and responsibilities.

Within the classroom, students in the upper elementary grades benefit from hands-on learning experiences. Students can build models to illustrate health lessons, such as showing how drugs affect the circulatory or respiratory system. Teachers can assign independent research projects that promote critical thinking about substance use. Students can prepare class projects that reflect real-life events, such as mock television interviews or press conferences. These are just a few examples of hands-on learning experiences. Can you think of others?

***Middle and Junior High School (Grades 7–9)***   The onset of adolescence creates new challenges for substance abuse prevention. The natural desire for peer acceptance may become a significant cause of anxiety and concern for the adolescent. As a result, the influence of peer pressure to use drugs may become intense. The desire to appear mature and independent rapidly emerges during the middle/junior high school years. Access to tobacco, alcohol, and other drugs is often relatively easy for many in this age group. Also, changing bodies and developing minds are very vulnerable to the damaging effects of psychoactive substances.

Adolescents often possess a sense of personal invulnerability ("It can't happen to me"), together with a great insecurity about personal attractiveness and social responsibility. For these reasons, emphasizing that alcohol, tobacco, and other drug use can immediately affect their appearance, coordination, thinking, and behavior can be an effective teaching strategy. Nothing gets the attention of junior high school students like knowing that they may look ridiculous, may smell bad, may not be capable of playing sports, may become unattractive, or may not develop physically and sexually. Suggestions that drugs can impair one's chances of getting into college and succeeding in a career begin to have a powerful impact at this age. And, particularly in view of the many other strains on today's families, young teenagers are likely to pay close attention to discussions of how drug use impairs family relationships.

Most adolescents understand that they are gradually gaining freedom; they should also understand that this means greater accountability for their actions. Accordingly, at this grade level, curricula should emphasize personal responsibility, awareness of the law, and penalties for law-breaking. As students begin dating, contemplate college and career, and anticipate a driver's license and other aspects of adulthood, the time is right for introducing training for adult responsibilities.

Because middle and junior high school students will probably be exposed to people who use drugs and who pressure them to do so, they need to be familiar with support resources. The curriculum should make students aware of what these services are and how they function. Students should learn that they are not responsible for creating or curing another's problem, but that there are responsible adults and services to which it is proper to turn to for help.

Middle and junior high school students often become involved in school-sponsored social events and activities. The organization and supervision of these activities (such as bands, athletics, clubs, and student organizations) should focus on making and keeping them drug-free. Students at this age also benefit from field trips, guest presentations, and research assignments. For example, students in these grades might visit a hospital, might hear presentations from personnel working with drug addicts, and might cooperate on developing classwide research projects involving different media.

**High School (Grades 10–12)**   Students in these grades are beginning the transition to adulthood, and it can be a confusing time for them. Even though they are obtaining licenses to drive and preparing for work and postsecondary education, most high-schoolers are still minors under the law. Alcohol and other drugs are illegal for them. Substance abuse prevention education faces the challenge of motivating these students to continue resisting illicit substances, and of helping them behave responsibly as they prepare to assume new roles in society.

Students in high school are in the process of establishing themselves in the world. Thus, it is essential that the lessons of substance abuse prevention education carry over into students' lives outside of class. Among the aspects of increasing responsibility that should be stressed are the importance of serving as positive role models for younger children, realizing one's responsibility in the workplace, and understanding how substance abuse affects personal growth and professional success.

Some curricula use high school students as peer leaders. Peer leaders make presentations to students in lower grades and serve as "buddies" to younger children. Peer leadership can be very effective in motivating older students. However, peer leaders need close supervision and monitoring by teachers and school personnel. Student leaders should be drug-free and well trained. They should be trained to refer any problems to teachers or other school officials. Properly supervised, peer leaders can help maintain communication and reduce the likelihood of tragedy during a critical period in students' lives.

**Special Education Students**   Physically and mentally, special education students may be more susceptible to pressure to use drugs than other children. They are vulnerable to exploitation, may have low self-esteem, and may feel an intense need for acceptance. For these reasons, they may not understand the risk without careful instruction. It is incumbent upon school personnel to teach them sound prevention principles and to make sure that they get their full share of prevention education.

Educators also need to recognize that many physically and mentally impaired students must rely upon medicines to treat their health conditions. They are psychologically sensitive to implications that there is something wrong with them because they rely on medication. They may also be very sensitive to substance abuse prevention education when their impairment is the product of, or is affected by, their parents' use of dangerous drugs.

## High-Risk Students

**High-risk students** are those who are at high risk of becoming a substance user or who are already abusing drugs. High-risk students include students who:

1. Drop out of school or suffer academic failure

2. Become pregnant

3. Are economically disadvantaged

4. Are children of an alcohol or other drug abuser

5. Are victims of physical, sexual, or psychological abuse

6. Have committed violent or delinquent acts

7. Have attempted suicide

8. Have substance-abusing friends

Curricula for high-risk students should present drug education early and in a form appropriate for a child's age and experience. Resistance training and lesson plans should pay attention to the total environment in which such children live. If they have not begun using drugs, prevention-oriented education can be useful. Recovering users can also benefit from a positively presented message about drug-free lifestyles. Children who are using drugs, recovering, or dealing with the addictions of family members and friends need to learn and be constantly reminded that addiction does not end when formal treatment ends; addiction cannot be cured, but can effectively be treated and controlled.

Both children who are recovering and those who are subjected to high-risk environments need support services outside the curriculum. **Support groups** are an effective method of in-school or out-of-school assistance for students and staff. These are confidential discussion and counseling sessions led by professionals or trained volunteers. Nonusers may find such groups helpful in dealing with friends who use drugs, and with home problems such as the addictions of parents or siblings. For recovering users, support groups can reinforce their determination to stay off drugs, while helping fulfill the terms of their conditional reentry to school.

## Infusion of Substance Abuse Prevention Education into the Curriculum

Schools often have limited time for prevention education in the curriculum. One solution to this problem is to infuse substance abuse prevention into other curricular subjects. Substance abuse prevention education can be integrated into virtually every other subject in the curriculum. For example:

❖ *Math* classes can use statistics to describe the financial and human costs of substance abuse.

❖ *Science* classes can explore the chemical characteristics and physiological effects of specific drugs.

❖ *Visual arts* and *English* classes can discuss media pressures and advertising techniques and explore ways to resist these pressures.

❖ *Social studies* classes can discuss the effects of substance abuse on society and individuals.

❖ *Physical education* classes and coaches can discuss the effects of anabolic steroids.

## Substance Abuse Problems

### Tobacco Use*

Most cigarette smokers begin smoking during their teen years. In fact, 80% of adult smokers started smoking before the age of 18. Every day of the year, more than 3,000 young people become regular smokers in the United States (see Figure 6-1). At least 4.5 million adolescents (age 12–17 years) in the United States smoke cigarettes. A substantial proportion of these young people will die of a smoking-related disease. More than 6.4 million children living today will die prematurely because of their decision as children or teenagers to smoke cigarettes.

*Nicotine*  When a person inhales cigarette smoke, the **nicotine** in the smoke is rapidly absorbed into the blood and starts affecting the brain within seven seconds. In the brain, nicotine activates the same reward

---

* Unless otherwise noted, the facts and statistics cited in this section are from the CDC's Tobacco Information and Prevention Source website (http://www.cdc.gov/ tobacco).

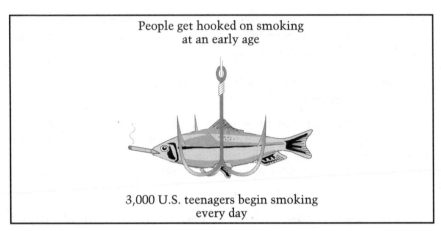

People get hooked on smoking
at an early age

3,000 U.S. teenagers begin smoking
every day

**FIGURE 6-1    Early onset of smoking**

system as do other drugs of abuse, such as cocaine or amphetamine, although to a lesser degree. Nicotine's action on this reward system is believed to be responsible for drug-induced feelings of pleasure and, over time, addiction. Nicotine also has the effect of increasing alertness and enhancing mental performance. In the cardiovascular system, nicotine increases heart rate and blood pressure and restricts blood flow to the heart muscle. The drug stimulates the release of the hormone epinephrine, which further stimulates the nervous system and is responsible for part of the "kick" from nicotine. It also promotes the release of the hormone beta-endorphin, which inhibits pain.

People addicted to nicotine experience withdrawal when they stop smoking. This withdrawal involves symptoms such as anger, anxiety, depressed mood, difficulty concentrating, increased appetite, and craving for nicotine. Most of these symptoms subside within three to four weeks, except for the craving and hunger, which may persist for months.

***Health Consequences of Smoking***   More than 440,000 people die in the United States each year as the result of cigarette smoking, making smoking the single most preventable cause of death (see Figure 6-2). This is more than 1,200 deaths per day (see Figure 6-3). Cigarette smoking kills more people than AIDS, alcohol abuse, illegal drug abuse, car crashes, murders, suicides, and fires—combined (see Figure 6-4). The smoking of cigarettes results in more than 6 million years of potential life lost each year .

Health studies have clearly documented that smoking cigarettes causes heart disease, lung and esophageal cancer, and chronic lung disease. Cigarette smoking contributes to cancer of the bladder, pancreas, and kidney. Studies have also demonstrated that women who use tobacco during

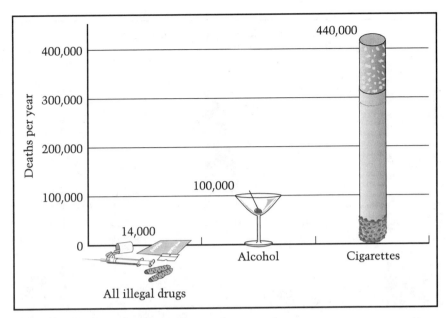

**FIGURE 6-2    Deaths per year from substance abuse**

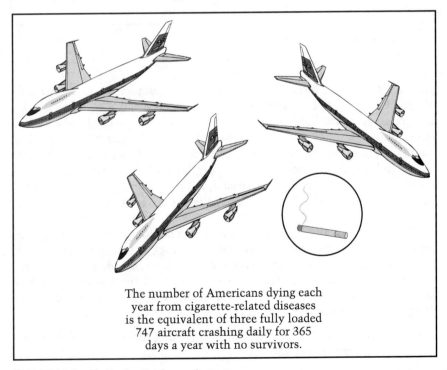

The number of Americans dying each
year from cigarette-related diseases
is the equivalent of three fully loaded
747 aircraft crashing daily for 365
days a year with no survivors.

**FIGURE 6-3    Daily deaths from cigarettes**

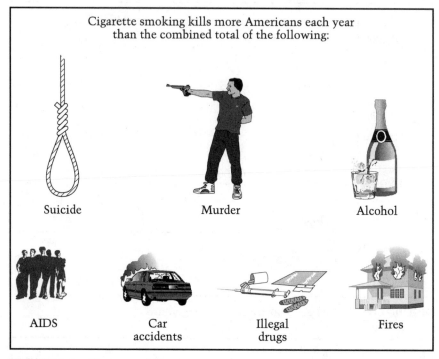

Cigarette smoking kills more Americans each year
than the combined total of the following:

Suicide          Murder          Alcohol

AIDS          Car          Illegal          Fires
             accidents      drugs

**FIGURE 6-4    Cigarettes kill . . .**

pregnancy are more likely to have adverse birth outcomes, including low-birthweight babies. Low birthweight is a leading cause of death among infants. Studies also indicate that nonsmokers are adversely affected by environmental tobacco smoke. Researchers have identified more than 4,000 chemical compounds in tobacco smoke; of these, at least 43 cause cancer in humans and animals. Each year, because of exposure to environmental tobacco smoke, an estimated 3,000 nonsmoking Americans die of lung cancer, and 300,000 children suffer from lower respiratory tract infections.

In addition to the long-term consequences of cigarette smoking (e.g., lung cancer, emphysema, coronary heart disease), smoking has short-term consequences for young people who smoke. These include respiratory and nonrespiratory effects, addiction to nicotine, and the associated risk of other drug use. Health effects of cigarette smoking for young people include the following consequences:

❖ Cigarette smokers have a lower level of lung function than those persons who have never smoked.

❖ Smoking reduces the rate of lung growth.

❖ Studies have shown early signs of heart disease and stroke in adolescents who smoke.

❖ Smoking affects young people's physical fitness, both performance and endurance, even among young people trained in competitive running.

❖ On average, someone who smokes a pack or more of cigarettes each day lives seven years less than someone who never smoked.

❖ The resting heart rates of young adult smokers are two to three beats per minute faster than nonsmokers.

❖ Among young people, regular smoking is responsible for coughs and increased frequency and severity of respiratory illnesses.

❖ The younger people start smoking cigarettes, the more likely they are to become strongly addicted to nicotine.

❖ Teens who smoke are 3 times more likely than nonsmokers to use alcohol, 8 times more likely to use marijuana, and 22 times more likely to use cocaine, and also are at increased risk of engaging in other risky behaviors, such as fighting and engaging in unprotected sex.

❖ Smoking is associated with poor overall health and a variety of short-term adverse health effects in young people and may also be a marker for underlying mental health problems, such as depression, among adolescents.

❖ Smoking at an early age increases the risk of lung cancer—for most smoking-related cancers, the risk rises as the individual continues to smoke.

❖ Teenage smokers suffer from shortness of breath almost three times as often as teens who don't smoke, and produce phlegm more than twice as often as teens who don't smoke.

❖ Teenage smokers are more likely to have seen a doctor or other health professionals for an emotional or psychological complaint.

***Cigarette and Cigar Smoking in Youth***     Results from the 2000 National Youth Tobacco Survey showed that 28.0% of high school students and 11.0% of middle school students reported smoking cigarettes in the past 30 days. Approximately one-half of current smokers in middle and high school reported that they usually smoke Marlboro cigarettes. African-American students are more likely to smoke Newport cigarettes than any other brand.[15]

Cigar use (in the past 30 days) was reported by 22.0% of high school boys and 7.3% of high school girls. Among high school students, the use of bidis and kreteks in the past 30 days was 4.1% and 4.2%, respectively.[15] **Bidis** are thin, unfiltered cigarettes produced in India that are wrapped in brown leaves and tied with a short length of thread. They come in different flavors, including strawberry, chocolate, almond, and root beer. They are sold in tobacco specialty stores, and frequently in health food stores as well. Although some people claim that bidis are a safe alternative to regular cigarettes, this is not true. Bidi smoke contains higher levels of carbon monoxide, nicotine, and tar than cigarette smoke. The fact that bidis are filterless means that more of the cancer-causing agent, tar, goes directly to the smoker's system. **Kreteks** are clove cigarettes that are sometime mistaken for bidis. They are made in Indonesia and contain tobacco and clove. The clove deadens sensation in the lungs, making it easier to inhale smoke deep into the lungs.

***Cigarette Smoking and Girls***    The U.S. surgeon general's report *Women and Smoking*, released in 2001, declared that the United States is in the midst of a "full-blown epidemic" of smoking-related disease in women.[16] Smoking has long been the leading cause of preventable death and disease among women. And, according to recent surveys, many women do not realize that lung cancer, once rare among women, surpassed breast cancer in the late 1980s as the leading cause of female cancer death. Cigarette smoking—once thought of as an almost exclusively male behavior—is now nearly as high among women as men (22% of women smoke, compared with 26% percent of men). Almost as many teenage girls smoke as teenage boys (32.8% of high school senior boys and 29.7% of high school senior girls report having smoked within the past 30 days). More than 22 million adult women and at least 1.5 million adolescent girls in the United States currently smoke cigarettes. As a result, smoking-related diseases cause the premature death of approximately 165,000 American women per year.

Cigarette smoking poses additional health risks to women besides lung cancer. Women who smoke or who live with a smoker face unique health effects related to reproductive health, including problems related to pregnancy, oral contraceptive use, menstrual function, and cancers of the cervix and bladder. There is also evidence that women who smoke have increased risks for liver and colorectal cancer and for cancers of the pancreas and kidney. In addition to causing lung and other cancers, lung disease, coronary heart disease, and stroke and increasing risk for osteoporosis, smoking affects a female's appearance. Long-term smoking causes the skin to age prematurely and lose its elasticity, the nails and teeth to turn yellow, and the breath to smell foul.

Females might be more susceptible to the addictive properties of nicotine and might clear nicotine at a slower rate from their bodies than males. In addition, females seem to be more susceptible to the effects of tobacco carcinogens than men.

Young females needed to be alerted to the facts that smoking can impair fertility and the production and implantation of ova and can contribute to early pregnancy loss. Further, smoking appears to cause irregular menstrual cycles and increased menstrual discomfort. Women who smoke also have an earlier menopause, which may increase their risk of osteoporosis, heart disease, and other conditions for which estrogen provides a protective effect. Cigarette smoking also increases the risk of pregnancy complications. Women who smoke are more likely to experience bleeding and to have low-birthweight babies. The risk of sudden infant death syndrome (SIDS) is also increased when a female smokes. Females who smoke and who have children put them at risk of serious health problems. Children exposed to their mother's secondhand smoke have more frequent infections, including colds and flu, ear infections, and lower respiratory infections such as bronchitis and pneumonia. Secondhand smoke has been shown to cause new cases of asthma, as well as to make existing cases of asthma worse.

*Smokeless Tobacco Use*    The use of **chewing tobacco** and **snuff** delivers nicotine to the central nervous system. Although nicotine is absorbed more slowly through the mouth than the lungs, the blood nicotine levels of smokeless tobacco users are similar to those of cigarette smokers. Like cigarette smoking, smokeless tobacco use can lead to dependency on nicotine and result in withdrawal symptoms. Nicotine is a psychoactive substance that causes changes in mood and feeling and can produce **euphoria** or exaggerated feelings of well-being. Therefore, smokeless tobacco products, like cigarettes, are addictive substances.

The fact that smokeless tobacco products can be addicting is of great concern because of the high prevalence of use among young people, particularly males. In some parts of the United States, 25% to 40% of adolescent males have reported current use of smokeless tobacco. Student athletes are at high risk of smokeless tobacco use.

Smokeless tobacco users are more likely than nonusing youth to have family members who use smokeless tobacco and are not as likely to encounter parental disapproval of the practice. Use by friends and among peers is an important influence on a young person's decision to chew tobacco or use snuff. In fact, pressure from peers is cited by young smokeless tobacco users as the primary reason for initiating use. However, continuation of use is most often attributed to enjoyment of the taste and "being hooked." The use and portrayal of use by role models (particularly professional athletes) is also a powerful influence.

Some youth and adults believe that smokeless tobacco is a safe alternative to smoking cigarettes because it is not likely to cause lung cancer. However, chewing tobacco and snuff contain potent carcinogens that have been shown to cause cancer in animals. These carcinogens include nitrosamines (at levels 100 times higher than at the regulated levels found in beer, bacon, and other foods), polycyclic aromatic hydrocarbons, and radiation-emitting polonium. Oral cancers occur several times more frequently in smokeless tobacco users than nonusers.

An inspection inside a snuff dipper's or tobacco chewer's mouth often reveals an abnormally thickened, wrinkled, and whitish patch of tissue. These **oral leukoplakias** occur at the site where the tobacco is held in the mouth as a result of direct irritation and contact with tobacco juice. Some leukoplakias transform into precancerous and cancerous lesions in the mouth, throat, esophagus, or on the tongue or lip.

Smokeless tobacco use can lead to serious dental problems because the gums tend to recede from the teeth in areas near where the tobacco is held in the mouth. The bare roots are then more susceptible to decay and more sensitive to cold, heat, air, certain foods, and chemicals. Smokeless tobacco contains sugar, which can increase tooth decay. Abrasion of the enamel of teeth, as well as staining of teeth, may occur as a result of tobacco use. Bad breath is another problem of chewing and "dipping."

The Smokeless Tobacco Education Act of 1986 banned radio and television advertisement of smokeless tobacco products. However, manufacturers of smokeless tobacco products have rebounded by fully using the print media, billboards, and promotions. Advertisements typically appear in outdoor and sports magazines. Also, tobacco companies sponsor sporting events and display their logos so that they receive television coverage. Free samples and other promotional items (e.g., T-shirts, hats, visors) are also widely distributed.

As a result of the Smokeless Tobacco Education Act of 1986, manufacturers of chewing tobacco and snuff are required to include warning labels on the packages of their products. These warnings are as follows:

❖ This product may cause mouth cancer.

❖ This product may cause gum disease and tooth loss.

❖ This product is not a safe alternative to cigarettes.

***Tobacco Use Prevention and Cessation Programs in Schools***    Rising cigarette smoking rates and the dangerous effects of smoking underscore the need to have aggressive tobacco prevention programs beginning in elementary school and continuing through high school. A useful guide for schools planning tobacco use prevention programs is "Guidelines for School Health Programs to Prevent Tobacco Use and Addiction," published by the Centers for Disease Control and Prevention.[17] This publication advocates that schools provide instruction about the short- and long-term negative physiologic and social consequences of tobacco use, social influences on tobacco use, peer norms regarding tobacco use, and refusal skills. These educational strategies are important because many tobacco use prevention programs have been limited to providing only factual information about the harmful effects of tobacco use. Other educational strategies used in schools attempt to induce fear in young persons about the consequences of use. However, these strategies alone do not prevent tobacco use, may stimulate curiosity about tobacco use, and may prompt some students to believe that the health hazards of tobacco use are exaggerated.

Successful programs to prevent tobacco use (as well as other substance abuse problems) address multiple psychosocial factors related to tobacco use among children and adolescents. The psychosocial factors that need to be addressed include the following:

❖ *Immediate and long-term undesirable physiologic, cosmetic, and social consequences.* Educators should help students understand that tobacco use can result in decreased stamina, stained teeth, foul-smelling breath and clothes, exacerbation of asthma, and ostracism by nonsmoking peers.

❖ *Social norms regarding tobacco use.* Educators should use a variety of educational techniques to decrease the social acceptability of tobacco use, highlight existing antitobacco norms, and help students understand that most adolescents do not smoke.

❖ *Reasons that adolescents say they smoke.* Educators should help students understand that some adolescents smoke because they believe it will help them be accepted by peers, appear mature, or cope with stress. Educators should help students develop other more positive means to attain such goals.

❖ *Social influences that promote tobacco use.* Educators should help students develop skills in recognizing and refuting tobacco-promotion messages from the media, adults, and peers.

❖ *Behavioral skills for resisting social influences that promote tobacco use.* Educators should help students develop refusal skills through direct instruction, modeling, rehearsal, and reinforcement, and should coach them to help others develop these skills.

❖ *General and personal skills.* Educators should help students develop necessary assertiveness, communication, goal-setting, and problem-solving skills that may enable them to avoid both tobacco use and other health-risky behaviors.

Schools should address these psychosocial factors at developmentally appropriate ages. Particular instructional concepts should be provided for students in early elementary school, junior high or middle school, and senior high school.

Successful tobacco use prevention programs develop and enforce a school policy on tobacco use. A school policy on tobacco use must be consistent with state and local laws. Further, the CDC recommends that a policy should include the following elements:

❖ An explanation of the rationale for preventing tobacco use (e.g., tobacco is the leading cause of death, disease, and disability)

❖ Prohibitions against tobacco use by students, all school staff, parents, visitors on school property, in school vehicles, and at school-sponsored functions away from school property

❖ Prohibitions against tobacco advertising in school buildings, at school functions, and in school publications

❖ A requirement that all students receive instruction on avoiding tobacco use

❖ Provisions for students and all school staff to have access to programs to help them quit using tobacco

❖ Procedures for communicating the policy to students, school staff, parents or families, visitors, and the community

❖ Provisions for enforcing the policy

To ensure broad support for school policies on tobacco use, representatives of relevant groups, such as students, parents, school staff, and school board members, should participate in developing and implementing the policy. Clearly articulated policies, applied fairly and consistently, can help students decide not to use tobacco. Policies that prohibit tobacco use on school property, require prevention education, and provide access to cessation programs rather than solely instituting punitive measures are most effective in reducing tobacco use among students.

A tobacco-free school environment can provide health, social, and economic benefits for students, staff, the school, and the district. These benefits include decreased fires and discipline problems related to student smoking, improved compliance with local and state smoking ordinances, and easier upkeep and maintenance of school facilities and grounds.

"Guidelines for School Health Programs to Prevent Tobacco Use and Addiction" stresses that schools should support cessation efforts among students and all school staff who use tobacco. Services to help children and adolescents using tobacco are rarely available within a school system or community. However, this is an important need, especially when tobacco use is disallowed by school policy.

Effective cessation programs for adolescents focus on immediate consequences of tobacco use, have specified attainable goals, and use contracts that include rewards. The programs provide social support and teach avoidance, stress management, and refusal skills. Further, students need opportunities to practice skills and strategies that will help them remain nonusers. Cessation programs with these characteristics may already be available in the community through the local health department or voluntary health agency (e.g., American Cancer Society, American Heart Association, American Lung Association). Schools should identify available resources in the community and provide referral and follow-up services to students. If cessation programs for youth are not available, such programs may be jointly sponsored by the school and the local health department, voluntary health agency or other community health providers, or interested organizations (e.g., churches or civic clubs).

More is known about successful cessation strategies for adults. School staff members are more likely than students to find existing cessation options in the community. Most adults who quit tobacco use do so without formal assistance. Nevertheless, cessation programs that include a combination of behavioral approaches (e.g., group support, individual counseling, skills training, family interventions, and interventions that can be supplemented with pharmacologic treatments) have demonstrated effectiveness. For all school staff, health promotion activities and employee assistance programs that include cessation programs might help reduce burnout, lower staff absenteeism, decrease health insurance premiums, and increase commitment to overall school health goals.

Sometimes medications may assist smokers in efforts to quit tobacco use. The primary medication therapy currently used to treat nicotine addiction is nicotine replacement therapy, which supplies enough nicotine to the body to prevent withdrawal symptoms but not enough to provide the quick jolt caused by inhaling a cigarette. Four types of nicotine replacement products are currently available. Nicotine gum and nicotine skin patches are available over the counter. Nicotine nasal spray and nicotine inhalers are available by prescription. On average, all types of nicotine replacement products are about equally effective, roughly doubling the chances of successfully quitting.[13]

Another medication approved by the Food and Drug Administration as an aid for quitting smoking is the antidepressant bupropion, or Zyban. The association between nicotine addiction and depression is not yet understood, but nicotine appears to have an antidepressant effect in some smokers. Paradoxically, though, buproprion is more effective for treating nicotine addiction in nondepressed smokers than in smokers who are depressed.[13]

## Alcohol

Alcohol is a central nervous system depressant. Alcohol hinders coordination, slows reaction time, dulls senses, and blocks memory functions. It affects virtually every organ in the body, and chronic use can lead to numerous preventable consequences, including serious injuries, alcoholism, and chronic disease. Heavy drinking can increase the risk for certain cancers, especially those of the liver, esophagus, throat, and larynx (voice box). It can also cause liver cirrhosis, immune system problems, brain damage, and harm to the fetus during pregnancy. In addition, drinking increases the risk of death from automobile crashes, recreational accidents, and on-the-job accidents, and increases the likelihood of homicide and suicide (see Figure 6-5).

Although it is illegal for anyone under the age of 21 to purchase, possess, and consume alcohol, many young people do drink. In addition to breaking the law, young people are particularly vulnerable to the various problems that alcohol can cause. Among young people, alcohol use is linked to troubles with law enforcement authorities and academics, property destruction, physical fighting, and a host of other problems. Alcohol lowers inhibitions and impairs judgment, which can lead to risky behaviors, including practicing unprotected sex. This can lead to acquiring HIV/AIDS as well as other sexually transmitted diseases and unwanted pregnancy. Driving ability is seriously hampered when combined with alcohol use. Approximately 40% of motor vehicle fatalities among teenagers are alcohol related. Many drownings and other injuries among young people are also alcohol related. Alcohol abuse is responsible for more than 100,000 deaths in the United States each year.[18]

Results from the 1999 Youth Risk Behavior Survey show that a large proportion of high school students are at risk of alcohol-related injuries and consequences. One-third of high school students (33.1%) nationwide report riding one or more times with a driver who had been drinking alcohol

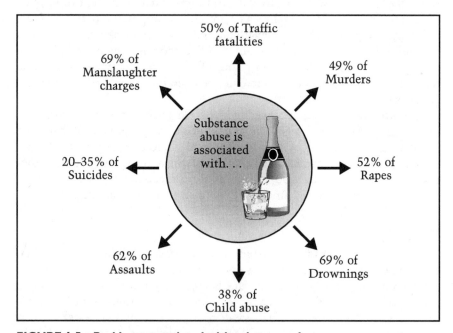

**FIGURE 6-5    Problems associated with substance abuse**

in the past month. Seventeen percent of male and 8.7% of female high school students reported that they drove a vehicle one or more times after drinking alcohol in the past month. One-fourth of students who were currently sexually active said that they had used alcohol or other drugs at last sexual intercourse.

Eighty-one percent of high school students have had at least one drink of alcohol during their lifetime, and 50.0% have drunk alcohol in the past month. Thirty percent of students have had five or more drinks of alcohol (episodic heavy drinking) on at least one occasion in the past month. Overall, male students (34.9%) were more likely than female students (28.1%) to report episodic heavy drinking.

*Alcoholism*   **Alcoholism** is best explained as a complex, progressive disease. It involves a progressive preoccupation with drinking that leads to physical, mental, social, and/or economic dysfunction. The complexity of alcoholism is due to various causes and factors—genetic, psychologic, familial, and social—many of which are not clearly understood. Alcoholism usually has the following characteristics:

❖ *Craving:* A strong need, or compulsion, to drink

❖ *Loss of control:* The frequent inability to stop drinking once a person has begun

❖ *Physical dependence:* The occurrence of withdrawal symptoms, such as nausea, sweating, shakiness, and anxiety, when alcohol use is stopped after a period of heavy drinking (these symptoms are usually relieved by drinking alcohol or by taking another sedative drug)

❖ *Tolerance:* The need for increasing amounts of alcohol in order to get "high"

Adolescents, in comparison to adults, appear to be more susceptible or vulnerable to alcoholism. The disease of alcoholism shows a more accelerated progression in adolescents than that observed in adults. By the time parents, health providers, or school personnel become aware of the problem, an adolescent may have a serious drinking problem.

**Signs and Symptoms of Youth Alcoholism and Problem Drinking**
Increases in youth alcoholism and problem drinking may be due partly to the following factors:

❖ Easy availability of alcoholic beverages

❖ Alcohol advertisements on television and in print media

❖ Exposure to parental and adult problem drinkers

❖ Toleration by parents of drinking and drunkenness

❖ Growing use of alcohol to cope with the pressures and conflicts of adolescence

❖ Cultural ambivalence about alcohol and drugs

❖ Few strict controls for the social use of alcohol or against the abuse of alcohol

It is important for educators to be aware of the signs and symptoms of youth alcoholism, which include:

❖ The tendency to drink in secret or to hide one's level of consumption

❖ Guilt about drinking

❖ Drinking in response to worry, depression, tiredness, and so forth

❖ Increasing tolerance to alcohol (need to increase consumption to achieve desired effect)

❖ Alcoholic blackouts (periods of alcohol-induced amnesia)

❖ Increasing the frequency and amount of drinking

❖ Continuance of drinking after others have stopped

❖ Lying about one's drinking

❖ Preoccupation with procuring and maintaining a supply of alcohol

❖ Gulping drinks

❖ Early-morning drinking

❖ Early-morning tremors

❖ Difficulty managing money

❖ Changes in eating behavior

❖ Withdrawal symptoms when efforts are made to stop drinking (these include restlessness, tremors, insomnia, depression, mental confusion, and in severe cases hallucinations and convulsions)

In addition to these warning signs of alcoholism, young alcoholics often demonstrate indirectly related behaviors that are observable by teachers and parents, such as:

❖ Impulsive behavior

❖ Lying to teachers and parents

❖ Declining grades

❖ Sudden decrease in handwriting skills

❖ Absences from and tardiness to school

❖ Decreased attention span

❖ Inability to cope with frustration

❖ Change from one peer group to another

❖ Irritability with others

❖ Suspiciousness of others

❖ Rebelliousness

❖ Difficulty completing projects and assignments

## Addiction in the Family

Addiction to alcohol or other drugs has tragic effects not only upon the addict but also upon the children of addicts. There are an estimated 28 million children of alcoholics in the United States. About one in five adult Americans lived with an alcoholic while growing up. An average of five students in every classroom come from a home with a parent who has a substance addiction.

Children raised in substance-abusing families have different life experiences than children raised in non-substance-abusing families. It is important, however, to realize that children raised in other types of dysfunctional families may have similar stressors as do the children raised in families of substance-abusing parents.

The impact of substance abuse and addiction is immense and affects the entire family. Excessive parental substance abuse contributes to a family environment of chaos, unpredictability, anxiety, tension, and denial, in which the primary needs of children are not met. Children of addicts often feel great responsibility and guilt for their parents' substance abuse behavior. They are told by parents or given subtle messages that "if they were better dad or mom wouldn't be so angry and drink so much."

Unpredictability results because children are confused by the difference between the intoxicated and sober behavior of a parent. Promises made by an intoxicated parent are likely to be forgotten when the parent is sober, or vice versa. Confusion and unpredictability also result when a certain action is praised one day and then ignored or punished the next.

Parental substance abuse breeds low self-esteem and insecurity about parents' love. Substance abuse by a parent is often equated with not being loved. "If Mommy really loved me, she wouldn't drink." Children may also be angry with a non-substance-abusing parent who does not protect them from the violent addicted parent.

Children of addicts parents have reason to fear for their own safety as well as that of their addicted parent. There are concerns about being in an accident when driving with an intoxicated parent or of having the home catch on fire because a parent passed out while holding a lit cigarette. They realize that a frequently intoxicated parent could lose control of the car while driving home late at night or become seriously injured in many other ways. Children are also terrified of the arguments between parents that typify the addict home. They may have suffered abuse at the hands of an addicted parent or are fearful that they will become victims of abusive behavior.

We will now take a closer look at how alcohol abuse affects the family. Many of the following observations made about an alcoholic family can also be made of families with other substance abuse problems.

***Effects of Growing Up in an Alcoholic Family***    There are three rules that characterize an alcoholic family: "don't talk," "don't trust," and "don't feel." Children learn to not talk about the alcoholism in the family to anyone outside and, therefore, they "don't talk." Because the reactions of the alcoholic parent cannot be predicted or trusted, they "don't trust." And as children see painful feelings avoided or numbed through the use of alcohol, they learn to "not feel," and use denial to escape emotional pain.

The stressful environment of an alcoholic family can lead to depression, insomnia, headaches, upset stomachs, and other physical manifestations. In addition, children of alcoholic parents are likely to develop learning disabilities, deviant and antisocial behavior, eating disorders, and drug and alcohol dependencies.

Children of alcoholics may be hampered by their inability to grow up in developmentally healthy ways. As a result, children of alcoholics are likely to:

❖ Become isolated and afraid of people, particularly authority figures

❖ Have difficulty bonding with teachers and other students at school

❖ Become approval seekers, losing their identities in the process

❖ Be frightened by angry people and/or personal criticism

❖ Live life from the viewpoint of helping others and seek people who need help

❖ Have an overdeveloped sense of responsibility

❖ Have difficulty expressing themselves

❖ Experience feelings of guilt when standing up for themselves

❖ Confuse love with pity

❖ Bury feelings

❖ Judge themselves harshly due to poor self-esteem

❖ Be terrified at the thought of abandonment

❖ Be perfectionistic

❖ Be excessively self-conscious

❖ Be reactors rather than actors

❖ Eventually become alcoholics, marry them, or both

To further cope and survive in their alcoholic environments, children often assume roles that represent particular and rigid ways of relating to other family members and the outside world. The four roles assumed by children in alcoholic families are discussed next, along with classroom strategies for dealing with children of alcoholics.

*Family Hero*    The **family hero** is often, but not always, the eldest child. The role of the hero is to make up for the deficits in the family, diverting attention from the alcoholic by achieving or overachieving in schoolwork, athletics, music, or other pursuits. They are often very responsible with a drive or compulsion to achieve. Perhaps they are attempting to show the world that the family must be problem-free and functional to have produced such an exceptional child.

These children often assume unfulfilled parenting responsibilities within the family. Family heroes are usually well-behaved children but may seem bossy or parental in their relationships with other children. They are frequently labeled the "teacher's pet" by other children. These children assume leadership roles and tend to "take charge" in group activities rather than participate as equal members or followers. They may volunteer often and have a strong need for attention and approval from adults. Family heroes are not likely to be recognized as needing attention from school personnel because they seem so well-adjusted and because of their achievements.

As adults, family heroes are prone to becoming compulsive oveachievers who have an insatiable drive to always be on top. Therefore, they tend to become workaholics and perfectionists. In addition, they are likely to suffer physical problems, probably related to the stress created from their constant striving to achieve and succeed. The adult family hero often relies on drugs and alcohol to sustain the highly straining lifestyle. Family heroes who are not dependent on alcohol or other substances often marry spouses who are chemically dependent, weak, sick, or otherwise dependent. When a family hero marries a chemically dependent person, he or she becomes the chief enabler of the chemically dependent partner.

Despite all the achievements, an adult family hero often feels a deep sense of failure, because the accomplishments and brilliant performances did not make the alcoholic parent stop drinking. She or he does not know how to relax or play, having spent years "mothering" and attending to the needs of parents, spouses, and others. A sense of failure also arises with the realization that the hero is continually meeting other peoples' needs while ignoring his or her own, is often taken advantage of, and does not know how to stop it.

The family hero needs to learn how to ask for help, how to follow and negotiate, how to identify and meet his or her own needs, how to relax and have fun, and how to balance work and play. To facilitate this, teachers can:

❖ Limit classroom responsibilities of the child

❖ Give positive attention at times the child is not achieving

❖ Give attention to the child when he or she participates as a follower rather than a leader in an activity

❖ Help the child understand that it is all right to make mistakes

❖ Suggest to the child that he or she pay attention to his or her own needs

❖ Teach relaxation techniques such as progressive relaxation, imagery, exercise, and biofeedback

❖ Do not allow the child to monopolize class discussions or always be the first to volunteer or answer a question

❖ Validate the child's worth based on being himself or herself, not on doing or achieving

❖ Help the child balance work and play by organizing and participating in social and recreational activities

**The Scapegoat**   Often described as the problem child because he or she displays rebelliousness, irresponsibility, breaking rules, talking back to parents and school workers, and acting out, the **scapegoat** relies strongly on peers and tends to blame others. Acting out is often through substance abuse, but may be through other delinquent or problem behaviors, such as criminal activity, sexual promiscuity, or other high-risk behaviors. The scapegoat serves to divert attention from the alcoholic parent, in essence, allowing the outside world to believe that the family is fine, but the scapegoat is just a problem child and troublemaker.

The scapegoat often comes to the attention of school personnel because of the manifested behaviors and attitudes. Children serving this role are very difficult and frustrating to have in class. They neglect schoolwork, are disruptive, talk back to teachers, and break rules. Teachers are likely to feel as if they have tried everything to deal with a scapegoat child, with no success, and to feel tremendous frustration about how to deal with the child.

Scapegoats are very vulnerable to addiction to alcohol and other substances as teenagers and adults. Engagement in substance abuse and other high-risk behaviors increases the likelihood of such consequences as early pregnancy, accidental death, suicide, disease, and trouble with the law.

The scapegoat needs to learn how to express anger in a constructive manner, to forgive himself or herself, and to take responsibility for his or her mistakes but not those of others. In addition, the scapegoat needs to learn activities that will bring positive attention and social skills that will allow friendships. Teachers can assist the scapegoat by:

❖ Stressing the importance of personal responsibility for the child's actions and not allowing the child to blame others

❖ Giving affirmations to the child when he or she takes responsibility

❖ Applying logical consequences when the child misbehaves

❖ Developing an understanding of the child's behavioral and attitudinal patterns, to avoid getting angry at the child's behavior

❖ Providing suggestions for developing social skills, and working with the school counselor to provide this training

❖ Not treating the child in a special manner

❖ Not taking the child's behavior personally

❖ Not agreeing with the child's blaming and complaints about others

*The Lost Child*   Fisher describes the lost child as follows:

> The lost child in the alcoholic family presents himself or herself as withdrawn and shy. Again, this child may not be referred to the school counselor because the lost child rarely misbehaves and his or her academic work is usually acceptable, although unremarkable. Teachers frequently ignore this child, because there are so many more demands from disturbing children. (pg. 176)[19]

The **lost child** may fade into the family and classroom "woodwork," never causing any trouble or calling attention to himself or herself, thereby being the one child in the family that the parents do not have to worry about. This child tends to be quiet, to have few friends, and to seldom cause problems. He or she likes to work alone at school and is often creative in nonverbal ways, such as art, music, and writing. The lost child typically daydreams and fantasizes to escape painful reality.

The difficulty that lost children have in interpersonal and social relationships remains as they become adults. Lack of social skills, combined with low self-esteem and shyness, contributes to dissatisfying interpersonal and marital relationships in adulthood. Inability to deal with conflicts sends the lost child into further social withdrawal and avoidance, resulting in loneliness that is often coped with inappropriately through substance abuse.

The lost child needs to realize that he or she is important and deserves attention, to get what he or she wants and needs, to recognize and own feelings, to initiate activities, and to make personal choices. Teachers can help lost children by:

- ❖ Taking an inventory of students in your classroom who are lonely or whose name you cannot consistently recall

- ❖ Making efforts to notice and attend to the child

- ❖ Finding out more about the child's interests and talents

- ❖ On a one-to-one basis encouraging the child's creativity, talents, and academic progress

- ❖ Assisting the child in developing relationships with other children in the classroom

- ❖ Having the child work in small groups frequently in order to build social trust and confidence

- ❖ Making a point of calling on the child in class, not allowing him or her to remain silent

- ❖ Not allowing other children in the class, siblings, or parents to take care of the child by talking and answering for him or her

- ❖ Redirecting fantasy and daydreaming activities into appropriate and creative channels, such as writing or artwork

- ❖ Not being overly sympathetic to the child

***The Mascot or Clown***   The **mascot** or family clown diverts attention from the alcoholic parent and reduces family tension by being cute or funny. In school, this child makes repeated and constant attempts to be funny or get attention and is often suspected of hyperactivity, and as a result comes to the attention of the school counselor or nurse.

The "job" of mascot becomes a full-time role that mascots do not seem to outgrow even as adults. There is the constant need to be the clown, yet unhappiness underlies continual attempts to be humorous or funny. Unfortunately, many mascots turn to alcohol and other drugs to deal with their deep feelings of sadness and depression.

The mascot needs to learn how to receive attention, praise, and help from others in appropriate manners, how to deal with conflict and solve problems, and to recognize and accept feelings. Classroom teachers can assist the mascot by:

- ❖ Giving attention to the child when he or she is not attempting to be funny or exhibiting attention-getting behaviors

- ❖ Reinforcing to the rest of the class the importance of not paying attention to the child's misbehavior

- ❖ Giving the child classroom jobs or tasks that require responsibility

- ❖ Discussing the importance of appropriate behavior with the child in brief, one-to-one discussions

- ❖ Encouraging an appropriate sense of humor

- ❖ Not laughing at the mascot's attempts to be funny

- ❖ Remembering that the mascot's behavior is an effort to mask fear and depression

*Al-Anon and Alateen*  **Al-Anon** is a fellowship of people who have been affected by the alcohol abuse of someone. Al-Anon members meet in small groups to harness the strength and hope of others who have lived with alcoholism. Al-Anon provides an opportunity in which individuals can learn from the experience of others who have lived in similar situations. **Alateen** meetings are similar to Al-Anon meetings except that Alateen is restricted to people under age 20 who live, or have lived, with someone who abuses alcohol. Alateen meetings include one or two Al-Anon sponsors. Young people who are living with a person with an alcohol problem, or who have lived with an alcohol abuser in the past, should be encouraged to attend an Alateen meeting. They will find other young people who have faced similar experiences. Further information about Al-Anon and Alateen can be obtained from the Al-Anon and Alateen website at http://www.alanon.alateen.org.

## Cocaine

**Cocaine** is a strong stimulant derived from the leaves of the coca bush. The coca bush grows in the Andean Mountain region of South America (Colombia, Peru, Bolivia). Coca leaves are processed into cocaine hydrochloride, a white crystalline powder that is inhaled through the nose ("snorted") or injected. When inhaled, cocaine's effects peak in 15 to 20 minutes and disappear in 60 to 90 minutes. When injected intravenously, the result is an intense high that crests in 3 to 5 minutes and wanes over 30 to 40 minutes. Another form of cocaine is "crack" cocaine. **Crack cocaine** is made by processing cocaine hydrochloride to a base state with baking soda and water. Crack cocaine looks like slivers of soap but has the general texture of porcelain. It is smoked in a pipe and produces an intense cocaine high.

Cocaine directly stimulates the reward centers of the brain, producing intense feelings of euphoria. When the euphoria and excitement of the initial cocaine high taper off, the user slides into a physiological depression, a "let-down" feeling, dullness, tenseness, and edginess. A user wants to take cocaine again in an effort to counteract these "let-down" feelings. This causes a cycle of using cocaine to achieve euphoria and to ward off the negative feelings associated with coming down from its effects.

Daily or binge users undergo profound personality changes. They become confused, anxious, and depressed. They are short-tempered and grow suspicious of friends, loved ones, and other associates. Their thinking is impaired; they have difficulty concentrating and remembering things. They experience weakness and lassitude. They neglect work and other responsibilities. They lose interest in food and sex. Some become aggressive, and some experience panic attacks. The more of the drug they use, the more profound their symptoms.

In some cases, where consumption of cocaine is frequent or the dose is high, or both, users suffer a partial or total break with reality, or cocaine psychosis. The cocaine psychotic has delusions and may become paranoid, sometime reacting violently against those he or she imagines are persecuting him or her. Many have visual, auditory, or tactile hallucinations (one of the most common is "coke bugs," or **formication**, the sensation of insects crawling under the skin). Cocaine psychosis can continue for days, weeks, or months. Severe cases require hospitalization and antipsychotic medications.

Cocaine use can cause chest pain and irregular heartbeat, and can worsen preexisting coronary heart disease and bring on a heart attack. Because cocaine increases acute blood pressure, it can cause blood vessels in the brain to rupture and cause strokes. Cocaine may also damage the walls of arteries. Those who inject cocaine, or any other drug for that matter, are at high risk of infection from contaminated needles. HIV, hepatitis B, and hepatitis C are some of the infections that can be spread from contaminated needles. Another serious risk associated with cocaine use is seizures. Cocaine has been known to induce epilepsy even in those with no previous signs of it.

## Methamphetamine

**Methamphetamine** is a powerful central nervous system stimulant. Methamphetamine is made easily in clandestine laboratories with over-the-counter ingredients (e.g., ephedrine, pseudoephedrine). Methamphetamine is commonly known as **"speed," "meth," "chalk," "crystal," "crank," "fire,"** and **"glass."** Methamphetamine comes in many forms and can be smoked, snorted, orally ingested, or injected. Immediately after smoking the drug or injecting it intravenously, the user experiences an intense rush, or "flash," that lasts only a few minutes and is described as extremely pleasurable. Snorting or oral ingestion produces euphoria, but not the intense rush obtained by smoking or injections. Snorting produces effects within 3 to 5 minutes, and oral ingestion produces effects within 15 to 20 minutes.

Methamphetamine produces pronounced effects on the central nervous system: increased activity and wakefulness, increased physical activity, decreased appetite, and a general sense of well-being. The effects of methamphetamine can last six to eight hours or longer. After the initial rush, there is typically a state of high agitation that in some individuals can lead to violent or irrational behavior.

As with similar stimulants (e.g., cocaine), methamphetamine most often is used in a "binge and crash" pattern. In an effort to obtain desired effects, users may take higher doses of the drug, take it more frequently, or change their method of drug intake. In some cases, users forego food and sleep while binging on the drug or on a "run." After the binge or run, a user "crashes." During the crash, the user may sleep for more than 24 hours and become depressed and hungry and feel intense craving for the drug.

Methamphetamine has toxic effects. It has been shown to damage nerve terminals in the dopamine-containing regions of the brain. High doses can elevate body temperature to dangerous, sometimes lethal, levels, as well as cause convulsions. Abuse can lead to inflammation of the heart lining, increased blood pressure, rapid and irregular heartbeat, and strokes in the brain. If methamphetamine is injected, there is increased risk of HIV, hepatitis B, and hepatitis C transmission. This is particularly true for individuals who inject the drug and share injection equipment.

Long-time users exhibit symptoms that can include violent behavior, anxiety, confusion, and insomnia. They also can display a number of psychotic features, including paranoia, auditory hallucinations, mood disturbances, and delusions (for example, the sensation of insects creeping on the skin, called *formication*). The paranoia can result in homicidal as well as suicidal thoughts.

In the 1980s, "**ice**," a smokable form of methamphetamine, came into use. Ice is a large, usually clear crystal of high purity that is smoked in a glass pipe like crack cocaine. The smoke is odorless, leaves a residue that can be resmoked, and produces effects that may continue for 12 hours or more.

In addition to the dangers of methamphetamine abuse, the manufacturing process presents its own hazards. The production of methamphetamine requires the use of hazardous chemicals, many of which are corrosive or flammable. The vapors that are created in the chemical reaction attack mucous membranes, skin, eyes, and the respiratory tract. Some chemicals react dangerously with water, and some can cause fire or explosion. Methamphetamine manufacturing results in a great deal of hazardous waste. The manufacture of one pound of methamphetamine results in six pounds of waste. This waste includes corrosive liquids, acid vapors, heavy metals, solvents, and other harmful materials that can cause disfigurement or death when contact is made with skin or breathed into the lungs. Lab operators almost always dump this waste illegally in ways that severely damage the environment. National parks and other preserved sites have been adversely affected.

## Heroin

**Heroin** is a narcotic drug that is processed from morphine, a naturally occurring substance extracted from the seed pod of the opium poppy. It is typically sold as a white or brownish powder or as the black, sticky substance known on the streets as "**black tar heroin.**" Although purer heroin is becoming more common, most street heroin is cut with other drugs or with substances such as sugar, starch, powdered milk, or quinine. Street heroin can also be cut with strychnine or other poisons. Because heroin abusers do not know the actual strength of the drug or its true contents, they are at risk of overdose or death. Heroin also poses special problems because of transmission of HIV and other diseases that can occur from sharing needles or other injection equipment.

Heroin is usually injected, sniffed/snorted, or smoked. Typically, a heroin abuser may inject up to four times a day. Intravenous injection provides the greatest intensity and most rapid onset of euphoria (seven to eight seconds), while intramuscular injection produces a relatively slow onset of euphoria (five to eight minutes). There is an increase in new, young users who are being lured by inexpensive, high-purity heroin that can be sniffed or smoked instead of injected. Heroin has also been appearing in more affluent communities.

Heroin is particularly addictive because it enters the brain so rapidly. With heroin, the rush is usually accompanied by a warm flushing of the skin, dry mouth, and a heavy feeling in the extremities, which may be accompanied by nausea, vomiting, and severe itching. After the initial effects, abusers will be drowsy for several hours. Mental function is clouded by heroin's effect on the central nervous system. Heart rate and blood pressure slow. Breathing is also severely slowed, sometimes to the point of death. Heroin overdose is a particular risk on the street, where the amount and purity of the drug cannot be accurately determined.

Heroin use can rapidly progress to addiction. As with abusers of any addictive drug, heroin abusers generally spend more and more time and energy obtaining and using the drug. Once addicted, the heroin abuser's primary purpose in life becomes seeking and using drugs. The drugs literally change the brain. Physical dependence develops with higher doses of the drugs. With **physical dependence,** the body adapts to the presence of the drug, and **withdrawal symptoms** occur if use is reduced abruptly. Withdrawal may occur within a few hours after the last time the drug is taken. Symptoms of heroin withdrawal include restlessness, muscle and bone pain, insomnia, diarrhea, vomiting, cold flashes with goose bumps ("**cold turkey**"), and leg muscle spasms. Taking methadone can prevent withdrawal. As a result, methadone is used in treating heroin addiction.

## Oxycodone

**Oxycodone** is a very strong narcotic pain reliever similar to morphine. It is an effective pain reliever for mild to moderate pain, chronic pain, and for treatment of terminal cancer pain. It is designed so that the oxycodone is slowly released over time, allowing it to be used twice daily. Oxycodone (also known by the brand name OxyContin) is abused for its narcotic effects. Rather than ingesting the pill as indicated, abusers use other methods of taking the drugs. Abusers crush oxycodone tablets in order to release all the narcotic in the drug at once and produce an intense, heroin-like high. Once the tablets are crushed, they are either snorted or dissolved in liquid for injection. The abuse of oxycodone is increasing in many parts of the United States. Many people have become addicted to this drug. Reports of thefts at pharmacies are increasing as a result of people stealing oxycodone and other narcotic pain relief pills such as hydrocodone (Vicodin, Lortab).

## Marijuana and Cannabis

**Marijuana** is the dried, shredded flowers and leaves of the hemp plant *Cannabis sativa*. There are hundreds of slang terms for marijuana, including "pot," "herb," "weed," "boom," "Mary Jane," and "chronic." It usually is smoked as a cigarette (called a *joint* or *nail*) or in a pipe or bong. In recent years, it has appeared in **blunts**, which are cigarettes that have been emptied of tobacco and refilled with marijuana. Some users mix marijuana into foods or use it to brew tea.

THC (which is short for delta-9-tetrahydrocannabinol) is the chemical that accounts for the major psychoactive effects of marijuana. THC is found most abundantly in the upper leaves, bracts, and flowers of the resin-producing variety of the plant. The dried leaves (marijuana) average from 3% to 5% THC. However, through special breeding marijuana may yield greater amounts of THC (7% or higher). **Hashish**, which is the dried and pressed flowers and resins, has up to 12% THC. **Hashish oil**, a crude extract of hashish, has up to 60% THC. THC tends to remain stored for long periods of time in the body. Complete elimination of THC can take up to 30 days.

A typical marijuana high may last two to three hours. The user experiences an altered perception of space and time. Marijuana adversely affects judgment, complex motor skills, and physical coordination. These effects make driving a car dangerous and increase the possibility of many types of accidents. Using marijuana can also impair one's judgment regarding decision making about sex. Sexual activity places young people at risk for unplanned pregnancy and sexually transmitted diseases, including HIV infection. Marijuana users are also likely to experience difficulty in thinking and problem solving. There is concern that regular use of marijuana by young people may impair psychological and physical maturation and development. Apathy, lack of concern for the future, and the loss of motivation have been seen in some heavy users.

There is much concern about the effects of smoking marijuana on the lungs, because it is usually taken through smoking. A marijuana smoker is likely to experience many of the same respiratory problems that tobacco smokers have. However, marijuana is typically inhaled more deeply and held in the lungs for a longer period of time than tobacco smoke. These inhalation practices are likely to increase the risk of respiratory problems. As a result, marijuana smokers may have daily cough and phlegm, symptoms of chronic bronchitis, and more frequent chest colds. There is concern that marijuana smoke contains carcinogens that could increase the risk of lung cancer.

Several thousand people are treated each year for marijuana dependency. Marijuana's effects on the brain and those produced by such highly addictive drugs as alcohol, heroin, cocaine, and nicotine are quite similar. Marijuana seems to affect the brain's reward systems in much the same way as these other addictive substances. These actions in the brain keep users desiring to repeat the use of marijuana. When heavy users of marijuana abruptly stop taking the drug, they are likely to feel anxiety and other negative emotions. Individuals may keep using marijuana in an effort to avoid these feelings. Many teenagers who seek treatment for drug dependency report being addicted to marijuana.

## Club Drugs

**Club drugs** is a general term for a number of illicit drugs, primarily synthetic, that are most commonly encountered at nightclubs and "raves." The drugs include MDMA, ketamine, GHB, Rohypnol, LSD, PCP, methamphetamine, and, to a lesser extent, psilocybin mushrooms. This section on club drugs discusses MDMA, LSD, PCP, and psilocybin mushrooms. Ketamine, GHB, and Rohypnol, which are popular on the club and rave scene, are discussed in the following section ("Date-Rape Drugs") because they are also used as date-rape agents. Methamphetamine was discussed earlier in this chapter.

One reason that these drugs have gained popularity is the false perception that they are not as harmful or as addictive as mainstream drugs such as cocaine and heroin. A serious danger surrounding many of these club drugs is that users are often unaware of what is contained in the pills that they acquire. Look-alike substances, such as paramethoxyamphetamine (PMA) and dextromethorphan (DXM), are sometime sold as MDMA. These substances can cause a dangerous rise in body temperature and have resulted in the death of some who unknowingly took them in pills they believed to be Ecstasy (MDMA). MDMA tablets may also contain other substances, such as ketamine, PCP, caffeine, ephedrine, or methamphetamine.

The use of synthetic drugs has become a popular method of enhancing the club and rave experience, which is characterized by loud, rapid-tempo "techno" music (140 to 200 beats per minute), light shows, smoke or fog, and pyrotechnics. Users of drugs such as MDMA report that the effects of the drugs heighten the user's perceptions, especially the visual stimulation. Quite often, users of MDMA at clubs will dance with light sticks to increase their visual stimulation. Legal substances such as Vick's nasal inhalers and Vick's VapoRub are often used to enhance the effects of the drugs. The culture surrounding clubs and raves creates a favorable environment for illegal drug trafficking. These drugs are showing up more frequently at high school parties and in rural areas.

*MDMA*   MDMA is the most popular of the club drugs. Most MDMA is manufactured and trafficked from Europe (primarily the Netherlands). There is widespread abuse of MDMA, most commonly known as "Ecstasy," in many areas of the United States. **MDMA, Ecstasy,** or **"e"** is a synthetic, psychoactive substance possessing stimulant and mild hallucinogenic properties. Known as the "hug drug" or "feel good" drug, it reduces inhibitions, eliminates anxiety, and produces feelings of empathy for others. In addition to chemical stimulation, the drug reportedly suppresses the need to eat, drink, or sleep. This enables club-scene users to endure all-night and sometimes two- to three-day parties. Although it can be snorted, injected, or rectally inserted, MDMA is usually taken orally in tablet form, and its effects last approximately four to six hours. When taken at raves, where all-night dancing usually occurs, the drug often leads to severe dehydration and heat stroke in the user since it has the effect of "short-circuiting" the body's temperature signals to the brain.

An MDMA overdose is characterized by a rapid heartbeat, high blood pressure, faintness, muscle cramping, panic attacks, and, in more severe cases, loss of consciousness or seizures. One of the side effects of the drug is jaw muscle tension and teeth grinding. As a consequence, MDMA users will often suck on pacifiers to help relieve the tension. The most critical, life-threatening response to MDMA is hyperthermia, or excessive body heat. Recent reports of MDMA-related deaths were associated with core body temperatures ranging from 107 to 109 degrees Fahrenheit. Many rave clubs now provide cooling centers or cold showers so participants can lower their body temperatures.

There is evidence that Ecstasy causes damage to the neurons (nerve cells) that utilize serotonin to communicate with other neurons in the brain, and that recreational MDMA users risk permanent brain damage that may manifest itself in depression, anxiety, memory loss, learning difficulties, sleep disorders, sexual dysfunction, and other neuropsychiatric disorders. In addition to the dangers posed by MDMA, incidents involving look-alike tablets containing substances such as PMA, methamphetamine, and methamphetamine/ketamine are increasing. Tablets containing MDMA in combination with other illicit drugs, such as phencyclidine (PCP), have also been encountered. Users are unaware of the dangers posed by these drugs and unknowingly ingest potentially dangerous or even lethal amounts. In 2000 alone, PMA was associated with three deaths in Chicago and six deaths in central Florida.

*LSD*   LSD (lysergic acid diethylamide) is a potent hallucinogenic drug. One liquid ounce contains about 300,000 human doses. It is a colorless, odorless, and tasteless compound. The liquid is dropped onto blotter paper ("blotter acid") or made into tiny colored pills ("microdots"). LSD is taken orally, and its effects generally last 8 to 12 hours.

Usually, the user feels the first effects of the drug 30 to 90 minutes after taking it. LSD's physiological effects include sweating, an increase in blood pressure and heart rate, and an enlargement (dilation) of the pupils of the eye. Other effects that a user may experience include increased body temperature, loss of appetite, sleeplessness, dry mouth, and tremors.

Users refer to their experience with LSD as a "trip." The effects of LSD are unpredictable. They depend on the amount taken; the user's personality, mood, and expectations; and the surroundings in which the drug is used.

LSD is perhaps best known for its effects in altering perceptions. Psychologically, a user may experience delusional thinking and hallucinations. **Hallucinations** are alterations of vision and other senses. Some users experience **synesthesia,** which is a crossing of the senses—seeing sounds or hearing colors. An LSD user may have opposite feelings at the same time, such as elation and depression or relaxation and tension. For many users, the sense of time is distorted, and hours may be perceived as much longer increments of time—perhaps days, weeks, or even years. The drug can alter perceptions to such an extent that the user engages in bizarre behavior. There have been instances in which users have jumped off a tall building or into a body of water. Another bizarre effect is the sensation that one's body is distorted or even coming apart. An LSD trip can be pleasant or terrifying; there is no way of predicting the outcome of a trip. A **"bad trip"** refers to an LSD experience accompanied by severe, terrifying thoughts and feelings. Fatal and serious accidents have occurred during bad trips.

Many LSD users experience flashbacks. A **flashback** is a recurrence of certain aspects of a person's LSD experience without the user having taken the drug again. Flashbacks occur suddenly, often without warning, and may occur within a few days or more than a year after LSD use.

*PCP*   On the street, **PCP,** (phencyclidine) has many names, including "angel dust," "PeaCe Pill," "cadillac," "crystal joints," "superpot," "superweed," "monkey weed," and "horse tranquilizer." PCP is often substituted for, and sold as, LSD and mescaline on the street.

PCP was first used in pill form, but now is most often snorted like cocaine or mixed with tobacco, marijuana, or parsley and then smoked.

Some users inject PCP into their veins, and others swallow it in a liquid form.

PCP has depressant, stimulant, hallucinogenic, and analgesic properties. Quite a combination! The effects of the drug on the central nervous system vary greatly. At low doses the most prominent effect is similar to that of alcohol intoxication, with generalized numbness and reduced sensitivity to pain. As the amount of PCP increases, the person becomes more insensitive and may become fully anesthetized. Large doses cause coma, convulsions, and death.

Common effects include flushing, excessive sweating, and a blank stare. The size of the pupils is not affected by PCP. At higher doses side-to-side eye movements (**nystagmus**), double vision, muscular incoordination, dizziness, nausea, and vomiting may occur. Also, tremors, jerky movements, and grand mal and prolonged seizures may follow high doses.

PCP's psychological effects are unpredictable. Any combination of the following may occur with use: mood fluctuations, distortions in thinking, exaggerated sense of well-being, exhilaration, sedation, drunkenness, delusions, auditory and visual hallucinations, and violent behavior.

In some users, PCP causes psychotic reactions that last for weeks or months. Some researchers believe that permanent brain damage can result from PCP use. The withdrawal effects associated with chronic PCP use include anxiety, depression, and short-term memory difficulties.

*Psilocybin Mushrooms*    Although they are not as popular as the synthetic drugs, **psilocybin mushrooms** are encountered at raves and clubs and increasingly are used by high school and college students. Mushrooms can be ingested alone or in combination with alcohol or illegal drugs. The mushrooms can be soaked or boiled in water to make tea, and often are cooked and added to other foods to mask their bitter taste. Although mushroom potency varies, they generally contain 0.2% to 0.4% psilocybin, and only a trace amount of psilocyn (a related hallucinogenic chemical). Psilocybin is broken down by the body to produce psilocyn, which may be the source of the mind-altering effects of the drug. The physical effects of the mushrooms appear within 20 minutes of ingestion, and last approximately six hours. These effects include nausea, vomiting, muscle weakness, yawning, drowsiness, tearing, facial flushing, enlarged pupils, sweating, and lack of coordination. Other physical effects include dizziness, diarrhea, dry mouth, and restlessness. Information published on a number of rave Internet sites indicates that, although mushrooms are used at clubs, they provide no energy for the dancer, and affect coordination. Most users experience profound relaxation and the lack of desire to move.

The psychological and physical effects of the drug include changes to audio, visual, and tactile senses. Colors reportedly appear brighter, and users report a crossing of the senses, such as seeing a sound and hearing a color. Users often report a sense of detachment from their body and a greater feeling of unity with their surroundings. Furthermore, the high is described as a more natural sensation than that supplied by synthetic hallucinogens. A large dose of the drug produces hallucinations and an inability to discern fantasy from reality. This sometimes leads to panic reactions and psychosis. No evidence of physical dependence exists, although tolerance does develop when mushrooms are ingested continuously over a short period of time. Individuals tolerant to LSD also show tolerance to mushrooms.

## Date-Rape Drugs

Certain drugs are being used to incapacitate individuals and thereby facilitate sexual assault. The drugs that are used most frequently as date-rape drugs are Rohypnol, GHB, and ketamine. These substances are typically slipped into a victim's beverage at a party or bar while a drink is left unattended or he or she is distracted. After ingestion, the victim feels disoriented and may appear drunk. This leaves the victim very vulnerable, and the perpetrator often volunteers to drive the victim home. Hours later, a victim may wake up in unfamiliar surroundings with little or no memory of what has happened.

*Rohypnol*   Rohypnol (flunitrazepam) is a powerful sedative-hypnotic in the same class of drugs as Valium. It is 10 times stronger than Valium. Rohypnol has never been approved for medical use in the United States. It is illegal to possess in the United States but is available as a prescription drug in several countries, including Mexico. Much of the Rohypnol that comes into the United States comes from Mexico. Rohypnol has been linked to several sexual assaults. It is known on the street as "roofies," "roachies," "rib," "forget pill," and "mind-erasers."

*GHB*   GHB (gamma hydroxybutyric acid) is another drug with high potential for abuse as a date-rape drug. GHB acts powerfully as a central nervous system depressant, taking effect within 15 minutes. Its effects are similar to Rohypnol, causing dizziness, confusion, overwhelming drowsiness, and unconsciousness. Victims often cannot remember events that occur after the drug is ingested. It is easily obtained and can be manufactured by amateur "basement" chemists. It comes in liquid form and can be easily slipped into drinks because it is colorless and odorless. However, it may be detected because it has a slightly salty taste. Several deaths are attributed to GHB abuse. GHB is also known by the following names: "Georgia Home Boy," "Grievous Bodily Harm" (GBH), "Liquid X," "Easy Lay," "G," and "Bedtime Scoop."

*Ketamine*   Ketamine is a legal drug in the United States that is approved for use as a veterinary anesthetic. It produces a dissociative effect similar to the drug PCP. Ingestion of ketamine causes hallucinations and feelings of being separated from one's body. Amnesia and dreamlike memories make it difficult for a date-rape victim to remember whether a sexual assault was real or imagined. An unsuspecting victim of date rape could easily be given a dangerous overdose of this drug. Taking too high a dose of ketamine can cause the heart to stop. The main source of ketamine for illegal use is through stealing the drug from veterinary clinics. "Special K," "K," "Vitamin K," and "Bump" are street names for ketamine.

*Alcohol*    Perpetrators of sexual assault now have new drugs to add to their arsenal of date-rape drugs. Yet alcohol has been used for many years as a date-rape agent. A majority of victims of date rape are drunk or have been drinking when the assault occurred. Alcohol is a central nervous system depressant. Drinking alcohol can impair judgment and cause disorientation. Drinking large amounts of alcohol can cause a person to pass out. These effects place a young person at high risk of being taken advantage of sexually.

*Protection Against Date-Rape Drugs*    A date-rape drug can be slipped into any type of beverage. For this reason, young people should be taught to not drink any beverage that they did not open for themselves. This may require a person to refrain from drinking from a container that is passed around or from a punch bowl. Young people should also be instructed to never leave a drink unattended. Drinks that were left unattended are best discarded rather than drunk. When offered a drink at a party or social event, the person should go to where the drink is opened, carefully watch it being poured, and then carry the drink himself or herself. Warn young people to avoid drinking a beverage that has an unusual taste or appearance (e.g., salty taste, excessive foam, unexplained residue). Also, warn young people not to accept rides home from strangers.

## Inhalants

Substances inhaled to induce psychoactive effects, such as euphoria or intoxication, can be classified into three basic groups: volatile solvents, aerosols, and anesthetics. The **volatile solvents** include the chemical components (e.g., toluene, acetone, benzene) of commercial products such as plastic (model) cement, fingernail polish removers, paint thinners, gasoline, kerosene, typewriter correction fluid, and lighter fluid. **Aerosols** are products discharged by the propellant force of compressed gas. Chemicals in the aerosol products and the propellant can be toxic. Many abused aerosols contain gases of chlorinated or fluorinated hydrocarbons, nitrous oxide, and vinyl chloride. Various aerosol products are abused, including hair sprays, spray paints, cooking sprays, and Freon gas. Many aerosols and volatile solvents are extremely poisonous and can damage body organs and systems.

**Anesthetics** include ether, chloroform, nitrous oxide, halothane, and related gases. Nitrous oxide ("laughing gas") is the most widely used; it is available as an anesthetic and commercially as a tracer gas to detect pipe leaks, as a whipped-cream propellant, and as a pressurized product to reduce preignition in racing cars.

Children commonly abuse the volatile solvents and aerosols. There are two major types of young inhalant abusers: experimenters, or transitional users, who either quit using or move on to other drugs, and chronic abusers. Chronic abuse is usually limited to those who have limited access to more popular mind-altering substances, such as the young and the very poor. Inhalant experimentation is widespread among the young. Chronic inhalant abuse is often related to parental alcoholism and neglect or abuse.

Frequently, the abused substance is emptied or sprayed into a plastic or paper bag, which is held tightly over the nose and mouth, and the fumes are inhaled. A cloth may be dipped in a liquid solvent, or the active solvent may be applied to the cloth, which is then held against the nose and/or mouth.

There are many hazards associated with inhalant abuse. Each inhaled substance carries different hazards. Because these substances are often poisonous, long-term (e.g., brain damage, hepatitis) or short-term damage to body tissues and organs is possible. Fatal overdoses occur when the central nervous system is depressed to the point that breathing stops. The risk of accidents is high because these substances often affect reasoning, orientation, and muscle coordination. Suffocation and asphyxiation can also occur.

## Anabolic Steroids

**Anabolic steroids** are synthetic derivatives of the male hormone testosterone. The full name is *androgenic* (promoting masculine characteristics) *anabolic* (building) *steroids* (the class of drugs). These derivatives of testosterone promote the growth of skeletal muscle and increase lean body mass. Anabolic steroids were first abused by athletes seeking to improve performance.

Today, athletes and others use anabolic steroids to enhance performance and also to improve physical appearance. Anabolic steroids are seldom prescribed by physicians today. Current legitimate medical uses are limited to certain kinds of anemia, severe burns, and some types of breast cancer.

Because these drugs produce increases in lean muscle mass, strength, and ability to train longer and harder, athletes in a variety of sports are attracted to these substances in hopes of enhancing athletic performance and improving physique. Young people are attracted to anabolic steroids in efforts to accelerate their physical development.

Anabolic steroids are taken orally or injected, and athletes and other abusers take them typically in cycles of weeks or months, rather than continuously, in patterns called cycling. **Cycling** involves taking multiple doses of steroids over a specific period of time, stopping for a period, and starting again. In addition, users frequently combine several different types of steroids to maximize their effectiveness while minimizing negative effects, a process known as **stacking.** Steroids are produced in tablet or capsule form for oral ingestion, or as a liquid for intramuscular injection. Those who inject anabolic steroids run the risk of contracting or transmitting hepatitis or the HIV virus that leads to AIDS.

Steroid users subject themselves to serious side effects and hazards, many of which yet remain unknown, particularly when high doses are used over long periods of time. Some side effects appear quickly, such as trembling, acne, jaundice (yellowish pigmentation of skin, tissues, and body fluids), fluid retention, and high blood pressure. Others, such as heart attack and strokes, may not show up for years.

A major concern of anabolic steroid use is the impact upon physical growth and development. Among adolescents, anabolic steroids can prematurely halt growth through premature skeletal maturation and accelerated pubertal changes.

In males, use of steroids can cause shrinking of the testicles, reduced sperm count, infertility, baldness, and development of breasts. In females, irreversible masculine traits can develop along with breast reduction and sterility. Females using anabolic steroids may also experience growth of facial hair, changes in or cessation of the menstrual cycle, enlargement of the clitoris, and deepened voice.

Aggression and other psychiatric side effects may result from anabolic steroid abuse. Many users report feeling good about themselves while on anabolic steroids, but researchers report that anabolic steroid abuse can cause wild mood swings, including manic-like symptoms, which lead to violent, even homicidal, episodes. Depression is often seen when the drugs are stopped and may contribute to steroid dependence. Users may suffer from paranoid jealousy, extreme irritability, delusions, and impaired judgment stemming from feelings of invincibility.

Signs of steroid use include quick weight and muscle gains (if steroids are used in conjunction with weight training); behavioral changes, particularly increased aggressiveness and combativeness; jaundice; purple or red spots on the body; swelling of feet or lower legs; trembling; unexplained darkening of the skin; acne; and persistent breath odor.

## Drug Injection and Blood-Borne Pathogen Risk

Increased HIV and hepatitis B and C transmission are likely consequences of drug abuse, particularly in individuals who inject the drug and share injection equipment. Infection with HIV and other infectious diseases is spread among injection drug users primarily through the reuse of contaminated syringes, needles, or other paraphernalia by more than one person. Drug abusers can then pass on these infections to sexual partners and children. In nearly one-third of Americans infected with HIV, injection drug use is a risk factor, making drug abuse the fastest growing vector for the spread of HIV in the nation.

## Key Terms

alcopops   199
normative education   203
peer tutors   205
peer counselors   205
wellness   217
high-risk students   220
support groups   220
nicotine   221
bidis   226
kreteks   226
chewing tobacco   227
snuff   227
euphoria   227
oral leukoplakias   228
alcoholism   233
family hero   237
scapegoat   238
lost child   239
mascot   240
Al-Anon   241
Alateen   241
cocaine   241
crack cocaine   241
formication   242
methamphetamine   242
speed   242
meth   242
chalk   242
crystal   242
crank   242
fire   242
glass   242
ice   243

heroin   244
black tar heroin   244
physical dependence   244
withdrawal symptoms   244
cold turkey   244
oxycodone   245
marijuana   245
blunts   245
THC   245
hashish   245
hashish oil   245
club drugs   246
MDMA   247
Ecstasy   247
e   247
LSD   248
hallucinations   248
synesthesia   248
bad trip   248
flashback   248
PCP   248
nystagmus   249
psilocybin mushrooms   249
Rohypnol   250
GHB   250
ketamine   250
volatile solvents   251
aerosols   251
anesthetics   251
anabolic steroids   252
cycling   252
stacking   253

## Review Questions

1. What trends have studies shown for young people using illicit drugs, marijuana, cocaine, and alcohol, and smoking cigarettes? What accounts for some of these trends?
2. Studies indicate that children most often begin to use drugs at about what age? What is the usual sequence of usage?

3. Give multiple examples of how the media entree young people to use alcohol and tobacco. Discuss the effectiveness of corporation-sponsored "don't smoke" or "drink responsibly" campaigns.

4. Discuss the strengths and weaknesses of the seven substance abuse prevention education strategies and programs discussed in this chapter.

5. Identify the 12 principles of effective substance abuse prevention programs outlined in the National Institute on Drug Abuse's publication.

6. Cite examples of school-based drug prevention programs that work. How does DARE compare with these programs?

7. What are the major components that should be included in substance abuse prevention curricula for grades K–3? Grades 4–6? Grades 7–9? Grades 10–12? Special education students?

8. Explain what high-risk students are. What should the substance abuse prevention curricula include for high-risk students?

9. Where and how can substance abuse prevention education be infused into the curriculum?

10. What are some important facts about tobacco use and young people?

11. What is nicotine and what are its effects?

12. Explain the various short-term and long-term health consequences of smoking and being exposed to tobacco smoke.

13. How many young people smoke cigarettes? Cigars? How do you explain the rise in smoking rates among young people and among girls?

14. Who is most likely to use smokeless tobacco, why might they use it, and what are the harmful effects of chewing?

15. Identify the psychosocial factors that need to be included in programs to prevent tobacco use.

16. Identify the seven recommendations by the Centers for Disease Control and Prevention for school policy on tobacco use.

17. Identify the components of effective tobacco cessation programs.

18. Identify the many problems associated with alcohol use, and some of the major findings of the 1999 Youth Risk Behavior Survey regarding students and alcohol.

19. Identify the usual characteristics of alcoholism and some of the signs and symptoms of youth alcoholism and problem drinking.

20. How many American adults lived with an alcoholic while growing up? What are the three rules that characterize an alcoholic family? Describe some ways children of alcoholics may be hampered and the roles they often assume in the alcoholic family.

21. Identify the administration, effects, hazards and any street names for the following drugs: cocaine, methamphetamine, heroin, oxycodone, marijuana, MDMA, LSD, PCP, psilocybin mushrooms, Rohypnol, GHB, ketamine, aerosols, and anabolic steroids.

22. What three diseases are likely consequences of drug abuse?

# References

1. Johnston, L. D., P. M. O'Malley, and J. G. Bachman (2002). *Monitoring the Future: National Results on Adolescent Drug Use. Overview of Key Findings, 2001* (NIH Publication No. 02-5105). Bethesda, MD: National Institute on Drug Abuse. Available at http://monitoringthefuture.org/pubs/monographs/overview2001.pdf.

2. Center for Science in the Public Interest (1998, September 4). "Kids Are as Aware of Booze as Presidents, Survey Finds" [Press release]. Washington, DC: Center for Science in the Public Interest.

3. Hacker, G. A. (2002, January 10). "Alcohol Advertising: Are Our Kids Collateral or Intended Targets?" *Booze News.* Available at http://www.cspinet.org/booze/alcohol_advertising_targets.htm.

4. Perry, C. L. (1999). "The Tobacco Industry and Underage Youth Smoking: Tobacco Industry Documents from the Minnesota Litigation." *Archives of Pediatric and Adolescent Medicine*, 153: 935–941.

5. Farrelly, M. C., C. G. Heaton, K. C. Davis, P. Messeri, J. C. Hersey, and L. Haviland (2002). "Getting to the Truth: Evaluating National Countermarketing Campaigns." *American Journal of Public Health*, 92: 901–907.

6. Bath, C. (2002). "The Evils of Alcohol Advertising." Speech delivered at Duke University. Available at http://www.campussafety.org/parents/rbath/dukespeech.html.

7. Sargent, J. D., M. L. Beach, M. A. Dalton, L. A. Mott, and J. J. Tickle (2001). "Effect of Seeing Tobacco Use in Films on Trying Smoking Among Adolescents: Cross Sectional Study." *British Medical Journal*, 323: 1–6.

8. Sargent, J. D., M. L. Beach, M. A. Dalton, L. A. Mott, and J. J. Tickle (2002). "Viewing Tobacco Use in Movies: Does It Shape Attitudes That Mediate Adolescent Smoking?" *American Journal of Preventive Medicine*, 22(3): 137–145.

9. Escamilla, G., A. L. Cradock, and I. Kawachi (2000). "Women and Smoking in Hollywood Movies: A Content Analysis." *American Journal of Public Health*, 90: 412–414.

10. Elias, M. (2002). "Teen Drinking Linked to Music Videos, TV." *USA Today.* Retrieved January 18, 2002, at http://depts.washington.edu/ecttp/alcohol/usarticle.htm.

11. Dusenbury, L., M. Falco, M. Lake, and A. Lake (1997). "A Review of the Evaluation of 47 Drug Abuse Prevention Curricula Available Nationally." *Journal of School Health*, 67(4): 127–132.

12. Botvin, G. (1996). "Preventing Drug Abuse Through the Schools: Intervention Programs That Work." Paper presented at the National Conference on Drug Abuse Prevention Research, Washington, DC. Available at http://165.112.78.61/MeetSum/C-ODA/Schools.html.

13. National Institute on Drug Abuse (1997). *Preventing Drug Abuse Among Children and Adolescents: A Research-Based Guide.* Available at http://www.nida.nih.gov/Prevention/Prevopen.html.

14. Lynam, D. R., R. Milich, R. Zimmerman, S. P. Novak, T. K. Logan, C. Martin, C. Leukefeld, and R. Clayton (1999). "Project DARE: No Effects at 10-Year Follow-up." *Journal of Consulting and Clinical Psychology*, 67(4): 590–593.

15. Centers for Disease Control and Prevention (2001). "Youth Tobacco Surveillance—United States, 2000." *Morbidity and Mortality Weekly Report*, 50(SS-4).

16. Centers for Disease Control and Prevention (2001). *Women and Smoking: A Report of the Surgeon General.* Atlanta, GA: CDC, Office on Smoking and Health. Available at http://www.cdc.gov/tobacco/sgr_forwomen.htm.

17. Centers for Disease Control and Prevention (1994). "Guidelines for School Health Programs to Prevent Tobacco Use and Addiction." *Morbidity and Mortality Weekly Report*, 43(RR-2).

18. Galanter, M. (1998). *Recent Developments in Alcoholism: Vol. 14.* New York: Plenum Press.

19. Fisher, G. L. (1989). "Counseling Strategies for Children Based on Rules and Roles in Alcoholic Families." *The School Counselor*, 36: 173–178.

# 7

# VIOLENCE, ABUSE, AND PERSONAL SAFETY

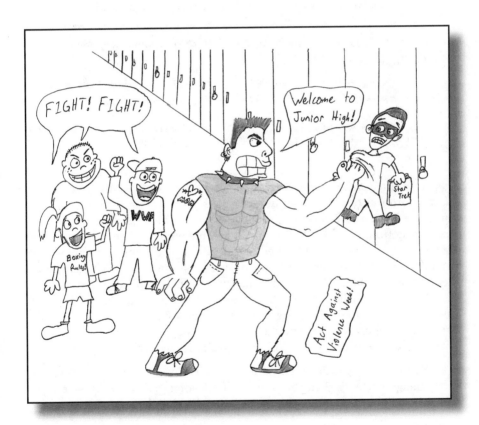

## *April 1999, Littleton, Colorado*

*Eric Harris and Dylan Klebold used assault weapons and homemade bombs to lay siege to their high school. The two boys killed 12 classmates and a teacher, injured 23 other teenagers, and then killed themselves.*

*Their friends said the two boys were constantly ridiculed and taunted at school. There was an unfounded accusation made by an anonymous classmate that Eric and Dylan had brought marijuana to school, prompting a search of their property.*

*There was another incident, even more humiliating than the search. "People surrounded them in the commons and squirted ketchup packets all over them, laughing at them, calling them faggots. That happened while teachers watched. They couldn't fight back. They wore the ketchup all day and went home covered with it."*

*According to the school's student body president: Eric and Dylan felt bullied and alienated, and in their minds it was "Payback time."*

Source: "Stories About Bullying" from the Bully B'ware Productions web page. This and other stories can be found at http://www.bullybeware.com/story.html.

According to the recent surgeon general's report on youth violence, no community, whether affluent or poor, urban, suburban, or rural, is immune from the devastating effects of youth violence.[1] In the decade extending from roughly 1983 to 1993, an epidemic of violent, often lethal behavior broke out in the United States, forcing millions of young people and their families to cope with injury, disability, and death. This epidemic left lasting scars on victims, perpetrators, and their families and friends.

Since 1993, when the epidemic peaked, youth violence has declined significantly nationwide, as signaled by downward trends in arrest records, victimization data, and hospital emergency room records. But the problem has not been resolved, as the following statistics depict:

❖ Youths' confidential reports about their violent behavior reveals no change since 1993 in the proportion of young people who have committed physically injurious and potentially lethal acts.

❖ Arrests for aggravated assault have declined only slightly, and in 1999 remained nearly 70% higher than pre-epidemic levels.

❖ In 1999, there were 104,000 arrests of people under age 18 for a serious violent crime—robbery, forcible rape, aggravated assault, or homicide.

❖ In 1999, there were 1,400 arrests for homicide committed by adolescents and, on occasion, even younger children (see Figure 7-1).

The homicide rate among 15- to 24-year-old U.S. males exceeds the rate in the following countries by . . .

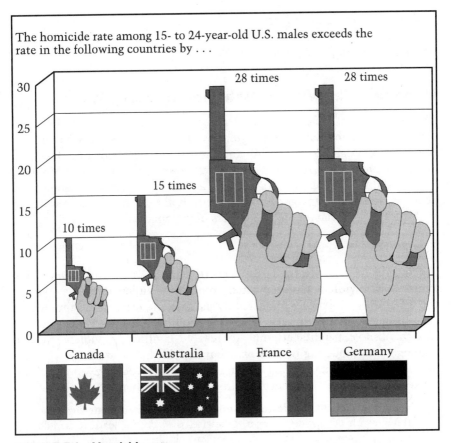

**FIGURE 7-1    Homicide rates**

❖ For every youth arrested in any given year in the late 1990s, at least 10 other youths were engaged in some form of violent behavior that could have seriously injured or killed another person.

The surgeon general's report stresses that this is no time for complacency. The epidemic of violence that swept the United States from 1983 to 1993 was fueled in large part by easy access to weapons, notably firearms. Today, with fewer people carrying weapons, including guns, to school and elsewhere, violent encounters are less likely to result in homicide and serious injury and therefore less likely to draw the attention of police. If the sizable numbers of youths still involved in violence today begin carrying and using weapons as they did a decade ago, this country may see a resurgence of the lethal violence that characterized the violence epidemic. Despite the present decline in gun use and in lethal violence, the proportion of young people involved in nonfatal violence has not dropped from the peak years of the epidemic. Thus, the headlines that you may have read proclaiming that the epidemic of youth violence that began in the 1980s is over are far from the truth. The reality is that youth violence is an ongoing, troubling, and pervasive problem.

# Understanding Violent Behavior in Young People

There are several factors to consider in understanding why children and adolescents exhibit violent behavior. Awareness of these factors enables educators and parents to develop and implement strategies to reduce and prevent violent behavior. This section reviews the following contributing factors—family, media, substance use, access to weapons, personal and peer characteristics, and gang involvement. It also examines early warning signs of violent behavior and the effects of violence on youth.

## Family Factors

Violence is often a learned response to conflict and frustration. This explains why violent children often come from violent families. Within these families, violence is modeled by parents and other family members as a problem-solving strategy. Therefore, children have ample opportunities to observe parents attempt to resolve conflict by violent means. Through this modeling of violent behavior, children learn to solve their personal conflicts and stress by violent means. Wodarski and Hedrick make the following comment regarding violent children:

> [V]iolent children do not learn empathic behaviors nor adequate cognitive strategies for dealing with anger. Likewise, they do not learn to handle stress in a prosocial manner. Thus, violent children are not prepared to deal with stress once they leave protected homes. (pg. 31)[2]

Lack of appropriate parenting is also often an important factor in the development of violent behavior. A lack of parental monitoring and discipline, poor supervision, inconsistent rule application, and aversive interactions are likely to be present within parent-child interactions of families of children exhibiting violent behavior. Family rejection also increases the likelihood of long-term violent behavior. Conversely, the National Longitudinal Study on Adolescent Health found that good parental and family relationships are associated with reduced risk of adolescent violent behavior.[3]

## Exposure to Media Violence

A large proportion of the media that children and adolescents are exposed to includes acts of violence. It is estimated that by the age of 18, the average young person will have viewed 200,000 acts of violence on television alone. Sixty-one percent of television programs contain interpersonal violence—and much of this violence is portrayed in an entertaining or glamorized manner with little to no depiction of realistic pain or harm. The suffering, loss, and sadness of victims and perpetrators are rarely shown. Rather, most violence in the media is used for entertainment in an attempt to provide immediate visceral thrills to those who view it.

American films are the most violent in the world. It is not uncommon for a young person viewing a major motion film to see numerous people shot, stabbed, crushed, punched, slapped, raped, maimed, or blown up during the course of the movie. It is clear that children learn to be violent by the steady diet of violence they consume from films and TV.

The amount of violence in the American media is constant and excessive. This overabundance is illustrated by a study examining the amount of violence on the major television networks. Of the 94 prime-time shows airing on ABC, CBS, NBC, and Fox networks during one week, 48 depicted at least one act of violence. On these shows were 276 violent incidents, which included such acts as pushing and slapping, assaults, rape, and killings—most of which could be classified as criminal.[4] On average, Fox showed a violent act every 10 minutes; NBC had the fewest violent incidents, at a rate of 1 every 21 minutes. Eight prime-time movies were broadcast during the week on the four networks; only one had no violence.

Children's shows and music videos often depict violence. In fact, the level of violence during Saturday morning cartoons is higher than the level of violence during the prime-time viewing hours. There are 3 to 5 violent acts per hour in prime time, versus 20 to 25 per hour on Saturday morning.

The high occurrence of violence on television greatly exceeds the actual rate of violent behavior in our society. This clearly dispels the myth that television programming is a reflection of what is going on in society. On the other hand, what is portrayed on television appears to be shaping behavioral patterns with respect to violence. Television often teaches children that violence is an acceptable response to anger or frustration.

It is not just television and movies that expose young people to violence. Much of the music that young people listen to contains lyrics with violent messages. The lyrics of many rap and heavy metal songs expose young people to themes such as suicide, sexual violence, murder, Satanism, and substance abuse. Many songs glorify violence and other harmful behaviors and have become increasingly explicit in the past two decades. "Gangsta rap" involves many references to violence, weapons, sex, and drug use, and several major rap artists have been charged with violent crimes in real life. The celebrity status of these rap artists seems to glamorize their violent behavior and condone the violent messages in their music. The popular music CD that led the sales charts and won several Music Television Video (MTV) Music Awards in the year 2000 featured songs about rape and murder with graphic lyrics and sound effects. Music videos, particularly those shown on MTV, often contain violence, sexism, suicide, and substance abuse. Watching music videos is a popular pastime for many preteens and teenagers; as a result, they are frequently exposed to violence through this medium. Another popular pastime for many children and adolescents is the use of video games that award points for violence against others. These games may condition young people to instinctively react to particular situations in a violent manner.

*Influence of Media Violence*    After the Jonesboro, Arkansas, school shooting in which two boys, aged 11 and 13, shot and killed 4 students and a teacher (and also shot and injured 10 others), *Time* magazine (April 6, 1998) said: "As for media violence, the debate there is fast approaching the same point that discussions about the health impact of tobacco reached some time ago—it's over. Few researchers bother any longer to debate that bloodshed on TV and in the movies has an effect on kids who witness it." According to the American Academy of Pediatrics (AAP), more than 3,500 research studies have examined the relationship between media violence and violent behavior; all but 18 have shown a positive relationship.[5] The strongest single correlate with violent behavior is previous exposure to violence. As a result, health care professionals are increasingly recognizing that exposure to media violence can cause violent behavior to occur.

The AAP alerts parents and those who work with children that media violence affects children by:[6]

❖ Increasing aggressiveness and antisocial behavior

❖ Increasing their fear of becoming victims

❖ Making them less sensitive to violence and to victims of violence

❖ Increasing their appetite for more violence in entertainment and in real life

Children and adolescents who view violence may mirror conflict resolution techniques they see on television and in movies. Viewing aggressive acts on television increases aggressive behavior among children, particularly among those children most inclined to aggression initially. In particular, there is a strong relationship between heavy television viewing and aggression during preschool years. Children whose parents use physical punishment are more likely to be aggressive themselves or to become more aggressive after exposure to television violence.

Children younger than 8 years cannot discriminate between fantasy and reality. As such, they are particularly vulnerable to adopting as reality the values and attitudes that are portrayed in the media they watch.

The AAP stresses that media violence is associated with a variety of physical and mental health problems for children and adolescents, including aggressive behavior, desensitization to violence, fear, depression, nightmares, and sleep disturbances. David Grossman, a military expert on the effects of violence, relates the following story told to him by a woman who called him when he was a guest on a radio call-in show:

> My 13-year old boy spent the night with a neighbor. After that night, he started having nightmares. I got him to admit what the nightmares were about. While he was at the neighbor's house, they watched splatter movies all night: people cutting people up with chain saws and stuff like that.
>
> I called the neighbors and told them, "Listen: you are sick people. I wouldn't feel any different about you if you had given my son pornography or alcohol. And I'm not going to have anything further to do with you or your son—and neither is anybody else in this neighborhood, if I have anything to do with it—until you stop what you're doing." (pg. 15)[7]

David Grossman commented on this story by saying, "That's powerful. That's censure, not censorship. We ought to have the moral courage to censure people who think that violence is legitimate entertainment."

## Substance Use and Abuse

Alcohol and drug use increase the potential for violent behavior and victimization by reducing behavioral inhibitions and facilitating aggressive responses. Alcohol and other drugs can make people feel more aggressive and powerful, yet less able to control themselves and less aware of the consequences of actions. The trafficking of drugs is also strongly associated with violent crimes.

## Immediate Access to Weapons

The immediate accessibility of a weapon is another critical factor that increases the potential for violent behavior affecting both the carrier and others. The proliferation of guns and the relative ease with which young people acquire them appear to be some of the most potent factors accounting for episodes of lethal youth violence. Carrying a weapon, especially a firearm, greatly increases the possibility for escalation of violence and potential for its use. Weapon-carrying behavior for some youths may be a defensive strategy in response to the profound fear of being a victim of a violent act. However, research has shown that weapon carrying among youth appears to be more closely associated with criminal activity, delinquency, and aggressiveness than with purely defensive behavior. Handgun ownership by high school youth is associated with gang membership, selling and using drugs, interpersonal violence, being convicted of crimes, school truancy, and either suspension or expulsion from school. Gun carrying among junior high students is also strongly linked with indicators of serious delinquency, such as having been arrested.[8,9]

Law enforcement officials note that firearms are easily accessible to many young people. Some have access to guns in their homes. They can be

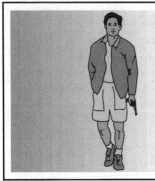

**Youth and Firearms**

- Firearm injuries are the second leading cause of death for young people aged to 24 years.
- For every child killed with a firearm, four are wounded.
- Of violent deaths in schools, 77% are caused by firearms.
- Nearly 90% of homicide victims aged 15 to 19 years are killed with a firearm.

**FIGURE 7-2    Firearm injuries**

readily borrowed from friends, bought by proxy, stolen, or even rented. On the street, guns can often be purchased by youth quite inexpensively.

The ready accessibility of firearms can be particularly dangerous for young people (see Figure 7-2). Harrington-Leuker explains that young people often use guns for solving seemingly trite problems: "a beef over something someone said, a fallout over a girl, a suspected slight, a pair of sneakers, a Raiders' jacket."[10] Guns are also increasingly being used by young people against older or larger children or teens who had a history of bullying or intimidating them. Thus, guns are used as an "equalizer," an equalizer that can readily be obtained by many youth.

Nearly 13% of school-age youth report knowing another student who has brought a gun to school.[11] The percentage of male high school students reporting carrying a gun in the past 30 days is 9%. A higher percentage of black male students (14.5%) carried a gun than Hispanic male (8.2%) and white male students (8%).[12]

## Personal and Peer Characteristics

It is common for young people who behave violently and aggressively to engage in other high-risk behaviors (e.g., alcohol abuse, illicit drug use, sexual promiscuity). Thus, youth who display violent behavior also share the following characteristics with youth engaging in other high-risk behaviors (e.g., substance abuse, sexual promiscuity):

❖ Early initiation of delinquent behavior

❖ Lack of parental support and guidance

❖ School failure

❖ Inability to resist peer influences

Violent children and adolescents often seem to not fit in with "mainstream" peers. They may feel rejected or isolated as a result of their displays of aggressive behavior. Or, they may have become aggressive in response to feeling left out or different. These feelings may be compounded by difficulties in learning. Early academic skill deficits and difficulty cause school failure and frustration. Thus, those experiencing this frustration do not "bond" to the school culture. Instead, they are more apt to bond with peers who are likewise experiencing school failure and who do not fit in with mainstream peers. Attachment to these peers often reinforces participation in violent behaviors and increases the likelihood of alienation from prosocial peers and institutions (e.g., school, church, youth groups). These factors also heighten the likelihood of gang involvement.

## Gang Involvement

Youth gang members are often actively involved in violent crime and behavior. Not only are gang members more likely to be involved in violent criminal activity as youth, but gang membership also prolongs one's involvement with violence into adulthood. Most youth gang members are male. However, there is concern that females are increasingly becoming involved in gangs.

Young people are attracted to gangs for many reasons. The primary attraction of gangs, however, is their ability to respond to youth needs that are not otherwise being met. For many youths, gangs become an extended family of sorts or even a surrogate family, where the banding together provides a sense of security. The gang also provides some youth with a sense of identity, belonging, power, and protection. Thus, young people lacking a sense of security are vulnerable to gang involvement. Among those feeling powerless and lacking control, gang activities become an outlet for their anger. Gangs may form among groups of recent immigrants and ethnic groups as a way of maintaining a strong ethnic identity.

## Early Warning Signs of Aggressive Rage or Violent Behavior Toward Self or Others*

It is not always possible to predict behavior that will lead to violence. However, educators and parents—and sometimes students—can recognize certain early warning signs. In some situations and for some youth, different combinations of events, behaviors, and emotions may lead to aggressive rage or violent behavior toward self or others. A good rule of thumb is

---

* This discussion and list of early warning signs is from the U.S. Department of Education, *Early Warning, Timely Response: A Guide to Safe Schools*, 1998. Available at http://www.ed.gov/offices/OSERS/OSEP/earlywrn.html.

to assume that these warning signs, especially when they are presented in combination, indicate a need for further analysis to determine an appropriate intervention.

We know from research that most children who become violent toward self or others feel rejected and psychologically victimized. In most cases, children exhibit aggressive behavior early in life and, if not provided support, will continue a progressive developmental pattern toward severe aggression or violence. However, research also shows that when children have a positive, meaningful connection to an adult—whether it be at home, in school, or in the community—the potential for violence is reduced significantly.

None of these signs alone is sufficient for predicting aggression and violence. Morever, it is inappropriate—and potentially harmful—to use the early warning signs as a checklist against which to match individual children. Rather, the early warning signs are offered only as an aid in identifying and referring children who may need help. School communities must ensure that staff and students only use the early warning signs for identification and referral purposes. Only trained professionals should make diagnoses in consultation with the child's parents or guardian.

The early warning signs below are presented with the following qualifications: They are not equally significant and they are not presented in order of seriousness. The early warning signs include the following:

❖ *Social withdrawal.* In some situations, gradual and eventually complete withdrawal from social contacts can be an important indicator of a troubled child. The withdrawal often stems from feelings of depression, rejection, persecution, unworthiness, and lack of confidence.

❖ *Excessive feelings of isolation and being alone.* Research has shown that the majority of children who are isolated and appear to be friendless are not violent. In fact, these feelings are sometimes characteristic of children and youth who may be troubled, withdrawn, or have internal issues that hinder development of social affiliations. However, research also has shown that in some cases feelings of isolation and not having friends are associated with children who behave aggressively and violently.

❖ *Excessive feelings of rejection.* In the process of growing up, and in the course of adolescent development, many young people experience emotionally painful rejection. Children who are troubled often are isolated from their mentally healthy peers. Their responses to rejection will depend on many background factors. Without support, they may be at risk of expressing their emotional distress in negative ways, including violence. Some aggressive children who are rejected by nonaggressive peers seek out aggressive friends who, in turn, reinforce their violent tendencies.

❖ *Being a victim of violence.* Children who are victims of violence—including physical or sexual abuse—in the community, at school, or at home are sometimes at risk themselves of becoming violent toward themselves or others.

❖ *Feelings of being picked on and persecuted.* The youth who feels constantly picked on, teased, bullied, singled out for ridicule, and humiliated at home or at school may initially withdraw socially. If not given adequate support in addressing these feelings, some children may vent them in inappropriate ways, including possible aggression or violence.

❖ *Low school interest and poor academic performance.* Poor school achievement can be the result of many factors. It is important to consider whether there is a drastic change in performance and if poor performance has become a chronic condition that limits the child's capacity to learn. In some situations—such as when the low achiever feels frustrated, unworthy, chastised, and denigrated—acting out and aggressive behaviors may occur. It is important to assess the emotional and cognitive reasons for the change in academic performance to determine the true nature of the problem.

❖ *Expression of violence in writings and feelings.* Children and youth often express their thoughts, feelings, desires, and intentions in their drawings and in stories, poetry, and other written expressive forms. Many children produce work about violent themes that for the most part is harmless when taken in context. However, an overrepresentation of violence in writings and drawings that is directed at specific individuals (family members, peers, other adults) consistently over time may signal emotional problems and the potential for violence. Because there is a real danger in misdiagnosing such a sign, it is important to seek the guidance of a qualified professional, such as a school psychologist, counselor, or other mental health specialist, to determine its meaning.

❖ *Uncontrolled anger.* Everyone gets angry; anger is a natural emotion. However, anger that is expressed frequently and intensely in response to minor irritants may signal potential violent behavior toward self and others.

❖ *Patterns of impulsive and chronic hitting, intimidating, and bullying behavior.* Children often engage in acts of shoving and mild aggression. However, some mildly aggressive behaviors, such as the constant hitting and bullying of others that occur early in children's lives, if left unattended might later escalate into more serious behaviors.

❖ *History of discipline problems.* Chronic behavior and disciplinary problems both in school and at home may suggest that underlying emotional needs are not being met. These unmet needs may be manifested in acting-out and aggressive behaviors. These problems may set the stage for the child to violate norms and rules, defy authority, disengage from school, and engage in aggressive behaviors with other children and adults.

❖ *Past history of violent and aggressive behavior.* Unless provided with support and counseling, a youth who has a history of aggressive or violent behavior is likely to repeat those behaviors. Aggressive and violent acts may be directed toward other individuals, be expressed in cruelty to animals, or include fire setting. Youths who show an early pattern of antisocial behavior frequently and across multiple settings are particularly at risk for future aggressive and antisocial behavior. Similarly, youth who engage in overt behaviors—such as bullying, generalized aggression, and defiance—and covert behaviors—such as stealing, vandalism, lying, cheating, and fire setting—also are at risk for more serious aggressive behavior. Research suggests that the age of onset may be a key factor in interpreting early warning signs. For example, children who engage in aggression and drug abuse at an early age (before age 12) are more likely to show violence later on than are children who begin such behavior at an older age. In the presence of such signs it is important to review the child's history with behavioral experts and seek parents' observations and insights.

❖ *Intolerance for differences and prejudicial attitudes.* All children have likes and dislikes. However, an intense prejudice toward others based on racial, ethnic, religious, language, gender, sexual orientation, ability, and physical appearance, when coupled with other factors, may lead to violent assaults against those who are perceived to be different. Membership in hate groups or the willingness to victimize individuals with disabilities or health problems also should be treated as early warning signs.

❖ *Drug and alcohol use.* Apart from being unhealthy behaviors, alcohol and other drug use reduces self-control and exposes children and youth to violence, either as perpetrators, as victims, or both.

❖ *Affiliation with gangs.* Gangs that support antisocial values and behaviors—including extortion, intimidation, and acts of violence toward other students—cause fear and stress among other students. Youth who are influenced by these groups—those who emulate and copy their behavior, as well as those who become affiliated with them—may adopt these values and act in violent or aggressive ways in certain situations. Gang-related violence and turf battles are common occurrences tied to the use of drugs that often result in injury and/or death.

❖ *Inappropriate access to, possession of, and use of firearms.* Children and youth who inappropriately possess or have access to firearms can have an increased risk for violence. Research shows that such youngsters also have a higher probability of becoming victims. Families can reduce inappropriate access and use by restricting, monitoring, and supervising children's access to firearms and other weapons. Children who have a history of aggression, impulsiveness, or other emotional problems should not have access to firearms and other weapons.

❖ *Serious threats of violence.* Idle threats are a common response to frustration. Alternatively, one of the most reliable indicators that a youth is likely to commit a dangerous act toward self or others is a detailed and specific threat to use violence. Recent incidents across the country clearly indicate that threats to commit violence against oneself or others should be taken very seriously. Steps must be taken to understand the nature of these threats and to prevent them from being carried out.

## Effects of Violence on Youth

Beyond the obvious threat that violence poses to children's personal safety, violence also poses another potential problem for youth. The threat of violence can adversely interfere with a child's development and learning potential. When children constantly confront the threat of violence at home, school, and/or in the community, they must learn to protect themselves by setting up defenses against their fears. These defenses take considerable emotional energy, robbing from the energy needed for other developmental tasks, including learning in school.

The presence of violence in the home is often associated with feelings of guilt and responsibility by children and consequent feelings of being bad or worthless. These feelings are not compatible with a child's potential for learning and commonly result in the feeling that one is incapable of learning. This, in turn, contributes to a lack of motivation to achieve in school.

Children who face the threat of violence, or who have suffered trauma from violence, have difficulty seeing themselves in meaningful future roles. Children who cannot perceive a positive and secure future for themselves are unable to give serious attention and energy to the tasks of learning and socialization. The unpredictablity of violence contributes to a sense of little or no control over one's life. Such a sense of helplessness interferes with the development of autonomy, which is essential for healthy growth and maturation.

## Bullying in Schools

Bullying is a form of violence that needs to be addressed because it is a prevalent form of violence among youth and can have long-lasting consequences. **Bullying** is the repeated infliction or attempted infliction of injury, discomfort, or humiliation on a weaker student by one or more students with more power. A wide range of physical or verbal behaviors of an aggressive nature are encompassed by the term *bullying*, including threatening, humiliating, insulting, teasing, harassing, abusing physically and verbally, and mobbing. Bullying differs from normal quarreling, teasing, childhood "rough play," or conflict because it is prolonged and there is a power differential between the bully and the victim (e.g., bullies are often physically larger and stronger). Bullies find enjoyment in harassing the same victims. Most bullying goes unreported because victims feel that nothing will be done and that they might receive greater retaliation the next time. Also, others watching bullying may fear reporting it because they might lose their social status or also become victims.

Bullying is common on school playgrounds, in neighborhoods, and in homes. A recent study investigated the prevalence of bullying among school children. Results indicated that 1 of 10 (10.6%) U.S. students in grades 6 through 10 has been bullied, and 13% have reported bullying others.[13]

Bullies tend to pick on those who appear vulnerable in one way or another. Students who are perceived as different in some way or who don't seem to fit in are at increased risk. Children who are fatter, skinnier, wear glasses or braces, have speech impediments, have a learning or physical disability, or differ in other personal characteristics are common victims of bullying. Victims are usually passive, anxious, sensitive, quiet, easily intimidated, avoid confrontation, and have a difficult time defending and standing up for themselves. They tend to have few friends they can rely upon to help them stand up to the harassment they receive. Gay, lesbian, and bisexual students and those perceived to be gay by their peers are often targeted by bullies for repeated verbal abuse and physical assault.

Victims of bullying suffer humiliation, insecurity, and loss of self-esteem. They may suffer physical injury as a result of the bullying. It is hard to concentrate on schoolwork if being bullied, and academic performance can suffer as a result. They may develop a fear of going to school and attempt to avoid school altogether. They may avoid public areas of the school, such as the cafeteria, restrooms, playground, or school buses, in order to stay clear of bullies. They might not participate in extracurricular activities because of the same fear. Students who are repeatedly victims of such abuse and assaults are at increased risk for mental health problems such as depression or suicide. Some retaliate to the enduring abuse in a violent way. Being a victim of severe bullying has been noted in the news media as a contributing factor in shootings at Columbine High School in Littleton, Colorado, in 1999, and Santana High School in Santee, California, in 2001, and in other acts of youth violence.[14] The psychological scars from being bullied often last into adulthood.

Children and adolescents who bully thrive on controlling and dominating others. They achieve a sense of accomplishment and esteem from causing weaker students distress or harm. They have often been victims of physical abuse or bullying themselves. Bullying is often the beginning of antisocial and rule-breaking behavior that can extend into adulthood.

Those who bully are also involved in other forms of antisocial behavior such as vandalism, shoplifting, skipping and dropping out of school, fighting, and the use of alcohol and other drugs. Bullying behavior in childhood or adolescence is also linked with participation in criminal behavior as adults.[14] Students who bully need intervention in an effort to prevent serious academic, social, emotional, and legal difficulties for the individual student and his or her family.

Schools should not condone or tolerate bullying. They can actively work to stop and prevent bullying behavior. School staff, students, and parents can work together to raise awareness about bullying, improve peer relations, intervene to stop intimidation, develop clear rules against bullying behavior, and support and protect victims. A highly effective bullying prevention program achieved reductions in bullying among elementary, middle, and junior high school students by instituting the following:[14]

- ❖ Determination of the nature and prevalence of the school's bullying problem by surveying students anonymously

- ❖ Increased supervision of students during breaks

- ❖ Schoolwide assemblies to discuss bullying

- ❖ Regular classroom meetings with students to discuss bullying

- ❖ Establishment and enforcement of classroom rules against bullying

- ❖ Staff intervention with bullies, victims, and their parents to ensure that the bullying stops

Lumsden makes some other suggestions for preventing and counteracting bullying:[15]

- ❖ Developing and distributing a written antibullying policy to everyone in the school community that sends the message that bullying will not be tolerated, and then fairly and consistently applying the policy (some states are now mandating policies)

- ❖ Mapping a school's "hot spots" for bullying incidents so that supervision can be concentrated where it is needed most

- ❖ Asking teachers to stand in the doorways of their classrooms during passing time so that the halls are well supervised

- ❖ Teaching bullies positive behavior through modeling, coaching, prompting, praise, and other forms of reinforcement

- ❖ Teaching students social skills, conflict management, anger management, and character education

- ❖ Using role-play situations in which counselors present students with provocative situations and help them recognize the difference between a "hot response" and a "cool response"

❖ Having students sign antiteasing or antibullying pledges

❖ Sending bystanders of bullying situations to after-school mediation

❖ Having students and their parents sign contracts at the beginning of the school year acknowledging that they understand it is unacceptable to ridicule, taunt, or attempt to hurt other students

❖ Teaching respect and nonviolence beginning in elementary school

## Violence and Abusive Behavior Prevention

Schools are a strategic setting for preventing violent and abusive behavior. Schools have the responsibility for providing a safe and violence-free environment for all school-age youth, school personnel, and others on school premises. Educators can also counter violence by providing students and families with violence prevention curricula. Intervention for troubled youth must also be addressed in such a way that there is adequate support in getting help for these youth.

It is important to note that the solution to violence does not just rest with schools. Solutions must be engineered that are communitywide and coordinated. This effort requires a shared responsibility between schools, families, courts, law enforcement, community agencies, community churches, business, and the broader community.

### Safe and Violence-Free School Environment

From California to New York, schools are grappling with how to protect children and school staff from violence. In the 1997–1998 school year, children as young as 11 years gunned down classmates and teachers in mass shootings at schools in Mississippi, Kentucky, Arkansas, and Oregon, leaving 13 dead and 45 wounded. In April of 1999, two high school students in Littleton, Colorado, planted approximately 30 pipe bombs, shot and killed 12 students and a teacher, and wounded 23 students before committing suicide. Episodes such as these have heightened violence as a major school concern across the nation—a concern that is no longer limited to large cities, but extends to suburbs, smaller cities, and rural areas as well.

Teachers are increasingly feeling threatened by the possibility of violence. The resulting fear has a negative impact on the ability of teachers to effectively teach students. It has been estimated that one in five teachers has been threatened by students.

Violence prevention begins by making sure the school campus is a safe and caring place. Compared to home and other settings, school is one of the safest places where young people spend their time. However, the tragic episodes of violence that have occurred on school campuses across the nation point out that no school and community can afford to be complacent about making and keeping schools safe. Schools must commit to policies that ensure a maximum effort to keep schools safe for students, staff, and others on school premises.

***School Security Measures***    As noted previously, guns and other weapons are readily accessible to many youth. Schools must ensure that weapons are not carried onto school premises and that students remain safe at school. When weapons are carried into schools, especially firearms, the potential for violent episodes to occur is heightened. In recent years, there have been far too many violent episodes involving weapons on school campuses that have led to tragedy.

Providing a safe and violence-free school requires school districts to consider such provisions and controls as locker searches, hiring security guards or police to patrol school premises, and possibly metal detectors that students must pass before entry.[16] Some schools have eliminated lockers altogether. Some have even eliminated book bags, providing instead one set of books to be used in class and another at home. Other schools require transparent book bags. Some schools employ uniformed security guards and/or install hallway cameras to monitor students. Some school systems have even created separate alternative schools for young people with a history of violent and abusive behavior. Although this option is attracting attention as a means to deal with violence, it is also controversial.

The 1999 school massacre in Littleton, Colorado, mentioned at the beginning of this section led many schools to make sweeping reforms and improvements in security procedures. Then the events of September 11, 2001, gave school officials more to worry about in terms of school security—possible terrorist attacks. In the wake of the World Trade Center and Pentagon attacks, some schools had bomb threats and anthrax scares to deal with. Although these turned out to be hoaxes, schools realized that they must be in a heightened state of alert for the possibility of terrorist acts in schools.

***Gun Free Schools Act***    Educators must be familiar with their state's laws regarding the carrying of firearms onto school premises. The **Gun Free Schools Act** requires that each state receiving federal funds under the Elementary and Secondary Act (ESEA) must have put in effect, by October 1995, a state law requiring local educational agencies to expel from school for a period of not less than one year a student who is determined to have brought a firearm to school. Each state's law also must allow the chief administering officer of the local educational agency to modify the expulsion requirement on a case-by-case basis. All local educational agencies receiving these funds must also have a policy that requires referral of any student who brings a firearm to school to the criminal justice or juvenile justice system.[17]

***Discipline and Dress Codes***    School officials may consider discipline and dress codes as strategies to curb violence. These codes must be crafted collaboratively by administrators, teachers, parents, and students and be reviewed by the district's legal staff so that they are in accordance with state law. An effective discipline and dress code clearly explains to students what behavior is acceptable and the policies for dealing with students who break the rules. Discipline and dress codes must be firmly, fairly, and consistently implemented and enforced. Every student, parent, and teacher must be given a copy of the discipline and dress code.

***Characteristics of a Safe Physical Environment***    The U.S. Department of Education's *Early Warning, Timely Response: A Guide to Safe Schools* suggests that school officials can enhance physical safety by doing the following:[17]

❖ Supervising access to the building and grounds.

❖ Reducing class size and school size.

❖ Adjusting scheduling to minimize time in the hallways or in potentially dangerous locations. Traffic flow patterns can be modified to limit potential for conflicts or altercations.

❖ Conducting a building safety audit in consultation with school security personnel and/or law enforcement experts. Effective schools adhere to federal, state, and local nondiscrimination and public safety laws, and use guidelines set by the state department of education.

❖ Closing school campuses during lunch periods.

❖ Adopting a school policy on school uniforms.

❖ Arranging supervision at critical times (e.g., in hallways between classes) and having a plan to deploy supervisory staff to areas where incidents are likely to occur.

❖ Prohibiting students from congregating in areas where they are likely to engage in rule-breaking or intimidating and aggressive behaviors.

❖ Having adults visibly present throughout the school building. This includes encouraging parents to visit the school.

❖ Staggering dismissal times and lunch periods.

❖ Monitoring the surrounding school grounds—including landscaping, parking lots, and bus stops.

❖ Coordinating with local police to ensure that there are safe routes to and from school.

❖ Identifying safe areas where staff and students should go in the event of a crisis.

The physical condition of the school building also has an impact on student attitude, behavior, and motivation to achieve. Typically, there tend to be more incidents of fighting and violence in school buildings that are dirty, too cold or too hot, filled with graffiti, in need of repair, or unsanitary.

***Identification of Warning Signs of School Violence***    Earlier in this chapter we presented several early warning signs of violence. An important aspect of effective violence prevention is having school personnel who are trained to recognize these signs. Schools should take special care in training all school personnel to understand and identify early warning signs. This is critical because these early warning signs can signal a troubled child and indicate that a student may need help. They may also indicate that the child is prone to violence toward self or others. When early warning signs are observed, teachers should be concerned, but should not overreact and jump to conclusions. In no way should early warning signs be used to exclude, isolate, or punish a child. Neither should children be inappropriately labeled or stigmatized because they have a set of early warning indicators.

When observing **early warning signs,** the educator's first and foremost responsibility should be to get early help for a child. Teachers and administrators are not professionally trained to deal with these issues. Professionals such as school psychologists, social workers, counselors, and nurses can help. Referrals to outside agencies or professionals may be necessary. Keep in mind that all referrals to outside agencies based on early warning signs must be kept confidential and be done with parental consent (except referrals for suspected child abuse or neglect).

Educators can increase their ability to recognize early warning signs by establishing close, caring, and supportive relationships with students. This requires getting to know students well enough to be aware of their needs, feelings, attitudes, and behavior patterns.

Unlike early warning signs, **imminent warning signs** indicate that a student is very close to behaving in a way that is potentially dangerous to self and/or others. Imminent warning signs require an immediate response. No single warning sign can predict that a dangerous act will occur. Rather, imminent warning signs usually are presented as a sequence of overt, serious, hostile, behaviors or threats directed at peers, staff, or other individuals. Usually imminent warning signs are evident to more than one staff member, as well as to the child's family. Imminent warning signs may include:

- ❖ Serious physical fighting with peers or family members

- ❖ Severe destruction of property

- ❖ Severe rage for seemingly minor reasons

- ❖ Detailed threats of lethal violence

- ❖ Possession and/or use of firearms and other weapons

❖ Other self-injurious behaviors or threats of suicide

When warning signs indicate that danger is imminent, safety must always be the first and foremost consideration. Action must be taken immediately. Immediate intervention by school authorities and possibly law enforcement officers is needed whenever a child:

❖ Has presented a detailed plan (time, place, method) to harm or kill others, particularly if the child has a history of aggression or has attempted to carry out threats in the past

❖ Is carrying a weapon, particularly a firearm, and has threatened to use it

In situations where students present other threatening behaviors, parents should be informed of the concerns immediately. Schools also have the responsibility to seek assistance from appropriate agencies such as child and family services and community mental health. These responses should reflect school board policies.

## Educational and Curricular Approaches to Violence Prevention

A variety of educational approaches are used in schools to prevent violence. Curricula have been developed for various grade levels that seek to increase knowledge about violence, encourage nonviolent attitudes, and to instill interpersonal skills that reduce the propensity for violent behavior. Various school-based educational interventions have been designed to modify such behavioral factors associated with violent behavior as weapon carrying, poor anger management, ineffective conflict management, poor communication skills, and substance use.

***Elements of Promising Violence Prevention Programs***    Several experts in the area of school-based violence prevention were interviewed to identify approaches that are most promising and effective. The researchers conducting the study identified the following nine critical elements of promising violence prevention programs:[18]

1. A comprehensive, multifaceted approach that includes family, peer, media, and community components was viewed by experts as critically important.

2. Programs should begin in the primary grades and be reinforced across grade levels.

3. Developmentally tailored interventions are important.

4. Programs should promote personal and social competencies (skills) such as anger management, decision making, active listening, effective communication, and resisting peer pressure.

5. Interactive techniques, such as group work, cooperative learning, discussions, and role-plays or behavioral rehearsal, facilitate the development of personal and social skills.

6. Ethnic identity/culturally sensitive material should be matched with the characteristics of the target population.

7. Staff development/teacher training ensures that a program will be implemented as intended by the program developers.

8. Activities designed to promote a positive school climate or culture should be elements of effective classroom management strategies promoting good discipline, because positive control in the classroom is essential to effective implementation of violence prevention programs.

9. Activities should be designed to foster norms against violence, aggression, and bullying.

The experts also identified the following six components of violence prevention programs that show little promise, could possibly increase aggressive behavior or violence, or can be counterproductive:

1. Using scare tactics that show pictures or videos of violent scenes

2. Adding a violence prevention program to a school system that is already overwhelmed

3. Segregating aggressive or antisocial students into a separate group for any purpose

4. Using instructional programs that are too brief and not supported by a positive school climate

5. Using programs that focus exclusively on self-esteem enhancement

6. Using programs that only provide information and do not help students develop skills to avoid and deal with conflict

The surgeon general's report on youth violence strongly advocates rigorous evaluation of prevention programs.[1] Although hundreds of prevention programs are being used in schools and communities throughout the country, little is known about the effects of most of them. The report states that nearly half of the most thoroughly evaluated strategies for preventing violence had been shown to be ineffective, and a few were known to harm participants. On the other hand, a number of youth violence intervention and prevention programs have demonstrated that they are effective, dispelling assertions that "nothing works." Most highly effective programs combine components that address both individual risks and environmental conditions, particularly building individual skills and competencies, parent effectiveness training, improving the social climate of the school, and changes in type and level of involvement with peer groups. In schools, interventions that target change in the social context appear to be more effective on average than those that attempt to change individual attitudes, skills, and risk behaviors. Involvement with delinquent peers and gang membership are two of the most powerful predictors of violence, yet few interventions have been developed to address these problems. Another factor relating to effectiveness is the quality of program implementation. Many programs are ineffective not because their strategy is misguided, but because the quality of implementation is poor.

***Personal and Social Skills Competencies Training***  Youth displaying aggressive and violent behavior usually have personal and social skill deficiencies in many areas. For this reason, educators should consider a skills training approach when selecting or developing violence prevention and reduction curricula and programs. Personal and social skills are best taught through approaches that incorporate modeling, role-playing, performance feedback, and adequate time for practicing the skills. Personal and social skills that youth may need training in could include any of the following:

- ❖ Initiating and carrying on a conversation
- ❖ Listening to others
- ❖ Introducing oneself to other people
- ❖ Giving compliments
- ❖ Saying thank you and showing appreciation
- ❖ Joining in activities and conversations
- ❖ Apologizing
- ❖ Asking for help
- ❖ Recognizing feelings
- ❖ Empathy for others' feelings
- ❖ Dealing with anger
- ❖ Resolving conflict
- ❖ Asking permission
- ❖ Negotiation
- ❖ Making a complaint
- ❖ Assertiveness
- ❖ Responding to teasing
- ❖ Dealing with embarrassment

❖ Dealing with being left out

❖ Dealing with peer and group pressure

❖ Responding to persuasion

❖ Setting goals

❖ Making decisions

***Conflict Resolution***     The inability to solve conflicts in an appropriate manner often leads to physical fighting or other forms of violent behavior. Many educators advocate teaching **conflict resolution skills** to children as a means of reducing their risk of perpetration of and victimization from violence. If children can effectively be taught to solve problems and conflicts in an appropriate manner, nonviolent patterns of behavior may be established that have potential of preventing violence and violent injury.

Conflict resolution skills are best learned by children when they are not caught up in the heat of their own conflicts and must be practiced over a wide range of contexts to be meaningful. Also, children need ample opportunity to practice these skills in a trusting and supportive environment. Such an environment helps children to talk about the conflicts they are having and provides a setting in which classmates can help each other with problem solving. For young children, puppets can be used for role-playing the range of conflict resolution skills, which includes defining the problem, negotiating, finding win-win solutions, and acting them out. In teaching conflict resolution, teachers can help students:

❖ Understand the problems that cause their conflicts in terms that make sense to them

❖ See that their conflicts have two sides and show the two viewpoints in the context of an immediate problem

❖ Realize what led up to a conflict and how each action taken affects the other person(s)

❖ See the whole problem and how their behavior contributed to it

❖ Retrospectively look at specific actions that led to a conflict and the effects of their actions

❖ Think of what will happen in a conflict if it is allowed to continue

❖ Think of potential solutions and think through negative and positive consequences of each, while taking into account both sides of the conflict

❖ Think of win-win solutions by suggesting various ways children can share positive solutions that worked for them in the past

❖ Provide opportunities to reflect on actions, acknowledge success, and give others ideas about how to solve conflicts

***Anger Management***    It is important to talk to young people about anger. Too often, children and adolescents come to believe that it is inappropriate to feel anger. Teachers can reinforce that anger is a normal emotion that can be expressed in constructive ways. It should be stressed to students that they are responsible for managing their anger.

Students need to become aware of how they experience and express their anger. They should recognize that there are physical responses to anger. Anger creates tension and stress. Building tension causes a release of hormones into the bloodstream that prepare the body for fight or flight. The heart beats faster, there is an increase in blood pressure, and breathing quickens. More blood is sent to the muscles, and these muscles become tense in anticipation of an emergency. Verbal responses to anger might include making sarcastic remarks, raising one's voice, and making put-downs. Recognizing these physical and verbal signals is important so that students can make decisions about how to respond to their anger before it takes over. They also need to become aware of which thoughts and/or situations trigger them to feel anger.

Self-control is an important aspect of anger management. Individuals respond behaviorally to anger in many different ways. Teachers need to emphasize that one's behavioral response to anger is a choice. Behavioral responses such as physical aggression or holding the anger in are usually destructive.

Like any other social skills, effective anger management skills can be learned. Skills training programs that incorporate modeling, role-playing, performance feedback, and adequate time for practice are most effective in helping students acquire anger management skills.

## Responding to Crises*

Effective schools create a violence prevention and response plan and form a team that can ensure it is implemented. The plan outlines how all individuals in the school and community (administrators, teachers, parents, students, bus drivers, support staff) will be prepared to spot the behavioral and emotional signs that indicate a child is troubled, and what they will need to do. The plan also details how school and community resources can be used to create safe environments and manage responses to threats and incidents of violence.

Because violence can happen at any time and anywhere, schools must be well prepared for any potential crisis or violent act. Crisis response is an

---

* This section is adapted from the U.S. Department of Education, *Early Warning, Timely Response: A Guide to Safe Schools*, 1998. Available at http://www.ed.gov/offices/OSERS/OSEP/earlywrn.html.

important component of a violence prevention and response plan. The two components that should be addressed in that plan are (1) intervening during a crisis to ensure safety and (2) responding in the aftermath of tragedy.

## Crisis Intervention Planning

**Crisis planning** prepares students and school staff for what to do when violence strikes. Crisis planning should include the following:

❖ Training for teachers and staff in a range of skills, from dealing with escalating classroom situations to responding to a serious crisis.

❖ Reference to district or state procedures. Many states now have recommended crisis manuals available to their local education agencies and schools.

❖ Involvement of community agencies, including police, fire, and rescue, as well as hospital, health, social welfare, and mental health services. The faith community, juvenile justice, and related family support systems also have been successfully included in such plans.

❖ Provision to the core team (the group of individuals who oversee the preparation and implementation of the prevention and response plan) to meet regularly to identify potentially troubled or violent students and situations that may be dangerous.

Effective schools also have made a point to find out about federal, state, and local resources that are available to help during and after a crisis, and to secure their support and involvement before a crisis occurs.

## Intervening During a Crisis to Ensure Safety

Weapons used in or around schools, bomb threats or explosions, and fights, as well as natural disasters, accidents, and suicides call for immediate, planned action and long-term, postcrisis intervention. Planning for such contingencies reduces chaos and trauma. The crisis response part of the plan also must include contingency provisions such as these:

❖ Evacuation procedures and other procedures to protect students and staff from harm. It is critical that schools identify safe areas where students and staff should go in a crisis. It is also important that schools practice having staff and students evacuate the premises in an orderly manner.

❖ An effective, foolproof communication system. Individuals must have designated roles and responsibilities to prevent confusion.

❖ A process for securing immediate external support from law enforcement officials and other relevant community agencies.

Just as staff should understand and practice fire drill procedures routinely, they should practice responding to the presence of firearms and other weapons, severe threats of violence, hostage situations, and other acts of terror. Schools can provide staff and students with such practice in the following ways:

❖ Provide inservice training for all faculty and staff to explain the plan and exactly what to do in a crisis. Where appropriate, include community police, youth workers, and other community members.

❖ Produce a written manual or small pamphlet or flip chart to remind teachers and staff of their duties.

❖ Practice responding to the imminent warning signs of violence. Make sure all adults in the building have an understanding of what they might do to prevent violence (e.g., being observant, knowing when to get help, and modeling good problem solving, anger management, and/or conflict resolution skills) and how they can safely support each other.

## Responding in the Aftermath of Crisis

Members of the crisis team should understand natural stress reactions. They should also be familiar with how different individuals might respond to death and loss, including developmental considerations, religious beliefs, and cultural values.

Effective schools ensure a coordinated community response. Professionals both within the school district and within the greater community should be involved to assist individuals who are at risk for severe stress reactions.

Schools that have experienced tragedy have included the following provisions in their response plans:

❖ *Help parents understand children's reactions to violence.* In the aftermath of tragedy, children may experience unrealistic fears of the future, have difficulty sleeping, become physically ill, and be easily distracted. These are a few of the common reactions.

❖ *Help teachers and other staff deal with their reactions to the crisis.* Debriefing and grief counseling are just as important for adults as they are for students.

❖ *Help students and faculty adjust after the crisis.* Provide both short-term and long-term mental health counseling following a crisis.

❖ *Help victims and family members of victims reenter the school environment.* Often school friends need guidance in how to act. The school should work with students and parents to design a plan that makes it easier for victims and their classmates to adjust.

❖ *Help students and teachers address the return of a previously removed student to the school.* Whether the student is returning from a juvenile detention facility or a mental health facility, schools need to coordinate with staff from that facility to explore how to make the transition as uneventful as possible.

## Child Abuse

The National Committee to Prevent Child Abuse reports that each year more than 3 million children are reported as victims of child abuse and neglect to child protective service (CPS) agencies in the United States.[19] Reports of child abuse have increased approximately 40% in the past 10 years. About 47 of every 1,000 children are reported as victims of child maltreatment.[20]

There are many forms of child abuse. **Physical abuse** is nonaccidental physical injury to a child. **Physical neglect** is the failure of a child's caretaker to provide adequate food, clothing, shelter, or supervision. **Emotional maltreatment** is belittling and rejecting the child—not providing a positive emotional atmosphere. **Sexual abuse** is the sexual exploitation of a child done for the gratification of an adult (or older child).

Teachers and school administrators are required by law to report suspected abuse to appropriate child protective agencies. Because mandatory reporting statutes vary from state to state, it is imperative that you become familiar with the specifics of the law within the state where you teach. Information about state child abuse laws is available from your school superintendent's office or your state attorney general's office. Teachers reporting suspected child abuse without malice are generally immune from prosecution for any civil or criminal damages that may result from the report.

Child abuse is frequently identified by school personnel in the classroom or school setting. This is possible because children spend a large part of their day in school, placing teachers and other school personnel in the position of being able to observe the signs and symptoms of abuse. The Carnegie Foundation for the Advancement of Teaching estimates that nearly 90% of teachers see abused or neglected children in their classrooms. However, teachers are often reluctant to report suspected cases of abuse. Reluctance may stem from a variety of reasons, including the following:

❖ Fear of getting involved in the situation

❖ Concern about interfering with private family relationships and child-rearing practices

❖ Anxiety about a parent's potential retaliation

❖ Wariness of alienating families

❖ Inadequate training regarding child abuse identification and reporting

These factors underscore the necessity of quality inservice and preservice training for school teachers regarding child abuse issues. Inservice and preservice training for teachers (as well as the entire school staff) should consist of the following:

❖ Identification and reporting of child abuse

❖ Coping with disclosures

❖ Legal and ethical issues

❖ Family dynamics

❖ Interviewing children

❖ Confidentiality

❖ Implications for child development

❖ Treatment approaches

## Child Sexual Abuse

Child sexual abuse usually involves the engagement of a child in sexual activity through the use of bribes, subtle deceits, threats, or outright force. While some child sexual abuse involves sexual intercourse, most cases of child sexual abuse do not. Child sexual abuse can take the form of genital handling, oral-genital contact, sexual abuse of the breasts or anus, or requiring a child to undress and/or look at the genitals of adults. Sexual abuse typically involves less force than adult rape. Children often comply with the wishes of their abusers because of their smallness of physical stature, their innocence, and the persuasive powers of abusers. Sexual contact between relatives is **incest,** often a part of sexual abuse.

In many cases, child sexual abuse is not limited to a single episode. Many children are repeatedly abused and victimized over periods of months or even years. Sexual offenders against children often have abused many children before they are discovered. Those who abuse children are most frequently individuals with whom the child is familiar or acquainted. Often the abuser is a parent or other family relative, neighbor, family friend, baby-sitter, or day-care worker. Child sexual abuse is more likely to occur in the home of the child victim than in any other place. A small percentage of sexual abuse cases involves strangers to the child. Yet, ironically, most child sexual abuse prevention programs focus upon "stranger dangers." Consequently, few children learn about the possibility of assault by a relative or friend.

Those who abuse children were very often abused themselves as children. Thus, there is a vicious cycle in which the abused grow up to be abusers. Interestingly, boys who are abused are far more likely to turn into eventual offenders, and girls are more likely to produce children who are abused by others (possibly because they tend to associate with males who are abusive).

Abusers also typically have low self-esteem and suffer from poor impulse control. Alcohol abuse is also common among abusers of children. It seems that more prevention efforts should be directed toward helping abused children to not become abusers themselves, in order to break this cycle of abuse. This would entail activities such as assertiveness training, self-esteem enhancement activities, parenting skills development, and substance abuse prevention and treatment.

It is imperative that educators understand that under no circumstances is child sexual abuse ever the fault of an involved child. At the same time, educators should understand that the following characteristics in children may make them more vulnerable to victimization:

❖ Children who are poorly supervised

❖ Children whose care is entrusted to someone who has a substance abuse problem

❖ Children with low self-esteem

❖ Children who have been taught to blindly obey adults

❖ Children who are hungry for affection

❖ Children who are lonely

Reported cases of child sexual abuse represent only the tip of the sexual abuse "iceberg." Because sexual abuse is largely a secretive act, most occurrences go unreported. Also, offenders are likely to force, bribe, coerce, threaten, or deceive child victims to prevent them from telling. As a result, it is difficult to determine with certainty the number of children who are sexually abused, and estimates vary widely. However, studies show that 20% to 27% of adult women and 5% to 16% of adult men report that they experienced some form of sexual abuse as children.[21]

In 1996, President Clinton signed **Megan's Law,** which compels each state to make private and personal information on convicted high-risk sex offenders available to the public and local law enforcement agencies. The law allows each state discretion in establishing the criteria for this disclosure of information. This law offers citizens information on the whereabouts of sex offenders that they can use in taking steps to protect their children from victimization. Parents must be informed when a sex offender is released from prison and moves into their local area. The law authorizes local law enforcement authorities to notify the public about high-risk and serious sex offenders who reside in, are employed in, or frequent a particular community. Sex offenders are responsible under law to register their address with the local police upon release from prison and when moving to a new residence. Yet, many provide false information and fail to notify authorities when changing residences. Some who give correct information travel outside of the area to prey on children living in other areas, where no one has been warned about them.

Megan's Law takes different forms in different states. States differ in terms of registration and reregistration requirements. Some states list information about sex offenders on the Internet, allowing parents to check the registry to see if anyone on it has moved into their area. On the other hand, a state like California does not make this information available on the Internet out of concerns regarding legal disputes. Instead, this state distributes a CD-ROM that citizens, except for registered sex offenders, can view at a local sheriff or police department. The CD-ROM identifies more than 64,000 convicted sex offenders. In some states, law enforcement officers can call every residence in an area to warn about a sex offender who has moved in.

### Effects of Child Sexual Abuse

Many serious initial and long-term emotional, behavioral, and physical effects can result from child sexual abuse. Some of the immediate or initial emotional effects are:

- Fear and anxiety
- Anger and hostility
- Guilt
- Depression
- Withdrawal

Initial behavioral effects include:

- Sleeping and eating disturbances
- Persistent, inappropriate sexual behavior with self, peers, younger children, or toys
- Detailed and precocious understanding of sexual behavior
- Regressive behaviors
- Inability to make friends
- Inadequate peer relations

❖ Overly compliant or acting-out behavior

❖ Pseudomature behavior

❖ Inability to concentrate

❖ Sudden decrease in school achievement and performance

❖ Running away from home

❖ Suicidal ideation or actual attempts

❖ An extraordinary fear of males (in girls)

❖ Overly seductive behavior

Initial physical effects include:

❖ Sexually transmitted diseases

❖ Frequent urinary infections

❖ Pregnancy

❖ Difficulty walking or sitting

❖ Pain or itching in genital area

❖ Bruises or bleeding in external genitalia

❖ Headaches, rashes, vomiting—all without medical explanation

All children do not react identically to child sexual abuse. The degree to which a child is harmed emotionally is dependent upon a number of factors, for example, the age of the child, the nature and duration of the offense, the relationship between the victim and the offender, and the manner in which the abuse is handled by others. There is a definite connection to being abused as a child and later psychological and emotional problems. However, it is not presently understood why some abused children escape serious psychological problems while others suffer enormous psychological consequences. It is known that those who were abused by more than one person as a child are more likely to experience later emotional problems than those who were abused by one person. When children are abused by adults between the ages of 26 and 50, their prognosis is also poorer than those abused by offenders of other ages.

Other possible long-term effects of child sexual abuse include:

❖ Lack of basic trust

❖ Low self-esteem

❖ Pervasive feelings of helplessness and depression

❖ Self-destructive forms of behavior

❖ Revictimization from rape or attempted rape as adults (this may be related to low self-esteem, lack of assertion, and a pervasive feeling that they deserve to be punished)

❖ Difficulties in sexual intimacy in relationships

❖ Confusion with sexual identity

❖ Difficulty becoming sexually aroused or, the opposite, engaging in sex compulsively

Some victims of child sexual abuse display symptoms of posttraumatic stress disorder. These symptoms include recurrent dreams or flashbacks to the abusive experience(s), a sense of emotional numbness, and feelings of estrangement from others.

## Recognizing and Reporting Child Sexual Abuse

There are many reasons why children do not tell supportive adults that they have been or currently are a victim of sexual abuse. Some common reasons are that the child:

❖ Is too young to understand or tell that he or she is being abused

❖ Is afraid of the offender

❖ Is concerned about rejection by those he or she reports the abuse to or by the offender

❖ Is worried that she or he will not be believed

❖ May find the sexual contact or activity pleasurable

❖ Is afraid that telling will result in a loss of love

❖ Is concerned about the effect that telling will have on her or his image or reputation

❖ May have been bribed or rewarded not to tell

❖ May receive no attention other than the sexual abuse

Most states require that school officials and employees report any suspected cases of child abuse or neglect. School personnel should follow the reporting procedures of their respective schools and districts in order to ensure proper reporting. As an individual suspecting abuse, you are legally responsible for making certain that the report is made to designated child protective agencies immediately. Your legal responsibility is not satisfied by mentioning or reporting it to an administrator or counselor. Those who report in good faith are immune from liability under protection of most state laws. School personnel should be familiar with the indicators of sexual abuse (see Box 7-1) in order to effectively recognize sexual abuse or possible abuse among students.

# Indicators of Child Sexual Abuse

## Physical Indicators

◆ Sexually transmitted disease in a child of any age
◆ Pregnancy at 11 or 12, especially with no history of peer socialization
◆ Evidence of physical trauma to or bleeding from the oral, genital, or anal areas
◆ Complaints of pain or itching in oral, genital, or anal areas
◆ Unusual or offensive odors
◆ Torn or stained clothing
◆ Extreme passivity during a pelvic exam

## Family Indicators

◆ Extreme paternal dominance, restrictiveness, and/or overprotectiveness
◆ Family isolated from the community and support systems
◆ Marked role-reversal between mother and child
◆ History of sexual abuse for either parent
◆ Substance abuse by either parent or by children
◆ Other types of violence in the home
◆ Absent spouse (through chronic illness, depression, divorce, or separation)
◆ Severe overcrowding
◆ Complaints about a "seductive" child
◆ Extreme objection to implementation of child sexual abuse curriculum

## Behavioral Indicators

◆ Unusual interest in and/or knowledge of sexual acts and language inappropriate to age or development level
◆ Seductive behavior with classmates, teachers, or other adults
◆ Acting-out sexual behavior
◆ Excessive masturbatory behavior
◆ Attempts to touch the genitals of other children, adults, or animals
◆ Wearing many layers of clothing, regardless of the weather
◆ Inappropriate dress, such as tight and/or revealing clothing
◆ Continual avoidance of bathrooms
◆ Reluctance to go to a particular place or be with a particular person

*continued*

*continued*

- ◆ Reluctance to go home and/or constant early arrival at school
- ◆ Excessive clinging, fear of being left alone
- ◆ Frequent absence and/or constant late arrival at school, especially if the notes are always written by the same person
- ◆ Sudden school problems; a marked decline in interest in school
- ◆ An abrupt change in behavior or personality
- ◆ An abrupt change in behavior in response to personal safety lessons
- ◆ Aggression, anger directed everywhere
- ◆ Anxiety, irritability, constant inattentiveness
- ◆ Regression, frequent withdrawal into fantasy
- ◆ Overcompliance, extreme docility
- ◆ Compulsive behaviors
- ◆ Appearing to have overwhelming responsibilities
- ◆ Suicidal threats or gestures
- ◆ Use of alcohol and/or other drugs
- ◆ Drastic change in appetite
- ◆ Sleep disturbances
- ◆ Running away from home or attempting to run away
- ◆ Denial of a problem with a marked lack of expression
- ◆ Lack of affect, extreme absence of expressiveness
- ◆ Depression, excessive crying
- ◆ Low self-esteem
- ◆ Lack of friends, poor relationships with peers
- ◆ Reluctance to undress for PE, continual avoidance of PE
- ◆ Indirect hints, allusions to problems at home, fishing for attention

## Handling Disclosure

Responding to a student's disclosure of sexual abuse presents a difficult and delicate situation for a teacher or school professional. The following guidelines from the Colorado Department of Health and Education can assist you in properly handling the disclosure.

**DO:**

- ❖ Believe the child
- ❖ Find a private place to talk
- ❖ Reassure the child that he or she has done the right thing by reporting
- ❖ Listen to the child
- ❖ Rephrase important thoughts—use the child's vocabulary
- ❖ Tell the child help is available

❖ Let the child know you must report to someone who can help him or her

❖ Report the incident immediately to appropriate persons or agencies

❖ Seek out your own support system

**DON'T:**

❖ Promise confidentiality

❖ Panic or express shock

❖ Ask leading or suggestive questions

❖ Make negative comments about the perpetrator

❖ Disclose information indiscriminately

In addition, reassure the child that he or she is not at fault and should not take the blame for the abuse. Determine the child's immediate need for safety and ensure that the child will be protected and supported. It is also important to discuss with the child what will happen when the report is made.

## Abuse Prevention

The keys to sexual abuse prevention are building childrens' sense of self-esteem, training for assertiveness, and teaching specific protective behaviors. Because elementary school children constitute half of all sexual abuse victims, the elementary school is the logical and vital place to start prevention efforts. Of course, these efforts should continue through twelfth grade. Because of the sensitive nature of this issue, it is essential that administrative support is sought and enlisted prior to initiation of prevention efforts.

Most of the current prevention efforts are victim-centered, for example, teaching children to avoid abuse. However, educators should also be concerned with teaching children not to be abusers. Therefore, prevention education for children should cover the following areas and topics (see also Box 7-2):

❖ Right to safety

❖ Parenting skills (children as future parents, as nurturers)

❖ Early childhood development

❖ Awareness of factors that lead to child abuse

❖ Family and community living skills

❖ Awareness of one's potential as a human being

❖ Strategies for building self-esteem

❖ Not confusing the desire for love and nurturing with the desire for sexual gratification

❖ Being gentle, loving, and kind is all right

❖ Respect for themselves and others

❖ Healthy ways to deal with stress, anger, anxiety, and all feelings

IN THE
CLASSROOM
*7-2*

# Preventing Child Sexual Abuse

There are many ways in which parents and educators can prepare children to avoid potential abuse situations, and to prevent an initial approach from becoming a sexual assault. These prevention strategies can be presented in a realistic, nonthreatening manner, just as one might give children other safety advice. While adults may worry that children will be frightened by discussions of sexual abuse, it appears that children who know what to look for and who to tell will be less fearful than those with sketchy or exaggerated information. For example, one child whose parents had not discussed this issue believed "sex maniacs take off your clothes, murder you, and cut you up into about a hundred pieces."

*Teach children that some parts of their bodies are private.*    It is important to provide children with correct terms for their genitals and the private areas of their bodies, just as they are given correct terms for other body parts. Such terms not only give them a vocabulary for discussing body functions, but also help them to recognize and report sexual abuse. Children should be informed that their breasts, buttocks, anus, and genitals (penis, vulva, vagina) are *private* parts. They may be helped to remember these areas by noting that they are parts of the body covered by their bathing suits. Point out that no one has the right to touch these private areas—even when one is wearing clothing—with the possible exception of a parent or teacher dressing a child or a health professional conducting an examination in a medical office. Children should also know that no one has the right to ask them to touch another person's private parts.

*Help children identify different types of touching.*    Rather than teaching children to be wary of certain individuals, adults should help children to discriminate between different types of touching. Parents and teachers can provide examples of *good, confusing,* and *bad touches. Good touches* make children feel positive about themselves and include the welcome hugs, kisses, and handshakes from relatives and friends. *Confusing touches* make the child feel a little uncomfortable, such as when a parent requests that a child kiss an unfamiliar relative or friend. *Bad touches* include hitting, prolonged or excessive tickling, or touches involving the private areas of the body.

Children should be given concrete examples of bad touches to ensure that they understand the concept. For example, adults might explain that, "It would be very bad for an adult to put her or his hand on the child's breasts, anus, vulva, or penis, or to ask the child to touch the adult's own vulva or

*continued*

penis. It would also be wrong for someone to take pictures of you without clothes on or to ask you to lie down in bed with her or him." Emphasize that adults may try to bribe, trick, or force children into *bad* types of touching.

***Teach children to say no to unwanted touches.*** Children should be told of their right to control who touches them. Teaching them when and how to say *no* is important in preventing the onset of abuse. *No* should be used whenever the child encounters unwanted touches or is offered special treats in exchange for certain behaviors. Children can be coached to respond to these situations with statements such as "No, don't touch me there! That part of my body is private!" or "No, I'm not allowed to do that." Practicing such phrases may help children to respond assertively when approached by a potential offender.

***Explain that bad touches could come from someone the child knows.*** Children often believe that an abuser is *weird, ugly, monster-looking,* or *wearing a dark coat.* Therefore, it is important to point out that bad touches may not only come from unattractive strangers, but from friendly, attractive relatives or people the child knows. Children may be told that, "Although most teenagers and adults are nice, there are some who have a hard time making friends. They may ask you to do things that aren't right, such as getting undressed or putting your hands in their pants." If children ask why an adult would do this, try to avoid saying "because she or he is mean or sick." These words have concrete meaning to the child and may not fit the situation the child encounters. For example, when one boy was told that abusers were "sick in the head," he looked for men with bandages on their heads. Adults can admit that they don't know why some people do these things, but they want to warn children about individuals who might try to touch them in uncomfortable ways.

***Encourage open communication and discourage secrets.*** Sexual offenders often instruct children to keep abusive behaviors secret, and may frighten children by threatening that telling will bring harm to the child, the child's parents, or the offender ("If you tell, I'll go to jail"). Offenders may also attempt to convince children that their behavior is normal or a reflection of the offender's love for the victim. Therefore, children should be encouraged to share all incidents that make them feel frightened or uncomfortable with a parent or a trusted adult. Children should be told that they never have to keep secrets from these significant adults, even if the abuser made them promise or threatened to hurt them in some way.

Adults should also inform children that they will not be angry or blame them if an abusive event occurs—even though they were warned about bad

*continued*

*continued*

touching—but want children to come to them with the information. They can explain that everyone makes mistakes, and that the inappropriate touching was not the child's fault. Children should be helped to understand that reporting an assaultive attempt or actual incident involving themselves or one of their friends will protect others and make it possible for the offender to receive help.

Although most adults believe children's accounts of abusive incidents, children may be prepared for the possibility that someone (for example, a grandparent or caregiver) may doubt the truth of their story. After acknowledging how hurt or sad a child might feel if this occurred, adults should emphasize the importance of telling another person so that the problem can be eliminated. Children may be asked to name several adults they could tell if they were to encounter bad or confusing touches.

***Teach children how to tell.***    Children may have difficulty informing adults about unwanted touches, especially if they involve a relative or family friend. Therefore, adults may help them to practice ways of reporting sexual abuse until they feel comfortable with the words. For example, if a child encountered unwanted touching, he might say, "Mr. Smith is touching my penis and the private parts of my body. I want him to stop."

***Use games and stories to reinforce prevention concepts.***    Games such as "What if . . ." are effective in helping children to think for themselves and to formulate a plan for responding to possible abuse. Adults might ask a child, "What would you do if a neighbor asked you to look at some kittens in his bedroom?" or "What would you do if a cousin put his hand on a private part of your body at a family picnic?" Parents and teachers may also tell stories about other children who have successfully avoided difficult situations, providing children with positive role models. For example:

> Timmy, age 4, was being cared for by his favorite babysitter, 16-year-old John. When John put Timmy in the bath, he tried to rub his penis over and over— even though it wasn't dirty. Timmy remembered what his mother had told him about bad touching and firmly told John not to touch his penis or private parts. The next morning Timmy told his parents about his "touching problem."

Opportunities to talk about sexual assault and play prevention games arise frequently. For example, parents may initiate "what if" games on general safety during dinner, interspersing questions about sexual assault with other safety predicaments. Discussions may also be motivated by news articles or televised reports of sexual assault. Currently, most of the curriculum materials which address the problem of sexual abuse in children are in coloring

*continued*

book or workbook format. Parents and teachers can use these materials for background information, and adapt them for use with children in more creative ways.

*Continue to discuss safety rules concerning strangers.* Although the majority of sexual assault cases involve adults familiar to the child, a significant number of offenses are perpetrated by strangers. Offers of candy, a ride in a car, or the chance to play with some puppies or kittens are common inducements used to obtain a child's company. While most parents do warn their children about the dangers of accompanying strangers, our own research indicates that many children do not understand the definition of *stranger*. Adults might explain that, "A stranger is a person you don't know, even if the person says she or he knows your mom and dad. Strangers often look and act very nice, so you can't spot them by the way they look."

Children should be warned to say, "No I'm not allowed to do (the stranger's request)," even if they feel that there is no harm intended. Permission should first be obtained from a parent or responsible caregiver. Parents, teachers, and crime prevention specialists may also convey specific safety tips about what a child should do and where a child should go (for example, to a neighbor's house or crime watch house) if bothered by a stranger.

*Encourage children to trust their own instincts.* Children cannot be protected from sexual assault by safety rules alone since specific rules may not apply to all potential abuse situations. Consequently, they should be encouraged to trust their own feelings and intuitions about people and places in order to protect themselves from possible harm. Adults can encourage children to rely on their *inner voice* which tells them that some requests from adults are unreasonable or inappropriate.

*Teach children about the positive aspects of sexuality.* In teaching children about sexual abuse, it is important to communicate that sexuality is not bad or wrong. Rather it is the trickery, bribery, coercion, and taking advantage of another person that is harmful. To balance the information provided about exploitive touch, adults should make special efforts to point out the positive, nurturing, and joyful aspects of sexual interactions between loving persons. Adults who demonstrate warmth, affection, and support for others provide children with positive role models for later intimate relationships.

## Prevention Programs for Children

Teachers may complement their staff and parent education efforts with classroom presentations on sexual abuse prevention and stranger awareness for young children. It is important, however, that parents be supportive of and

*continued*

*continued*

informed about these classroom activities. Parent meetings on sexual abuse prevention provide an excellent opportunity for review of curriculum materials intended for classroom use.

The most effective curriculum units for preschoolers and elementary school children employ high interest, nonthreatening materials such as puppets, skits, and stories. These units ensure that children learn (1) the private areas of their bodies, (2) the difference between good and bad touches, (3) children's right to say no to touches they don't like, (4) the importance of telling a trusted adult about unwanted touch, and (5) that sexual assault is never the child's fault. Curriculum materials should include many examples of nonstranger sexual abuse.

The Coalition for Child Advocacy has developed one of the few weeklong prevention programs designed specifically for preschool children. Early sessions focus on helping children to identify different feelings. A general safety film, "Who Do You Tell?" gives children the chance to consider who they could inform if they had uncomfortable feelings about being touched by a specific adult. Later sessions ensure that children understand the private parts of their bodies, and allow them to rehearse ways of avoiding potential sexual abuse.

Programs for kindergarten and elementary school children emphasize similar prevention concepts, with activities appropriate for the child's developmental level. Role play activities are one means of helping elementary age children to think about how they might handle approaches from abusers. Incomplete stories, as exemplified below, are another technique which may familiarize teachers with children's understanding of the problem and may spark discussion about prevention strategies.

> One hot day Sara was invited to run through the sprinklers of the man who lived next door. After a little while the neighbor asked her to sit on his lap. As he began to tell Sara a story, he rubbed his hand between her legs. Sara didn't like it and wiggled free. She ran home without saying goodbye. Should Sara tell someone? Who?

Source: S. Koblinsky and N. Behana, "Child Sexual Abuse: The Educator's Role in Prevention, Detection, and Intervention," *Young Children*, September: 6–10, 1984. Reprinted with permission.

# Rape

**Rape** is the act of forcing or coercing someone to have sexual relations against her or his will. Rapes that occur to victims younger than the age of consent are **statutory rape,** whether or not force is involved. The rate of rapes in the United States has increased more in recent years than any of the other major crimes. Further, experts estimate that only 1 of every 5 to 20 rapes is reported. Not all rape victims are female; males are also frequently rape victims.

There are different types of rape. **Acquaintance rape** involves individuals who know each other casually prior to the rape, including coworkers, neighbors, and friends. **Date rape** occurs between two people who are spending time together with the possibility of building a closer relationship. **Marital rape** occurs between spouses. **Stranger rape** occurs between a victim and offender who had no prior relationship.

Many myths and erroneous perceptions associated with rape persist. These include the following:

❖ Victims "ask for" rape by their clothing, behavior, or actions.

❖ Males cannot be raped.

❖ Old or unattractive women do not get raped.

❖ Any victim can resist a rapist if she or he really tries.

❖ Victims can only be raped by someone they do not know.

❖ Rapists are mentally ill or sexually perverted.

❖ Victims secretly want to be raped.

❖ Nice people do not get raped.

❖ Rapes almost always occur in dark alleys or deserted places.

❖ The incidence of rape is overreported.

❖ Some victims deserved to get raped.

No one is immune to rape. Rape can happen to anyone regardless of age, social class, educational level, occupation, or race. The most common age range of rape victims is the 13–19 year age group, with 14 and 15 being the most frequent ages. This finding underscores the importance of rape prevention activities within the secondary schools. School-based rape prevention programs, directed toward both male and female students, must emphasize:

❖ Counteracting sex role stereotyping

❖ Acquaintance and date rape

❖ Communication skills

❖ Peer violence and pressure

❖ Assertiveness behavior

❖ Decoding mass media images and values that sanction violence and aggression, especially against women

❖ Dispelling readily accepted myths about rape

Rape prevention programs should also inform students of such precautions as follow:

❖ Admit that you could be a candidate for rape.

❖ Be especially cautious of first dates, blind dates, or of people you meet at a party.

❖ Be careful not to establish predictable patterns of movement to and from school or other activities—alter routes frequently.

❖ Do not walk alone at night.

❖ Walk briskly and with a sense of purpose.

❖ Avoid informing telephone callers that you are home alone.

❖ Place emergency telephone numbers near the telephone, or better yet, commit them to memory.

❖ Keep doors and windows locked securely.

❖ Take self-defense classes to assist in preventing assault.

## Date Rape

Does rape occur only if the attacker is a stranger? Certainly not! Anytime one person forces another to have sexual intercourse, it is rape. Unfortunately, it is not uncommon for females in our society to have an experience in which a male dating partner forced sex against their will. The aftermath of date rape can be devastating. Victims may experience any or all of the following:

❖ Anxiety

❖ Sleeplessness

❖ Nightmares and/or flashbacks

❖ Guilt and feelings of responsibility

❖ Lowered self-esteem

❖ Questioning of personal judgment

❖ Feeling ashamed

❖ Sense of humiliation

❖ Altered attitude toward sex

❖ Pregnancy and related decision making (who to tell? who to trust? abort? adopt out? raise the child? leave school? leave work?)

❖ Catching AIDS or another sexually transmitted disease

❖ Physical and/or verbal battering

To help prevent date rape, secondary curriculums should teach students to be cautious of the following dating behaviors or characteristics of dating partners:

❖ Lack of respect for women

❖ Generalized hostility or anger toward women

❖ Lack of concern for partner's feelings or wishes

❖ Obsessive jealousy

❖ Extreme competitiveness

❖ Attempts to induce feelings of guilt if sexual advances are rejected

❖ Becoming violent or abusive while drinking

❖ Physical roughness

❖ View females as primarily responsible for preventing rape

❖ Maintaining traditional belief about womens' roles

In addition, school programs can collaborate with community agencies in the prevention of date rape and dating violence by helping adolescents to:[22]

❖ Manage conflict in relationships, including dating

❖ Withdraw from a conflict that is getting out of control

❖ Deal with jealousy, rejection, and use of alcohol or other drugs in dating relationships

❖ Understand sexual signals and communication

❖ Understand the extent of dating aggression and date rape

❖ Recognize abuse and sexual coercion

❖ Become skillful at resisting violence and rape

❖ Develop assertiveness skills

❖ Obtain self-defense training

❖ Debunk rape myths

❖ Understand the legitimacy of saying no to unwanted sexual interaction

## Key Terms

bullying  269
Gun Free Schools Act  273
early warning signs  275
imminent warning signs  275
conflict resolution skills  279
crisis planning  281
physical abuse  283
physical neglect  283
emotional maltreatment  283

sexual abuse  283
incest  284
Megan's Law  285
rape  297
statutory rape  297
acquaintance rape  297
date rape  297
marital rape  297
stranger rape  297

## Review Questions

1. Summarize the surgeon general's report on youth violence, including trends and current problems.
2. Identify family factors common in children and adolescents exhibiting violent behavior.
3. Explain how the media play a role in violent behavior.
4. Handgun ownership by high school youth is associated with what six things?
5. Identify the four characteristics that youth displaying violent behavior share with youth engaging in other high-risk behaviors.
6. Identify some of the reasons young people are attracted to gangs.
7. Identify the 16 early warning signs of aggressive rage or violent behavior toward self or others.
8. Discuss the prevalence of bullying in today's schools, its causes and effects, and the proposed means of preventing and counteracting it.
9. Explain how schools can have safe and violence-free school environments. Discuss school security measures, the Gun Free Schools Act, and discipline and dress codes.

10. Identify how school officials can enhance physical safety.

11. Explain what teachers should and should not do if they identify early warning signs that a child might be prone to violence. Identify the imminent warning signs for violent behavior.

12. Identify and explain the nine elements of promising violence prevention programs. Identify the six components that show little promise in violence prevention programs.

13. Identify some of the personal and social skills in which youth may need training.

14. Explain how a teacher might teach conflict resolution and anger management in the classroom.

15. Identify some of the problems schools must plan for to ensure safety. Identify some of the provisions school safety planning should include.

16. What percentage of adult women and adult men report they experienced some form of sexual abuse as children? What is Megan's Law?

17. Identify some of the initial emotional, behavioral, and physical effects of child sexual abuse. Identify some of the possible long-term effects of child sexual abuse.

18. Explain how teachers should report child sexual abuse, including the *dos* and *don'ts* in handling the disclosure.

19. Identify ways educators can help prevent child sexual abuse.

20. Define and differentiate the following terms: *statutory rape, acquaintance rape, date rape, marital rape,* and *stranger rape.*

21. Identify some of the myths associated with rape.

22. Identify the behaviors that secondary curricula should teach students to be cautious of in dating behaviors or partners.

## References

1. Office of the Surgeon General (2001). *Youth Violence: A Report of the Surgeon General.* Washington, DC: U.S. Department of Health and Human Services. Available at http://www.surgeongeneral.gov/library/youthviolence/report.html.

2. Wodarski, J. S., and M. Hedrick (1987, Fall). "Violent Children: A Practice Paradigm." *Social Work in Education,* 28–42.

3. Resnick, M. D., et al. (1997). "Protecting Adolescents from Harm: Findings from the National Longitudinal Study on Adolescent Health." *Journal of the American Medical Association,* 278(10): 823–832.

4. Hansen, B. (1993, July 6). "Distorted Viewing: TV's Reflection of Life." *USA Today,* 3D.

5. American Academy of Pediatrics (2001). "Media Violence—Policy Statement." *Pediatrics,* 108(5): 1222–1226.

6. American Academy of Pediatrics (2001). "Some Things You Should Know About Media Violence and Media Literacy" [Factsheet]. Available at http://www.aap.org/advocacy/childhealthmonth/media.htm.

7. Grossman, D. (2002). "Trained to Kill." *Christianity Today,* 42(9): 30. Available at http://www.courttv.com/choices/grossman.html.

8. Page, R. M., and J. Hammermeister (1997). "Weapon-Carrying and Youth Violence." *Adolescence*, 32(127): 505–513.

9. Simon, R. R., J. L. Richardson, C. W. Dean, C. P. Chou, and B. R. Flay (1998). "Prospective Psychological, Interpersonal, and Behavioral Predictors of Handgun Carrying Among Adolescents." *Journal of the American Medical Association*, 88(6): 960–963.

10. Harrington-Leuker, D. (1992). "Blown Away by School Violence." *American School Board Journal*, 179: 20–26.

11. Chandler, K. A., C. D. Chapman, M. R. Rand, and B. M. Taylor (1998). *Students' Reports of School Crime: 1989 and 1995* (NCES No. 98-241). Washington, DC: U.S. Departments of Education and Justice. Available at http://nces.ed.gov/pubs98/crime/index.html.

12. Centers for Disease Control and Prevention (2000). "Youth Risk Behavior Surveillance—United States, 1999." *Morbidity and Mortality Weekly Report*, 49(SS-05).

13. Namel, T. R., M. Overpeck, R. S. Pilla, W. J. Ruan, B. Simons-Morton, and P. Scheidt (2001). "Bullying Behaviors Among U.S. Youth: Prevalence and Association with Psychosocial Adjustment." *Journal of the American Medical Association*, 2085: 2094–2100.

14. Ericson, N. (2001, June). "Addressing the Problem of Juvenile Bullying" (OJJDP Fact Sheet No. 27-FS-200127). Washington, DC: U.S. Department of Justice, Office of Juvenile Justice and Delinquency Prevention.

15. Lumsden, L. (2002, March). "Preventing Violence." *ERIC Digest*, 155. ERIC Clearinghouse on Educational Management. Available at http://ericcass.uncg.edu/virtuallib/bullying/1068.html.

16. "Preventing School Violence: No Easy Answers." (1998). *Journal of the American Medical Association*, 280(5): 404–406.

17. Dwyer, K., D. Osher, and C. Warger (1998). *Early Warning, Timely Response: A Guide to Safe Schools*. Washington, DC: U.S. Department of Education. Available at http://www.ed.gov/offices/OSERS/OSEP/Products/earlywrn.html.

18. Dusenbury, L., M. Falco, A. Lake, R. Brannigan, and K. Bosworth (1997). "Nine Critical Elements of Promising Violence Prevention Programs." *Journal of School Health*, 67(10): 409–414.

19. National Committee to Prevent Child Abuse (1998). "Child Abuse and Neglect Statistics." Available at http://childabuse.org/facts97.html.

20. Wang, C. T., and D. Daro (1998). *Current Trends in Child Abuse Reporting and Fatalities: The Results of the 1997 Annual Fifty State Survey*. Chicago: National Committee to Prevent Child Abuse.

21. National Committee to Prevent Child Abuse (1996). "Child Sexual Abuse." Available at http://childabuse.org/fs19.html.

22. Page, R. M. (1997). "Helping Adolescents Avoid Date Rape: The Role of Secondary Education." *The High School Journal*, 80(2): 75–80.

# 8

# DEPRESSION AND SUICIDAL BEHAVIOR

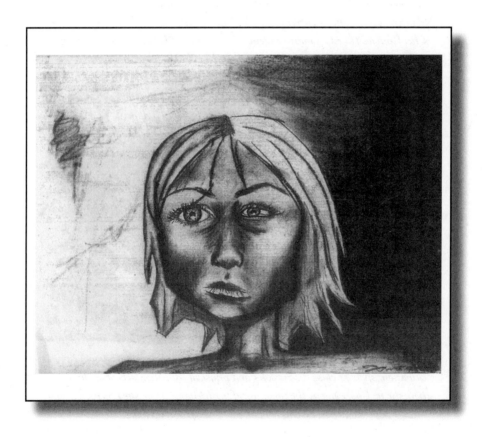

# *Brooke*

*Brooke is a member of your class. She is not particularly gifted academically; learning has never been easy for her. It takes her much longer and requires more concentration to understand concepts than many of her classmates. On occasion, certain classmates have made fun of her difficulties in learning. Feelings of inferiority are common for Brooke when she compares her performance to her classmates'. These feelings are heightened when she dwells on the accomplishments of her older sister.*

*Her older sister, Rachel, attends a prestigious private college in another city. When Rachel was a senior she was awarded a full four-year scholarship from the college she is currently attending. Rachel was very outgoing in high school and well liked by most students and teachers. She was an active member of several clubs and student body vice-president during her senior year.*

*Brooke's mother died of breast cancer just two years ago, leaving behind Brooke, Rachel, and two younger brothers, ages 6 and 8. Brooke's father is a professor of chemistry at a local university. He has had a difficult time adjusting to the death of his wife, drinking heavily at times and becoming absorbed in his work at the university. Unfortunately, his drinking occasionally causes him to be unreasonably angry and harsh toward his children.*

*Life at home is difficult for Brooke. She has little time for herself. She must come home quickly after school to attend to the needs of her younger brothers and father. The house still feels strangely cold and empty without her mother's presence. Most of Brooke's recollections of her mother are pleasant, but the memories of her mother's slow, painful death still torment Brooke. She believes she is somewhat responsible for her mother's suffering during her last days. Brooke is also torn with guilt because of the anger she feels toward her mother for leaving her.*

*As Brooke's teacher, you observe that during the past few months Brooke cries frequently, usually without apparent reason. She looks tired and often falls asleep during class. She tends to withdraw from activities requiring active participation, such as class discussions and physical education activities. In addition, she no longer enjoys the company of her friends. Lately, she has been giving away her personal possessions—her watch, rings, and necklaces.*

## Questions

1. Identify sources of emotional distress in Brooke's life.
2. Are there any signs that Brooke is depressed?
3. What actions may Brooke be considering?
4. What steps would you take if Brooke were in your class?

It is not easy growing up in today's world. Adolescence is a time of extraordinary change and stress. Young people are faced with pressures and complex decisions. Too many young people feel that they are not able to cope with pressures or feel that no one cares enough to help them. Sadly, some become desperate enough to take their own lives.

Suicide does not have to happen. Educators can help it from happening. This chapter will help you become more aware of the signs of depression and suicide risk. You will also learn specific actions that you can take to stop suicide.

## Understanding Depressive Disorders in Children and Adolescents*

A **depressive disorder** is an illness that involves the body, mood, and thoughts. It affects the way one eats and sleeps, the way one feels about oneself, and the way one thinks about things. A depressive disorder is not the same as a passing blue mood. It is not a sign of personal weakness or a condition that can be willed or wished away. People with a depressive illness cannot merely "pull themselves together" and get better. Without treatment, symptoms can last for weeks, months, or years. Appropriate treatment, however, can help most people who suffer from depression.

Only in the past two decades has depression in children been taken very seriously. The depressed child may pretend to be sick, refuse to go to school, cling to a parent, or worry that the parent may die. Older children may sulk, get into trouble at school, be negative and grouchy, and feel misunderstood. Because normal behaviors vary from one childhood stage to another, it can be difficult to tell whether a child is just going through a temporary "phase" or is suffering from depression. Sometimes the parents become worried about how the child's behavior has changed, or a teacher notices that a student doesn't seem to be himself or herself.

Depressive disorders can have far-reaching effects on the functioning and adjustment of young people. Among both children and adolescents, depressive disorders confer an increased risk for illness and interpersonal and psychosocial difficulties that persist long after the depressive episode is resolved; in adolescents there is also an increased risk for substance abuse and suicidal behavior. Unfortunately, these disorders often go unrecognized by families, school personnel, and health care professionals alike. Signs of depressive disorders in young people are often viewed as normal mood swings typical of a particular developmental stage. In addition,

---

* This section was adapted from the following two publications from the National Institute of Mental Health: *Depression in Children and Adolescents* (NIH Publication No. 00-4744), available at http://www.nimh.nih.gov/publicat/depchildresfact.htm; and *Depression* (NIH Publication No. 00-3561), available at http://www.nimh.nih.gov/publicat/depression. cfm#ptdep1.

health care professionals may be reluctant to permanently "label" a young person with a mental illness diagnosis. Yet early diagnosis and treatment of depressive disorders are critical to healthy emotional, social, and behavioral development.

The National Institute of Mental Health (NIMH) reports that studies have found that up to 2.5% of children and 8.3% of adolescents in the United States suffer from depression. NIMH also reports that research indicates that the onset of depression is occurring earlier in life today than in past decades. Further, depression that occurs early in life often persists, recurs, and continues into adulthood. Depression in youth may also predict more severe illness in adult life. Depression in young people often co-occurs with other mental disorders, most commonly anxiety, disruptive behavior, or substance abuse disorders, and with physical illnesses, such as diabetes.

## Types of Depressive Disorders

Depressive disorders include major depressive disorder (unipolar depression), dysthymic disorder (chronic, mild depression), and bipolar disorder (manic-depressive disorder).

*Major Depressive Disorder*   **Major depression** is manifested by a combination of symptoms that interfere with the ability to work, study, sleep, eat, and enjoy once pleasurable activities. Such a disabling episode of depression may occur only once, but more commonly occurs several times in a lifetime. The criteria used to diagnosis major depression and its key defining features in children and adolescents are the same as they are for adults. However, recognition and diagnosis of this disorder may be more difficult in youth for several reasons. The way symptoms are expressed varies with a young person's developmental stage. In addition, children and young adolescents with depression may have difficulty in properly identifying and describing their internal emotional or mood states. For example, instead of communicating how bad they feel, they may act out and be irritable toward others, which may be interpreted simply as misbehavior or disobedience. Parents are even less likely to identify major depression in their adolescents than are adolescents themselves.

The following list includes symptoms of major depressive disorder common to adults, children, and adolescents. Five or more of these symptoms must persist for two or more weeks before a diagnosis of major depression is indicated:

❖ Persistent sad or irritable mood

❖ Loss of interest in activities once enjoyed

❖ Significant change in appetite or body weight

❖ Difficulty sleeping, or oversleeping

❖ Psychomotor agitation or retardation

❖ Loss of energy

❖ Feelings of worthlessness or inappropriate guilt

❖ Difficulty concentrating

❖ Recurrent thoughts of death or suicide

The following signs may be associated with depression in children and adolescents:

❖ Frequent, vague, nonspecific physical complaints such as headaches, muscle aches, stomachaches, or tiredness

❖ Frequent absences from school or poor performance in school

❖ Talk of or efforts to run away from home

❖ Outbursts of shouting, complaining, unexplained irritability, or crying

❖ Being bored

❖ Lack of interest in playing with friends

❖ Alcohol or substance abuse

❖ Social isolation, poor communication

❖ Fear of death

❖ Extreme sensitivity to rejection or failure

❖ Increased irritability, anger, or hostility

❖ Reckless behavior

❖ Difficulty with relationships

While the recovery rate from a single episode of major depression in children and adolescents is quite high, episodes are likely to recur. In addition, youth with dysthymic disorder are at risk for developing major depression. Prompt identification and treatment of depression can reduce its duration and severity and the associated impairment in functioning.

**Dysthymic Disorder (or Dysthymia)**    A less severe type of depression, **dysthymia**, involves long-term, chronic symptoms that do not disable, but keep one from functioning well or from feeling good. Many people with dysthymia also experience major depressive episodes at some time in their lives. This less severe yet typically more chronic form of depression is diagnosed when depressed mood persists for at least one year in children and adolescents and is accompanied by at least two other symptoms of major depression. Dysthymia is associated with an increased risk for developing major depressive disorder, bipolar disorder, and substance abuse. Treatment of dysthymia may prevent the deterioration to more severe illness. If dysthymia is suspected in a young person, there should be referral to a mental health specialist for a comprehensive diagnostic evaluation and appropriate treatment.

***Bipolar Disorder***     Although rare in young children, **bipolar disorder**—also known as manic-depressive illness—can appear in both children and adolescents. Bipolar disorder, which involves unusual shifts in mood, energy, and functioning, may begin with either manic, depressive, or mixed manic and depressive symptoms. It is more likely to affect the children of parents who have the disorder. Twenty percent to 40% of adolescents with major depression develop bipolar disorder within five years after depression onset.

***Seasonal Affective Disorder***     **Seasonal affective disorder (SAD)** occurs in certain people who are especially vulnerable to depression on a seasonal basis. They become depressed during winter months and then feel much better in spring and summer when the days are longer and the amount of sunlight increases. SAD has been recognized in children and adolescents, but it is more commonly diagnosed in adults. Gazing into intense fluorescent lights (phototherapy) helps many people who suffer from SAD during the winter months.

## Risk Factors

In childhood, boys and girls appear to be at equal risk for depressive disorders; however, during adolescence, girls are twice as likely as boys to develop depression. Children who have major depression are more likely to have a family history of the disorder (often a parent who experienced depression at an early age) than those suffering with adolescent- or adult-onset depression. Adolescents with depression are also likely to have a family history of depression. Other risk factors include the following:

❖ Stress

❖ Cigarette smoking

❖ Loss of a parent or loved one

❖ Break-up of a romantic relationship

❖ Attentional, conduct, or learning disorders

❖ Chronic illnesses, such as diabetes

❖ Abuse or neglect

❖ Other trauma, including natural disaster

## He Always

He always wanted to explain things,
But no one cared.
So he drew.
Sometimes he would draw and it wasn't anything.
He wanted to carve it in stone or write it in the sky.
He would lie out on the grass and look up at the sky;
And it would be only the sky and him and the things inside him that needed
    saying.
And it was after that, he drew the picture.
It was a beautiful picture.
He kept it under his pillow, and would let no one see it.
And when it was dark, and his eyes were closed, he could see it.
And it was all of him,
And he loved it.
When he started school he brought it with him.
Not to show anyone, but just to have it with him like a friend.
It was funny about school,
He sat in a square, brown desk
Like all the other square, brown desks,
And he thought it should be red.
And his room was a square, brown room
Like all the other rooms.
And it was tight and close
And stiff.
He hated to hold the pencil and chalk,
With his arm stiff and his feet flat on the floor,
Stiff.
With the teacher watching and watching.
The teacher came and spoke to him.
She told him to wear a tie like all the other boys.
He said he didn't like them,
And she said it didn't matter.
After that they drew.
And he drew all yellow and it was the way he felt about morning;
And it was beautiful.
The teacher came and smiled at him.

*continued*

*continued*

"What's this?" she said, "Why don't you draw something like Ken's drawing?"
"Isn't that beautiful?"
After that his mother bought him a tie.
And he always drew airplanes and rocketships like everyone else.
And he threw the old picture away.
And when he lay out alone looking at the sky,
It was big and blue and all of everything.
But he wasn't anymore.
He was square inside and brown
And his hands were stiff,
And he was like everything else.
And the things inside him that needed saying didn't need it anymore.
It has stopped pushing;
It was crushed,
Stiff,
Like everything else.

Source: The source of this poem is unknown. It was supposed to have been given to a twelfth-grade English teacher by a student who committed suicide two weeks later.

## Assisting Young People Who Are Depressed

Depression is one of the most overlooked and untreated disorders of children and adolescents. It can be difficult to recognize depression in young people, particularly because they are likely to mask their feelings with behaviors not usually identified with depression, such as aggression, sexual promiscuity, academic failure, abuse of alcohol and other drugs, running away, and accident-proneness.

Depression has many faces and symptoms, making identification confusing and often complex. The presence of one or several of the following indicators warrants investigation for possible depression:

❖ Feelings of sadness, hopelessness, and worry

❖ Negative feelings of self-worth

❖ Inability to concentrate or easily distracted

❖ Inattentiveness and listlessness

❖ Decreased academic performance or drop in grades

❖ Frequent absences from school

❖ Daydreaming

❖ Withdrawn or sullen behavior

❖ Social isolation

❖ Quick reaction with tears to any kind of pressure

❖ Inability to maintain energy level or complete ordinary tasks

❖ Complaints of tiredness

❖ Decreased appetite

❖ Disruptive behavior inside and outside the classroom

❖ Low frustration tolerance

❖ Frequent complaints of physical symptoms or illness

Accurate, early recognition of these signals is essential for effective intervention. Unrecognized depression may escalate to suicidal thoughts and attempts. Because teachers are on the "front line" they may be the first to observe signs of depression. Suspected depression should be discussed with parents and a trained health professional such as a school counselor, psychologist, or nurse. Severely depressed children and adolescents need professional counseling and treatment.

Depressed children need a supportive relationship with the classroom teacher and integration into normal class processes. Supportive relationships with other students are also helpful. Depressed children have many strengths that can be mobilized and released when they feel that they have a friend.

By attending to the problems of depression, teachers can provide lasting and significant benefits to the lives of their students. Schlozman presents the following advice for classroom teachers concerning childhood and adolescent depression:[1]

❖ While making allowances for normal fluctuation in mood, teachers should be vigilant in watching out for signs and symptoms of depression in their students. They may be the first to notice when a student begins to act depressed.

❖ When a student is displaying signs and symptoms indicative of depression, a teacher should meet with the guidance counselor or school psychologist to discuss options for further investigation or referral. Teachers and counselors should make appropriate referrals through the school's proper channels for doing so.

❖ Teachers need to be aware that depressed students often feel as if they have little to contribute. A teacher can help by showing confidence, respect, and faith in a depressed student's abilities and by not doing things in the classroom that would raise the student's anxiety. For example, when a teacher asks questions for which there is no clearly correct answer, a depressed student may be more likely to participate in a classroom discussion.

❖ Another way to increase a depressed student's confidence is to have the student assist younger or less able students in some way.

❖ Help young people who are depressed in forming a connection with a trusted teacher or other adult. This is often central to a young person's recovery from depression.

❖ When depressed students have difficulty discussing their feelings, it might be helpful for them to identify with literary or historical figures and use them to explore their own feelings.

It is critical that educators recognize that none of the suggestions for helping depressed students in the classroom should substitute for the appropriate diagnostic evaluation and treatment of depression. Several tools that are useful for screening children and adolescents for possible depression can be used by counselors and mental health and health care professionals. They include the Children's Depression Inventory (CDI) for ages 7 to 17, and, for adolescents, the Beck Depression Inventory (BDI) and the Center for Epidemiologic Studies Depression (CES-D) Scale. When a young person screens positive on any of these instruments, a comprehensive diagnostic evaluation by a mental health professional is warranted. The evaluation should include interviews with the young person, parents, and, when possible, other informants such as teachers and social services personnel. Treatment for depressive disorders in children and adolescents often involves short-term psychotherapy, medication, or both, and interventions involving the home or school environment.[2]

Antidepressant medications, especially when combined with psychotherapy, can be very effective treatments for depressive disorders in adults. Using medication to treat mental illness in children and adolescents, however, has caused controversy. Many doctors have been understandably reluctant to treat young people with psychotropic medications because, until fairly recently, little evidence was available about the safety and efficacy of these drugs in youth. Some of the newer antidepressant medications, specifically the selective serotonin reuptake inhibitors (SSRIs), have been shown to be safe and effective for the short-term treatment of severe and persistent depression in young people, although more research to confirm this is needed.[2]

# Self-Injury

Some young people engage in acts of self-injury. **Self-injury,** also known as *self-harm* or *self-mutilation*, includes deliberate attempts to cause harm to one's own body; the injury is usually enough to cause tissue damage. Any method used to harm oneself might be used in self-injury, such as cutting, hair pulling, skin picking, burning, biting, bone breaking, head banging, self-poisoning, self-strangulation, or limb amputation. Self-injury is not generally an attempt at suicide, but it probably has resulted in deaths when sustained injuries were serious enough to cause fatality. It appears to be more common in girls than in boys.

Why would a young person intentionally harm himself or herself? Self-injury might be used to help someone relieve intense feelings such as anger, sadness, loneliness, shame, guilt, and emotional pain. It is believed that those who cut themselves do so in an attempt to release intense emotional feelings. Some young people troubled by a sense of emotional numbness report that seeing their own blood when they cut themselves helps them to feel alive because they usually feel dead inside. Others report that they injure themselves because dealing with the physical pain is easier than dealing with emotional pain. Self-injury is also used by some as a way to punish themselves for the guilt, shame, and blame that they carry for an abuse that they have suffered. Some harm themselves out of a sense of self-hatred for themselves and their body. Sometimes, self-injury is an attempt to get attention or a cry for help. But there are self-injurers who go to great extremes to keep their self-injurious behavior a secret. Whatever means is used for self-injury and whatever the reasons behind it, there is usually a release from built-up feelings and emotions. However, the emotional release is only temporary.

Many young people engaging in acts of self-injury have a troubled past. Many have a history of sexual or physical abuse, have emotionally absent parents, come from broken homes, or have substance-abusing parents. It is speculated that these factors could contribute to a young person's using self-injury as a way to cope with or block out the emotional pain resulting from these situations.

The act of cutting or other forms of self-injury are signs of disturbance or emotional difficulty that needs to be recognized. For some, self-injury is a last resort or a coping mechanism keeping them from committing suicide. They are choosing self-injury instead of death. Self-injury often becomes a habit, and some mental health experts describe it as an addiction. One woman who struggled with cutting said that "there was nothing like seeing your own blood dripping off your arm or leg and knowing you control it." Some say they are addicted to the blood, some to the scars, and some to the pain or a mixture of all three. The compulsion to self-injure becomes increasingly more dangerous. A young person self-injures and feels emotional release. Then, the next time he or she is feeling depressed or angry, his or her thoughts turn to self-injury. If the person succumbs to the urge, he or she is perpetuating a cycle of addiction.

Young people suffering from this dangerous behavior need to understand that accepting help is not a sign of weakness, but a sign of strength. Many adults do not understand how to react to someone who is injuring himself or herself. Educators and adults need to not react with shock, but with understanding. They need to understand that self-injury is a coping mechanism. They need to support a young person suffering from self-injury and to help him or her find help from mental health professionals who are trained to deal with this problem. The road to recovery may be long; hopefully, through the recovery process the self-injurer will find understanding from informed adults.

## Youth Suicide

Youth suicide is a serious public health problem. It is the third leading cause of death among adolescents and young adults. Nearly 5,000 American teenage and young adult (ages 15–24) deaths are recorded as suicide each year.[3] There are also reports of suicide deaths among younger youth, including children under the age of 10. Many additional youth suicides go unreported, so the total is probably much higher than these numbers indicate. Suicidal deaths may be disguised by family members or physicians as accidents, homicides, or other causes of death. Therefore, suicide statistics are understandably inaccurate because of the social stigma society has placed on suicide. Overall, more than 30,000 Americans die of suicide each year.[4] (See the *Did You Know?* box for further suicide facts.)

DID
YOU
KNOW?

### Suicide Facts

◆ More people die from suicide than from homicide in the United States. In 1998, there were 1.7 times as many suicides as homicides.

◆ Overall, suicide is the eighth leading cause of death for all Americans, and is the third leading cause of death for young people between 15 and 24 years of age.

◆ Suicide rates have increased over past decades among persons between the ages of 10 and 19, among young black males, and among elderly males.

◆ Nearly 60% of all suicides are committed with a firearm.

◆ Suicide took the lives of 30,575 Americans in 1998.

◆ In 1998, more than 90% of all suicides in this country were among whites, with white males accounting for 73% of all suicides. However, during the period from 1979–1992, suicide rates for Native Americans (a category that includes American Indians and Alaska Natives) were about 1.5 times the national rates. There was a disproportionate number of suicides among young male Native Americans during this period, as males 15 to 24 years of age accounted for 64% of all suicides by Native Americans.

◆ Suicide among black youths, once uncommon, has increased sharply in recent years. Although white teens still have a higher rate of suicide, the gap is narrowing.

Source: Centers for Disease Control and Prevention, "Suicide in the United States," 2002. Available at http://www.cdc.gov/ncipc/factsheets/suifacts.htm.

Adolescent boys complete suicide at a higher rate than girls. However, adolescent girls make more suicide attempts than boys. This appears to be because boys tend to rely on methods more likely to be lethal (e.g., guns and hanging), whereas girls are more likely to attempt suicide by swallowing drugs or poisons or slashing their wrists.

The use of firearms for suicide by young people is increasing at a faster rate than any other method. In fact, firearm suicides largely account for the dramatic increase in the adolescent suicide rate. The availability of guns in the home appears to increase the risk for suicide among adolescents. This is important also because most youth suicide attempts occur at home.

## Causes of Youth Suicide

The causes of youth suicide are complex and numerous, and there is no one reason that adolescents choose suicide (see *Did You Know?* on page 316). Adolescence is a period of particular vulnerability to thoughts about suicide. Physiological changes and sexual maturity, increasing independence, a new consciousness of self, and the process of questioning given values characterize adolescence. Rapid changes occur and the self-image is often insecure and fragile. Teenagers undergo so many changes so rapidly that they tend to feel a loss of control over their lives. As a result, teenagers are often lonely and feel that they are the only ones going through these changes. The fear of being ridiculed or taken lightly is extreme. These fears may explain why adolescents are often secretive and unapproachable. They have a tendency to shelter their thoughts rather than open themselves to misunderstanding or ridicule. A derisive or mocking remark made by either a peer or adult can be extremely destructive during this turbulent time of life.

Psychological and emotional pain is likely to seem hopeless and unending to a young person.[5] Feelings of hopelessness and depression are leading causes of youth suicidal ideation and behavior. In general, young people have not solved or coped successfully with many of life's problems, nor felt the relief or satisfaction that follows. Regretfully, many are reluctant to share their fears, concerns, and problems with adults. It is a common adolescent perception that adults cannot understand what teenagers are feeling. They either turn to peers or keep their concerns inside. When they find no relief from the pain, suicide may seem the only escape.

The loss of a parent is a major stressful event and a risk factor for suicidal thoughts and/or behavior. Loss of a parent may occur through death, separation, or divorce. Such a loss can lead young people to feel rejected by the deceased or absent parent. Others feel guilty for not having prevented the death or divorce. Quite often feelings of rejection and guilt coexist in the same young person. These are difficult emotions to deal with and cause great emotional pain.

DID
YOU
KNOW?

## Factors Contributing to the Rising Rate of Adolescent Suicide

Many factors are frequently cited as being related to the rising rate of adolescent suicide, including the following:

◆ A high level of social and academic competition and pressure
◆ Violence that children and adolescents are exposed to: real violence—such as rape, murder, and child abuse—and created violence on television, in videos, movies, and music
◆ The lack of socially acceptable ways for youngsters to express anger
◆ The lack of connection to religion
◆ The increase in abuse of alcohol and other drugs
◆ The special sensitivity of many kids to social isolation
◆ Elevated occurrence of depressive illness in adolescents
◆ The increase in the absolute number of adolescents in society and the associated increased competition for diminished resources
◆ The pressures on kids to grow up too quickly
◆ The increasing mobility of the American family
◆ High incidence of family fragmentation
◆ Greater availability of firearms

Source: R. M. Page, "Youth Suicidal Behavior: Completions, Attempts, and Ideations," *The High School Journal*, 80(1): 60–65, 1998.

Alienation from the family is a major cause of youth suicide. The changing nature of the family (e.g., increase in single-parent households, divorce rate, and number of mothers working) augments the likelihood of a breakdown in communication, of emotional conflicts, and of stress. To cope with stress and conflict, youths often withdraw from the family. Failure to achieve and pressures to live up to high parental expectations are additional reasons for alienation from the family. Severe punishment and child abuse can lead to alienation, low self-esteem, and suicidal behavior. Young people desperately need warm, supportive families who accept them as valuable and significant members.

Substance abuse and suicide are closely related. Adolescents and some children turn to alcohol and other psychoactive substances in an effort to reduce the emotional pain they suffer. These substances reduce inhibitions and magnify suicidal impulses, thus increasing the risk of suicide.

Our contemporary society is highly mobile and fast paced, which makes it difficult for many young people to establish roots. Moving from neighborhood to neighborhood, city to city, or state to state is difficult and can contribute to feelings of alienation and loneliness. Further, the news media keep young people informed of frightening world conditions and may create a great sense of distress and loss of control. It is not uncommon to develop a "doomsday" attitude such as, "We will not live to the age of our parents because we will be destroyed by a nuclear bomb, crime, air pollution, or acid rain." Adolescents may see no reason to go on living because there is nothing to look forward to.

Youths feel the pressures to succeed, and fear failure. These fears of failure are magnified when family, peer, or school expectations are excessive or unrealistic. Suicide is an effort to escape from such demands.

It has been widely reported that gay and lesbian youth are two to three times more likely to commit suicide than other youth, and that 30% of all attempted or completed youth suicides are related to issues of sexual identity. There are no empirical data on completed suicides to support such assertions, but there is growing concern about an association between suicide risk and bisexuality or homosexuality for youth, particularly males. Increased attention has been focused on the need for empirically based and culturally competent research on the topic of gay, lesbian, and bisexual suicide.[6]

***Causes Among Preteen Children***  Among preteen children, the causes of attempted suicide include a pattern of bad treatment at home, rebellious behavior in reaction, and then fear of punishment; jealousy of parents' affection for one another and guilt for such feelings; desire to punish others with grief over the suicide; difficulty at school; instability at home; real or perceived lack of love; physical defects, illness, or social deprivation that makes the child feel unloved; aggressive parents who provoke increased aggressive feelings; breakup of the home from separation, divorce, abandonment, or death of a parent; fear of being imprisoned for antisocial behavior; unhappiness in love; and wounded pride.

In a survey of elementary school counselors who reported having made contact with students who were considering suicide, family problems were ranked as the greatest contributing factor to the suicide attempts.[7] The family problems most likely to surface were divorce, separation, and parental alcoholism. Peer acceptance and pressure to achieve academically were also reported by the counselors as contributing factors in the suicide attempts of elementary school children. Sixty-eight percent of the elementary school counselors in the survey indicated that they had come into contact with one or more students who were considering suicide, yet only 17% of the schools had guidelines for staff to follow when a child exhibits suicidal behaviors. These percentages underscore the importance of suicide prevention and intervention programs within elementary schools.

It is important to realize that many young children do not conceptualize death. Even 10-year-olds may not see death (or suicide) as final and irreversible.

*Causes Among Teens*     Teenagers list the following motives for attempting suicide: shame, pangs of conscience, anger, quarreling, passion, being fed up with life, physical suffering, and worry. Personal factors include feelings of inferiority because of physical defects, mood swings produced by hormonal changes of adolescence, anxiety over pubertal changes, perception of a sexual abnormality, an undue guilt response to sexual intimacy, difficulty in making social adjustments, familial tendency toward psychological imbalance, personality disorders, psychosis, and low intelligence. Environmental factors include a broken home, unaffectionate parents, neglect, mental instability among household members, friction with siblings, feelings of being a burden or being unwanted, school difficulty, and friction with peers or teachers.

The instability of adolescents, the multiple stressors affecting this age group, and their immature coping mechanisms leave them vulnerable to impulsive decision making. Loss of child-parent dependence, failure at school, lack of success, or a feeling of being a burden at home may be precipitating factors.

## Suicidal Ideation and Attempts

The Youth Risk Behavior Survey provides information on the extent of **suicidal ideation** and **suicidal attempts** among high school students.[8] More than 1 in 5 (19.3%) high school students report having seriously considered attempting suicide in the past year. Female students (24.9%) were more likely than male students (13.7%) to have considered attempting suicide. More serious suicidal ideation was observed among 14.5% of students nationwide who, during the year preceding the survey, had made a specific plan to attempt suicide. Overall, 8.3% of students reported attempting suicide one or more times in the past year. This was true for more females (10.9%) than males (5.7%). The percentage of students reporting attempting suicide in the past year that resulted in an injury, poisoning, or overdose that had been treated by a doctor or nurse was 2.6%.

An attempted suicide must be taken very seriously. In addition to being a potentially lethal event, it is a risk factor for completed suicide and often an indicator of other problems such as substance abuse, depression, or adjustment and stress reactions.[9] Unfortunately, many youth suicide attempters do not receive medical or psychological treatment following their attempt. Suicide researchers estimate that the number of adolescent suicide attempts may be as high as 50 to 200 times that of completed suicides.[10]

A study of fatal and nonfatal suicide attempts among Oregon adolescents revealed some interesting facts.[11] Approximately 80% of suicide attempts in female adolescents involve the ingestion of drugs, compared with 57% among male adolescents. Males who attempt suicide are more likely to do so by hanging, suffocation, cutting or piercing, or with firearms. The proportion of fatal suicide attempts to nonfatal suicide attempts is nearly 100-fold higher among male adolescents compared with female adolescents. Nearly 80% of suicides among adolescents occur in their residences. The most attempts occur during the spring months (March, April, May) and the least during the summer months (June, July, August). Attempts occur most frequently on Mondays and least frequently on Saturdays.

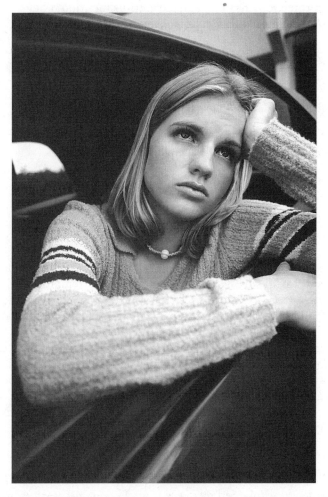

Most suicides are planned rather than committed on impulse. Educators should be alert for verbal, behavioral, situational, and depressive symptoms.

## Warning Signs of Suicide

Many signs may indicate suicidal thoughts or behavior in young people. These signs can be grouped in four categories: verbal, behavioral, situational, and depressive symptoms. Educators should be alert for these signs in the children and adolescents they work with.

*Verbal Signs*    Quite often direct or indirect statements about suicidal intentions or wishes are dismissed or overlooked as not being serious statements. Yet, in fact, they do indicate suicidal intentions and should be treated seriously. One of the most dangerous misconceptions about suicide is that people who talk about killing themselves rarely do it. Actually, more than three-fourths of all suicide victims mention it beforehand. Most suicides are planned rather than committed on impulse. Statements like these may indicate suicidal intentions:

- ❖ I wish I were dead.
- ❖ I'm going to kill myself.
- ❖ People (or my family) would be better off without me.
- ❖ Nobody needs me.
- ❖ If (such and such) happens, I am going to kill myself.
- ❖ I just can't go on living anymore.
- ❖ You won't have to worry about me anymore.
- ❖ How do you donate your body to science?
- ❖ Why is there such unhappiness in life?

*Behavioral Signs*    The most serious and predictive sign of suicide is a previous unsuccessful suicide attempt. Any suicide attempt should be considered serious. It is common for some youths to make weak attempts in order to gain attention. Yet, if these attempts are ignored or not regarded as serious, they may turn to more lethal methods.

"Setting one's affairs in order" is another behavioral sign that needs serious attention and is strongly suggestive of suicidal thoughts. This includes activities such as making arrangements to be a donor of vital body organs and giving away prized possessions. Any changes in behavior should be questioned, whether positive or negative. Behavioral signs include the following:

- ❖ Poor adjustment to a recent loss
- ❖ A suicide note that is left in advance
- ❖ A sudden, unexplained recovery from a severe depressive episode
- ❖ Alcohol and other drug abuse
- ❖ Extreme changes in mood or behavior

❖ Excessive irritability

❖ Feelings of guilt

❖ Unexplained crying (particularly if male)

❖ Truancy or running away from home

❖ Academic difficulty or poor schoolwork

❖ Aggressive behavior

❖ Promiscuity

❖ Self-mutilation

❖ Resignation from clubs or other groups

❖ Repeated episodes of accidental injury

❖ Social isolation or withdrawing from friends

***Situational Signs*** The most important situational signal is family strife. Family disruption by death of a parent or sibling, separation, or divorce is associated with suicidal behavior. Disruption or disorder in the family is frequently associated with alcohol or other drug abuse among parents. Suicidal behavior by an immediate family member is more prevalent among youth suicide attempters than among those who have not attempted suicide. Therefore, suicidal behavior by other family members may serve as a model for coping with stress. Young people growing up with these family models may be more likely to resort to suicide in response to stress. Other situational signs include the following:

❖ Loss of a job

❖ Loss of a boyfriend or girlfriend

❖ A fight with a peer

❖ A fight or serious disagreement with a parent

❖ Chronic illness

❖ Survival of an illness with a disability

❖ A move to a new city

❖ Academic failure

❖ Being caught for a crime, such as shoplifting or vandalism

***Depressive Symptoms*** Depression is strongly associated with youth suicide. Educators should be alert for the signs associated with depression discussed earlier in this chapter. Feelings of hopelessness are particularly highly correlated with suicidal ideation and behavior. Therefore, any signs of depression and hopelessness require serious attention.

## Prevention and Intervention

Often suicidal behavior is a cry for help with problems that seem impossible to solve. Showing that you care and listening are the most critical preventive measures that you can employ. Take warning signs and threats seriously and establish a sense of trust. A student's trust in a teacher often requires confidentiality. This places a great responsibility on the teacher to determine if the situation warrants informing parents or others. When intervention is necessary, the teacher can advise the student on how to get professional help. It is helpful when teachers serve as a liaison between the school and the professional help.

Daily contact with and knowledge of their students put teachers in an excellent position to detect the warning signs of suicide. Any suspicions about suicide cannot be ignored. It is best to calmly ask a student, "Are you thinking about suicide?" This direct approach helps lower a student's anxiety and lets him or her know that someone cares enough to simply listen.

By being a concerned listener, you help a young person know that he or she is being taken seriously. Listening conveys to the young person that you care and that he or she is not alone. Failure to listen may be perceived as a sign of an individual's sense of worthlessness.

Do not act shocked if a student discloses to you that he or she is thinking about suicide. Help the individual to realize that he or she is not so different because of thinking of suicide in response to problems or stresses. Thoughts of suicide are normal; however, suicidal actions are not. Disclosure of suicidal thoughts must be taken seriously. Do not dismiss them lightly. **Take appropriate action.**

**Do not attempt to deal with a suicidal person alone.** Enlist the support and help of parents, school counselors and other mental health professionals, clergy, and friends. It is very difficult for students to obtain professional assistance on their own. Therefore, teachers serve a critical role in the referral process. Trust your suspicions that a student may be contemplating suicide and take the appropriate action.

**Do not allow yourself to be sworn to secrecy by a suicidal student.** You may be confronted by a student who says "I have something important to tell you, but first you must promise not to tell anyone else." Your response should be, "If someone is hurting you or you are considering hurting yourself, I cannot promise that I will not tell anyone else. If it is a personal matter, I will not tell anyone and I will help and support you. However, if it is a problem for which you need assistance from others, I will help you get the help you need." Young people are often relieved that you are willing to help with their problem and that you are comfortable talking about it.

In discussing their problems and situation, take a positive approach and help them to see the alternatives to suicide. It is important that they realize that there are choices. Share some strategies that work for you in dealing with stressful situations, failure, loss, and disappointment. Ask them to share with you some strategies that have worked for them in the past. Convey that suicidal thoughts are normal and that they do not need to act upon those thoughts. Suicide is a normal thought, not a normal behavior.

It is important that depressed and unhappy youth understand that most problems solve themselves over time. Help them to get out of the thought pattern that things get worse and worse. Emphasize the temporary nature of most problems. Explain that the immediate crisis will pass in time and that time will help in the healing. Tell them that suicide is a permanent solution to a problem that is usually temporary.

Help the young person develop a network of support. Identify people that he or she can be with and talk with. Sometimes a **contract for life** helps. A contract for life is a formal, written agreement in which suicidal people state that they will ask for help before they hurt themselves. A contract for life should be dated and signed. Never let a contract for life expire without formal acknowledgment. Young people who pose an **immediate suicide risk should never be left alone.**

The continued increase in youth suicides suggests that not enough is being done to curtail this important problem. More schools and school personnel should become involved in suicide prevention and intervention programs. Educators must become more effective in identifying and helping potential suicide victims. In order to develop effective programs, teachers, school administrators, school staff members, parents, and community agencies must become more actively involved. We must reach out to identify and help potential suicidal youth. We must not fail our students.

---

IN THE
CLASSROOM
*8-2*

### Classroom Activities Dealing with Suicide

The following are examples of teaching activities that deal with suicide. This subject is usually addressed at the high school level. These activities help students review the warning signs of suicide, the proper steps to take in prevention and intervention, and the importance of life.

#### Chalk Line

Draw a horizontal line across a chalkboard. Tell the class that this line represents the time line of a person's life. Have the students identify the gender of the person and name the person. Divide the class into three groups. Have one group come up with important events that take place in the "chalk person's"

*continued*

*continued*

school years. Have the second group identify events in the person's young adult years, and have the third group identify events for midlife and beyond. Give the groups a few minutes to work independently to determine their life events. Then have the first group come up to the chalk line and mark in the important events, followed by the second group, and finally the third group. Don't be surprised if students mark in both good and bad events. Let them have fun with it. When they are finished say, "I'm sorry, this was to have been Jane Doe's life, but on (give a specific date and time indicating she died as a teenager) she committed suicide." Draw a very heavy line showing time of death. At this point the students will most likely become very quiet as they think about all that this fictitious person would have missed out on. This activity can be useful in introducing the topics of suicide and how life should be celebrated.

## Letters

Assign students to write a letter to an imaginary friend who is contemplating suicide.

## Speaker

Invite a suicide hotline crisis worker or other mental health specialist to talk with your class about suicide prevention and intervention.

## Brainstorm

Have students brainstorm the warning signs of suicide. Discuss how and why each sign makes suicide a likely possibility.

## Dos and Don'ts

In small groups, have students compile lists of "Dos and Don'ts" in helping suicidal students. Have each group share its lists with the rest of the class.

## Role-play

Have students role-play situations in which they practice suicide intervention and prevention. Examples of role-play situations include pretending to be a worker at a suicide hotline or responding to a friend who is contemplating suicide. Be sure to guide students in active listening skills and enlisting the help of adults.

## Key Terms

depressive disorder   305
major depression   306
dysthymia   307
bipolar disorder   308
seasonal affective disorder
  (SAD)   308

self-injury   312
suicidal ideation   318
suicidal attempts   318
contract for life   323

## Review Questions

1. Explain the difference between depressive disorders and "the blues."
2. Why is depression sometimes difficult to recognize in students?
3. How prevalent is depression among children and adolescents?
4. Identify the types of depressive disorders and their signs and symptoms.
5. What are the risk factors for childhood and adolescent depression?
6. In what ways do young people mask their feelings of depression?
7. How can educators help young people who are depressed?
8. Explain why some young people engage in acts of self-injury and what educators can do to help.
9. What are some of the causes of youth suicide? More specifically, what are the causes among preteen children? Teenagers?
10. How many high school students report having seriously considered attempting suicide in the past year? What percentage, made a specific plan to attempt suicide? What percentage reported attempting suicide one or more times in the past year?
11. Who is most likely to attempt suicide? Who is most likely to succeed in killing themselves?
12. Where do most suicide attempts occur and when?
13. Give several examples of verbal, behavioral, and situational signs of suicide.
14. Discuss some of the dos and don'ts of dealing with students who are suicidal.

## References

1. Schlozman, S. C. (2001). "The Shrink in the Classroom: Too Sad to Learn." *Educational Leadership*, 59(1): 80–83. Available at http://www.ascd.org/readingroom/edlead/0109/schlozman.html.
2. National Institute of Mental Health (2000). "Depression in Children and Adolescents: A Fact Sheet for Physicians" (NIH Publication No. 00-4844). Bethesda, MD: National Institutes of Health. Available at http://www.nimh.nih.gov/publicat/depchildresfact.cfm.
3. National Center for Health Statistics (1998). "Deaths: Final Data for 1996." *National Vital Statistics Report*, 47(9): 53.

4. National Center for Injury Prevention and Control, Centers for Disease Control and Prevention (1998). "Fact Sheet on Suicide." Available at http://www.cdc.gov/ncipc/dvp/suifacts.htm.

5. Page, R. M. (1991). "Loneliness as a Risk Factor in Adolescent Hopelessness." *Journal of Research in Personality*, 25: 1889–1895.

6. U.S. Public Health Service (1999). *The Surgeon General's Call to Action to Prevent Suicide*. Washington, DC: U.S. Department of Health and Human Services. Available at http://www.surgeongeneral.gov/library/calltoaction/calltoaction.htm.

7. Nelson, R. E., and B. Crawford (1991). "Suicide Among Elementary School-Age Children." *Elementary School Guidance and Counseling*, 25: 123–128.

8. Centers for Disease Control and Prevention (2000). "Youth Risk Behaviors Surveillance—United States, 1999." *Morbidity and Mortality Weekly Report*, 49(SS-05).

9. Page, R. M. (1996). "Youth Suicidal Behavior: Completion, Attempts, and Ideations." *The High School Journal*, 80(1): 60–65.

10. Garland, A. F., and E. Ziegler (1993). "Adolescent Suicide Prevention: Current Research and Social Policy Implications." *American Psychologist*, 48: 169–182.

11. Centers for Disease Control and Prevention (1995). "Fatal and Non-Fatal Suicide Attempts Among Adolescents—Oregon, 1988–1993." *Morbidity and Mortality Weekly Report*, 44(16): 312–315.

# 9

# DEATH AND DYING

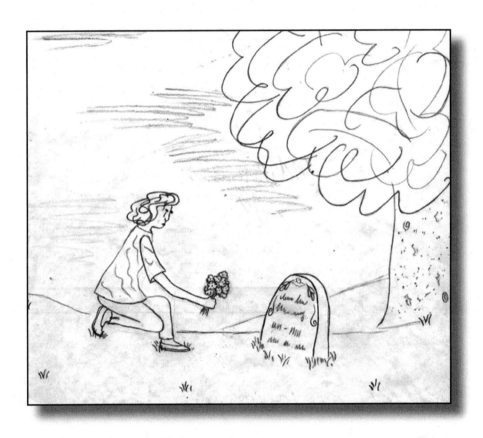

# When a Student Dies . . .

*Early in the fall, 13-year-old Mary was out of school with "the mumps." Weeks later, after much suffering, she developed a gum infection. In mid-November, the diagnosis was changed. Mary had leukemia. As a second-year teacher of trainable mentally impaired students, I had never before faced a crisis of this magnitude. I began to search for answers for myself as well as for my students.*

*From my knowledge of the five stages of death and dying as described by Elisabeth Kübler-Ross, I knew that denial would be my first reaction to this tragic news. I was therefore determined to face the facts realistically. It wasn't until much later that I became aware of the ways in which I did, in fact, deny Mary's impending death. I concentrated only on the disease itself, rather than its inevitable consequences. Even when talking with the family, I never permitted any of their foreshadowing to penetrate the barrier.*

*I found that I had a great need to help in a situation in which I felt helpless. I felt empathy for the parents of all terminally ill children—their fears, their apprehension, and their sense of uselessness as doctors, nurses, and technicians increasingly assume the necessary decision-making roles and eventually become solely responsible for the child's care. Mary's family fought long and hard to have Mary come home from the hospital. Her homecoming was their only solace. They needed to be taking care of Mary as much as she needed them to take care of her.*

*As my barrier of denial began to retreat, it was replaced by anger. I was angry that an innocent child was to be taken from persons who loved her. I was angry that she was being taken from me and that I should have to experience such a trauma. I was even angry at every 13-year-old who was healthy and strong.*

*Finally, however, I began to accept Mary's fate. Instinctively one day, I took out her notebook and threw it away. When the students questioned me, I answered truthfully that Mary would not be using it any more. After my students had left for the day, I phoned Mary's parents. Mrs. Smith was glad that I had called—Mary had died the night before. She described the final surge of life's energy and the moments before death shared by mother and father, brothers and sisters. I could say nothing. I hung up and cried.*

*I managed to inform the appropriate school personnel and then was overwhelmed by a sense of panic and confusion. At the request of Mary's family, the parents of my students had not been told that she had leukemia. How was I now to tell them of her death? More distressing, how would I tell my students?*

These questions remained unresolved until our school social worker referred me to a friend of hers, who was a grief therapist. We discussed Mary, my students, my fears. She explained that I would not be able to help others understand or cope with this crisis until I was able to accept it myself. She helped me realize that the only proper vehicle of communication was honesty. I had to be genuine in expressing my feelings. My students needed to know that it was all right to feel sad and even to cry. I was their role model. She also stressed that it was important not to treat the family as "lepers." They would need my friendship more than ever.

The next morning I met briefly with our social worker and program coordinator. The three of us then met with the general education students who worked as aides in my classroom. Finally, I returned alone to my classroom to talk with my own students. We gathered our chairs around the record player and talked about our favorite songs. I asked the class whether they remembered Mary's favorite album, and they told me that it was "Annie." As we played the record, we talked about the fact that Mary had been very, very sick. I emphasized the extreme nature of her disease so that the students would not associate every illness with death. I asked what might happen if someone was very sick. No one offered an answer. "Might that person die?" I probed. We then discussed our own experiences with death. Scott's dog had died, and Howard said that his grandmother had died. I added, "What do you think might have happened to Mary? Yes, she died, too."

Next, I explained that it was o.k. to feel sad, because we loved Mary and would miss her very much. Howard began to cry. I said, "Sometimes we need other people to help us out when we are sad. Do you feel like you might need a hug right now?" We held each other for a moment, and then Howard assured me he would be all right.

Scott's eyes filled with tears as he told us, "We'll get a new Mary." But when questioned, he realized we could not. The other students sat quietly as in disbelief. They did not understand death, but they understood the sadness.

We wanted to do something to remember Mary, so the class decided to draw pictures. We remembered lots of fun times we had had with our friend, and then we went back to our desks to an array of paper and crayons. I walked around the room and asked the students to explain their drawings. I wanted to keep them, but I felt that it was more important for the students to take them home to give their parents a starting point for discussion. I called each parent so they would know what had happened and could talk about it with their child.

I was now on my way to <u>acceptance.</u> There was still one need that I had not yet satisfied: my need to "help" the family. I told myself over and over again that

*I must call on the Smiths, but I could not bring myself to go. I was, in fact, treating them as "lepers." My visit to their home was the hardest part of the whole experience for me. It was Mrs. Smith who finally asked about the children's reactions to the news, which opened the door to sharing our feelings.*

*Many school staff members and parents wanted to make contributions to the Leukemia Foundation. My need to help was now channeled into a new direction. I began a fund in Mary's name. We contributed a total of $200 to the Leukemia Foundation, and a plaque was prepared for our school in memory of Mary. The plaque reads, "Let me win, but if I cannot win, let me be brave in the attempt. In loving memory of Mary Smith, January 16, 1980." The quotation is the theme of the National Special Olympics, in which Mary had participated.*

*In helping to guide my students through a tragedy, I also learned to cope with my own feelings. I developed a healthier attitude toward death and dying. My students were my counselors, as I was theirs, and Mary's memory is still very much alive in each of us.*

Source: M. S. Lubetsky and M. J. Lubetsky, "When a Student Dies," *Teaching Exceptional Children*, 15: 27–28, 1982. Reprinted with permission.

Not too many years ago, dying and death were very much a natural part of the total family life cycle. Families lived together, often with several generations in the same household. The dying process took place within the family circle, as did the death itself and the funeral in many cases. Young people were able to view the processes of dying, death, grief, and bereavement as natural parts of the total life cycle.

This is not true today, because the processes are typically removed from the family experience. In many instances, the act of dying has lost its dignity and normalcy and has become institutionalized, dehumanized, and mechanized—and young people have been excluded from the experience altogether. The resulting void of experience must be filled if society is going to gain a proper perspective toward the value of life. (pg. 49)[1]

In spite of September 11, 2001, and popular movies and TV shows about death and the afterlife, most children, adolescents, and adults are shielded from the realities of death. We are not as familiar with death as our predecessors. In the beginning of the twentieth century, the average life expectancy in the United States was slightly more than 47 years. Infant, child, and maternal mortality was high. As a result, children were intimately acquainted with death and dying. It was commonplace for children to have a parent (or grandparent, who resided nearby or with the family) or sibling die during their childhood, to care for a dying family member, to have a family member die in their home, to be present at the time of death, and to make preparations for and attend the funeral. It is interesting to note that about one-half of the poems printed in *McGuffey's Fifth Eclectic*

*Reader* clearly refer to death and dying. This reader was one of the most commonly used books in educating children until the 1930s.

Now, more than 7 of 10 people die over the age of 65. Also, 7 of 10 die in institutions, such as hospitals or nursing homes, often removed from the family and the rest of society. Further, many children are excluded (by parents or caretakers) from the funerals and viewings of family members. As a result, death is often alien to both children and adults. Richard Lansdown has remarked, "Death has become a foreign country where we don't know how to behave."[2]

## Children's Understanding About Death and Dying

For most children, an understanding about death follows an orderly sequence. This sequence begins with total unawareness in very early childhood and progresses through stages to the point where death is conceptualized as final and universal and where abstract thinking about death occurs. Mature concepts about death develop in a progressive, developmental sequence that generally follows Piaget's model of conceptual development. However, many children attain mature death concepts at younger ages than suggested by Piaget. The comprehension of death concepts such as irreversibility, universality, and cessation of function has been found to vary widely among the chronological ages of children.

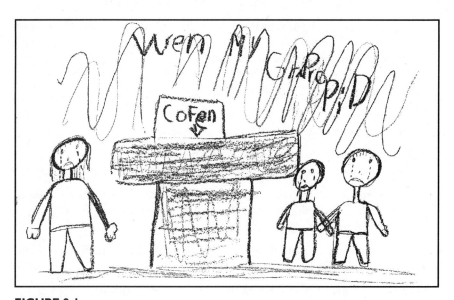

**FIGURE 9-1**
When children are simply asked to draw pictures about death, many different perceptions and experiences emerge. This child's grandfather had recently died. Notice the detail of the tears and coffin, and also the missing feet on the people who can't walk away from the pain.

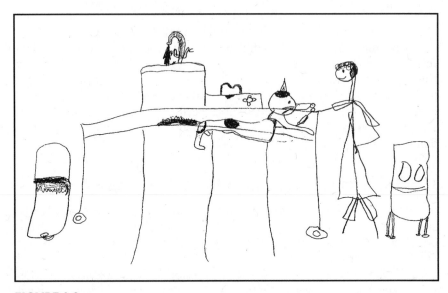

**FIGURE 9-2**
This child drew about her pet being put to sleep. The child had mixed feelings about this procedure. Notice the smile on the person and the intensity of the water coming out of the faucet.

Here are 10 needs Butler found children have concerning death:[3]

1. To learn how to mourn; that is, to go through the process of giving up some of the feelings they have invested in the deceased and go on with the living, to remember, to be touched by the feelings generated by their memories, to struggle with guilt over what they could have done, and to deal with their anger over the loss.

2. To mourn small losses, such as animals, in order to deal better with the larger, closer losses.

3. To be informed about a death. When they are not told but see parents upset, they may invent their own explanations or blame themselves.

4. To understand the finality of death. Because abstract thinking is difficult for young children, they may misunderstand adults who say a deceased person "went away" or is "asleep."

5. To say good-bye to the deceased by participating in funerals or viewings, even if only for a few minutes.

6. Opportunities to work out their feelings and deal with their perceptions of death through talking, dramatic playing, reading books, or expressing themselves through the arts.

7. Reassurance that their parents will take care of themselves and probably won't die until after their children are grown. It is important that

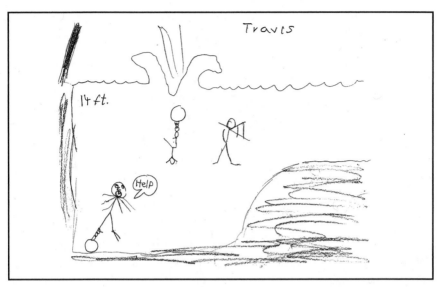

**FIGURE 9-3**
This child's depiction of death possibly reveals a fear of drowning.

they know that sometimes children die, but only if they are very sick or if there's a bad accident. It is equally important that they understand that almost all children grow up and live to be very old.

8. To know that everyone will die some day. It may be hard for adults to be honest about this fact, but if denied, children won't be prepared for dealing with death during their lives.

9. To be allowed to show their feelings: to cry, become angry, or laugh uncontrollably. The best approach is to empathize with their feelings.

10. To feel confident that their questions will be answered honestly and not avoided and that adults will give them answers they can understand.

## Preschool-Age Children

Children 3 to 5 years of age tend to see death as gradual and happening only to the very old, and as a departure that is reversible—as they have seen portrayed in cartoons. Many children believe there is a magical power that will bring a deceased person back to life. They are very curious about death, which is likely to lead to questions that parents and teachers may find unsettling.

When a deceased person continues to stay away, a child may become angry or hurt. A child may feel that he or she is responsible, believing that a thought or behavior may have caused the death. This evolves as a result

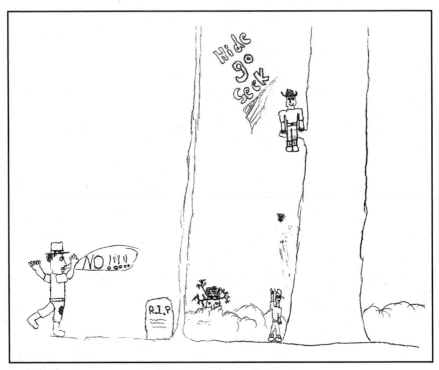

**FIGURE 9-4**
This child had had no real experience with death and depicted it with cartoons and Halloween images.

of the child's egocentric thinking. Fears of abandonment and anxiety also occur.

Concern about the dead person's physical well-being after death is common. A child is typically concerned with how the dead person will stay warm and get food after burial.

In the mind of a young child, death is associated with a cessation of body functions. A person or animal is considered to be dead when there is no longer any breathing or voluntary movement.

## Middle Childhood

Early in the middle childhood period (from about first to third grade), death is often personified as a monster, ghost, skeleton, or other predatory form. Because of this conception, children think death can be fought and overcome by magic. As a result, children consider themselves to be immortal and believe that only those who are weak or old are susceptible to death.

At about 9 or 10 years of age, children are able to conceptualize that death is final and not reversible. Although death is still an abstract thought, they come to realize that they too will die. Such realizations can create fears and concerns about dying. Interest in details about dying and the state of the body after death is heightened and questions are stimulated.

It is common for children to believe that a deceased person can see and hear them. As a result, children may feel pressure to "be perfect" for the deceased. Misunderstandings about death can accelerate fears about dying. The religious beliefs of the family concerning death gain new importance to children as they come to understand the finality of death.

## Adolescence

Adolescents are capable of comprehending that death is final, irreversible, and universal. This understanding brings concern about their own mortality. They often defend against the resulting anxiety by denying the possibility of their own death—except as an abstract event in a remote future. Denial serves as a buffer against this anxiety and contributes to an illusion of invulnerability and immortality. These illusions may contribute to risk-taking behaviors such as speeding and reckless driving and drug use.

Adolescents can also formulate abstract ideas about the nature of death. Piaget refers to this developmental period as "the period of formal operations." As such, young people can make generalizations about death beyond what they experience. They formulate their own theologies about life after death as they examine the religious views of their parents and others.

# Childhood and Adolescent Bereavement

Many children in elementary schools are confronted with the death of a family member, close friend, classmate, or a pet. Yet, few children have received any preparation for dealing and coping with these losses. Further, society tends to deny and avoid dealing with death. According to Bertoia and Allan:

> Every individual eventually faces the death of a loved one. For most, this experience is painful and difficult to share. Those wishing to offer support are often uncertain about what to say to a bereaved person and are uncomfortable with the thought of their own death. This discomfort results in their avoiding the topic and often the bereaved person. The message such behavior creates is that death is a taboo subject, and therefore, the bereaved individual attempts to deal with it alone, often internalizing the pain and developing behavioral or emotional difficulties later. Many adults are even more uncomfortable dealing with this topic when it relates to a child, and so ignore the issue, leaving the child to cope in isolation with only his or her imagination. (pg. 30)[4]

Bereaved children face the arduous tasks of coming to terms with death, grieving, and resuming the appropriate progression toward development of personality. Sensitive and skilled school personnel can help children accomplish these tasks. However, most teachers are either not comfortable or inadequately trained to offer appropriate support to bereaved children. These teachers cannot help children resolve their grief in a healthy manner and may even complicate the grieving process.

The process of acceptance of a death or loss is often referred to as **grief-work.** The death of a loved one, such as a parent or sibling, often requires two or more years before grieving is completed. A child's reactions to death depend on his or her age and cognitive developmental level, but resemble adult patterns of mourning. Typically, the initial responses are denial, anger, and anxiety. Later, these feelings are replaced by periods of sadness, despair, and depression. When these feelings are worked through, acceptance of the death emerges.

## Death of a Parent

About 6 of every 100 children experience the death of one or both parents before the age of 18. The death of a father is twice as likely to occur as the death of a mother. Most parental deaths are sudden. Therefore, children and surviving family members have little opportunity for anticipatory grieving or preparation for the death. Also, a surviving parent is in a state of shock, which makes it very difficult to obtain parental assistance and support with the child's grief.[2]

Responses to the death of a parent may include a host of emotions and behaviors. The death may frighten, stun, shock, bewilder, or overwhelm a child. Also, feelings of guilt, anger, loneliness, helplessness, and abandonment or rejection may occur. Behavioral responses that typically result are aggression, hostility, and noncooperation. Withdrawal and regressive behaviors also occur. Sometimes there are disturbances in school performance.

Although a major distress, most children survive the death of a parent without long-lasting effects upon their mental health. The support and care that a child receives from adults after a parent's death is a crucial factor in the healthy acceptance of the death.

When a parental death is sudden, school personnel will need to provide support to the child immediately upon return to school. When a child is isolated or feels rejected because of the death, class discussions may help. Class discussions also help other children overcome fears that such a loss will happen to them. When a child did not have an opportunity to say good-bye to a deceased person, the need to do so remains (this often happens when a child was shielded from the death and not allowed to attend the funeral). Counselors can assist by helping a child write a letter or draw a picture to say good-bye to a loved one. Further, children should be allowed to express their feelings about the death freely. Later psychiatric problems often result from incomplete grief-work. School personnel can play a key role in initiating and assisting children in their grief-work.

School personnel should be alert for the following behaviors in a bereaved child. According to Brenner, a combination of two or more of these behaviors may indicate the need for additional support, counseling, or therapy:[5]

❖ Deep and persisting fears that other loved ones will die or that the child himself or herself will die

❖ Repeated expressions of wanting to die in order to be with the dead parent

❖ Angry and violent outbursts combined with feelings of guilt for the parent's death

❖ Attempted role reversal from depending on the surviving adult to taking care of him or her

❖ Continual movement, inability to be quiet or to express sad feelings

❖ Marked reduction in activity by a formerly very active child

## Death of a Sibling

The loss of a sibling during childhood is a very traumatic experience. A sibling's death may be more difficult to accept and understand than a parent's death. Because the deceased sibling is close in age, the death represents the reality of a child's or adolescent's mortality. Further, the surviving sibling's need for support may be ignored by others in light of the needs of parents.

Parents' reactions to the sibling's death profoundly influence a child's quest for acceptance of the death. Some parents react by overprotecting surviving children, taking excessive precautions to make sure children are free from any risks. In such cases, a child may have difficulty developing independence due to these efforts to restrict the child's vulnerability to perceived danger. This can seriously thwart a child's normal development process.

Some parents may come to idealize the dead child. Consequently, surviving siblings may feel inadequate by comparison to the deceased sibling. Some parents try to recover the loss by unconsciously pressuring a remaining child to take on the personality or behavior of the dead one.

The siblings of a terminally ill child must deal with the stress of witnessing the pain and discomfort of their dying brother or sister. As the parents must focus upon the overwhelming needs of the dying sibling, other children in the family feel the loss of attention and companionship of their parents. An additional stressor faced by surviving siblings is that parents expect them to be well behaved and to take care of their own needs. Feelings of guilt are common to survivors because they are allowed to go on living while a sibling must die.

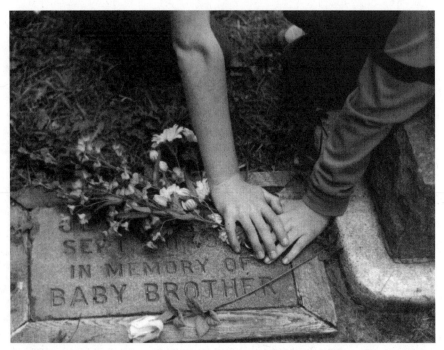

The death of a sibling may be more difficult to accept and understand than a parent's death.

When a sister or brother is actively involved in circumstances which lead to a sibling's death, extreme feelings of guilt are likely. Professional help is necessary to gain an understanding of the death and to come to the point that they can forgive themselves. Another concern focuses upon the reactions of the other family members to this sibling. Some have difficulty trusting and forgiving the child. Some direct anger toward the child as other family members deal with the death.

In response to the death of a sibling, it is common to experience feelings of shock, confusion, numbness, depression, anger, and loneliness. Thoughts about the dead sister or brother linger. It is common for the surviving siblings to have had thoughts about suicide, to have experienced sleeping and eating disturbances, or to report hallucinations in which a deceased sibling either spoke to them or reappeared to them.

## Death of a Pet

The death of a pet is often a child's first experience with death. When a pet dies, children are likely to grieve and feel significant pain. This loss represents an opportunity in which children can learn about death and the societal rituals (e.g., funerals). Children need extra support in dealing with their loss.

# Providing a Supportive Environment for the Terminally Ill Child

The presence of a terminally ill school-age child or adolescent in school involves and affects many. In addition to the terminally ill child and his or her family, school personnel and students can provide support as they cope with the situation.

Whenever possible, dying children are encouraged to continue to attend school for as long as possible. School provides frequent opportunities for creative expression and art activities, which provide natural outlets for working through the dying process. Schoolwork is often something that terminally ill youngsters can do, so it provides a means of performing successfully. This can be extremely important as a source of maintaining feelings of self-worth. School also allows a terminally ill young person to fulfill social needs.

Of course, the physical limitations of a terminal illness make full-time school attendance difficult, if not impossible. Absences are necessary for treatments and on days when a child feels too ill to attend school. The alterations in physical appearance and physical limitations of an illness also affect school attendance. Therefore, arrangements for partial days and homebound teaching support are usually necessary.

When the illness progresses to the point that school attendance is no longer possible, it helps if small groups of classmates visit the child. This maintains contact between the child and his or her class, which can be very supportive to a terminally ill child.

## The Teacher's Role

The classroom teacher can play a special role in the life of a terminally ill child. Bryant describes this role below:

> Remember that as a teacher you have a special place. You represent the child's normal world; you are an oasis for him. The doctors and nurses bring shots and machines; the parents hover with tears and anguish. You, however, know the child's work-a-day world. You are part of his business and social community. You, more than many, can maintain a semblance of his former world by your visits, news of the classroom, and occasional work assignments. Your interaction with a dying child can keep him among the living a little longer. (pg. 65)[6]

## The Classmates' Role

Throughout the terminal illness, the child needs to continue to feel included as a member of the class. When possible, classmates should be informed about the terminal illness and guided to deal with the situation in a constructive manner. Bertoia and Allan explain why this is important:

By including the child as part of the class throughout the treatment phase and during the course of an illness, the class as a whole can deal with the situation in a positive manner. Generally, class members will become very supportive of the child in class and protective on the playground. When the teacher or child explains something about the disease to class members, their fear of getting the same thing is diminished and the sick child is not isolated. Because family members are frightened by names such as "cancer" or "AIDS," general terms such as "blood disease" can be used. The counselor should get permission from the child's family if the proper name is to be used. Classmates will understand when standards do change and seem unfair because the sick child cannot complete as much work in the assigned time. Class discussions about feelings and behaviors help clarify what is happening in the classroom. (pg. 34)[4]

Questions that classmates have about the illness or the eventual death of their terminally ill classmate should never be ignored. It is important that children have the opportunity to ask questions and to have them answered. Further, the parents of classmates should be informed that their child was exposed to a death so they can recognize behaviors or other characteristics that indicate their child's grief and mourning. The parents can then help their children in their grief-work.

## Understanding the Dying Child

Children with terminal conditions come to understand death at younger ages than their same-age healthy peers. Dying children often demonstrate remarkable knowledge about the seriousness of their condition despite attempts by physicians and parents to conceal the child's impending death. Therefore, children do need to be informed that their condition is fatal.

Terminally ill children feel a great deal of anxiety regarding their illness and their future. However, open communication about the illness by medical personnel and family members is associated with lower stress and anxiety levels, increased relief about their concerns, and improved ability to cope among dying children.

Dying children begin to experience many losses in their lives. They are often separated from their family and school environment for long periods of time as they receive medical care. In the dying process, they may lose hair or undergo disfiguring surgery. Particularly to an adolescent, these changes in physical appearance result in severe blows to self-esteem.

Although school-age children lack the cognitive ability to grieve the loss of their future, adolescents do not. Preparatory grief can be overwhelming and debilitating. The process of **preparatory grief** typically follows five distinct stages. These stages were originally described by Dr. Elisabeth Kübler-Ross in the influential book *On Death and Dying*. The first stage is **denial** ("No, not me. It can't be true"), which works as a buffer to reduce the initial shock of news of a terminal illness. **Anger** and resentment follow as the realities of the illness can no longer be ignored.

**Bargaining** with a supreme being for full recovery or more time is attempted in order to delay or prevent the inevitable. When it is realized that the death is inevitable, a sense of deep **depression** sets in. It should be recognized that this sense of depression and loss is a normal part of preparatory grief, not a mental disorder. With adequate support and time, the dying adolescent works thorough the previous stages and comes to **acceptance.** Acceptance is neither a happy or sad time, but a period of accepting her or his fate. The depression and pain are mostly gone, and it is a time for rest and reflection.

There is an enormous need for communication when a child is dying. Preparatory grief is best facilitated when there are supportive adults who understand it and will provide a good listening ear. Teachers and school personnel can greatly facilitate this process by understanding why a dying young person feels and behaves in a particular manner, and then responding to his or her needs.

## Responding Appropriately to Death

During your teaching career, it is likely that you will have to deal with death in the classroom. Whether a student, fellow teacher, member of the community, or family member of a student dies, it can affect your entire school. This section provides additional insights into how to respond appropriately to death.

### Death of a Schoolmate

School personnel either deal with the death (or impending death) of a child in a direct manner or attempt to ignore it. Ignoring the death may seem justified on the basis that talking about it will upset the children in the school. In the following excerpts, Keith and Ellis provide this example of a school that ignored the death of a fourth-grade boy who was accidentally shot by a schoolmate.

> In the case of Jamie, where the child's death was ignored, officials abruptly removed the dead child's belongings, including the child's desk. The rest of the children's reaction to the event was fear. No questions were asked. A book, which had belonged to the dead child, was accidentally opened by one of the children in the classroom. The child who opened the book saw the dead boy's name, screamed, and dropped the book. Even though most of the materials of the dead boy had magically disappeared during the night, the classmates carried his memory with them. The students spoke of Jamie's disappearance and the rumors of death they had heard. During snack breaks, recess, and other times, the children would gather and talk of the boy who had disappeared. The reactions of the adults appeared to communicate that Jamie's disappearance was a magical, terrible event so horrible that no one could speak of it. The classroom effect consisted of

restless behavior, an inability to concentrate, and a slight decrease in learning. (pg. 26)[7]

The teacher in this case also experienced considerable difficulty:

> The counselor requested a series of interviews with the teacher who gradually acknowledged that she was having trouble helping her class master the death of their classmate. She related her personal, painful experiences with death and how upset she had felt upon learning of the death of the child in her class. As they talked, she became more upset, because the death of this child apparently made her relive previous personal experiences she had faced with the loss of important persons in her life. The teacher's repression of her feelings had sufficed until she was faced with the death of her pupil. (pg. 26)[7]

It is apparent that the children's reactions to the death of a schoolmate can be hindered by the behavior of school personnel. The most powerful hindrance is the teacher's denial of children's capacities to deal with death. Studies reveal that teachers who are open to the painful feelings aroused by death are the best facilitators, as they help their classes deal with death as a unit to explore together.[7] Some children need counselors or outside agencies, but the most effective method of handling children's reactions to the death of a schoolmate is within the classroom. The classroom was found to provide the best environment for children to deal with the trauma of a fellow student's death.

Immediately upon the news of a student's (or teacher's) death, a meeting should be held. The meeting should include the involved teacher(s), principal, school counselor, and school nurse to make a plan of action for talking to classmates about the death, removing the dead student's belongings, working with the family, and for some form of memorial activity.

School personnel should be designated to inform schoolmates of the death, to discuss the death with them, and to answer questions. It is preferable if the classroom teacher, who has an ongoing relationship with the students, is involved in these discussions. When the teacher is too uncomfortable to lead the discussion, it helps if she or he is present while someone else, such as a counselor, leads the discussion. Children should be encouraged to ask questions, and teachers should remain open for questions and comments beyond this initial discussion. Many questions and concerns will surface in the days and weeks that follow, and teachers should be prepared to deal with them as they arise. Teachers have to acknowledge their feelings about loss so they can be emotionally available to help their students. By displaying emotions, teachers validate those of their students and provide a model for grieving.

The grief-work of schoolmates is facilitated by planning and participating in memorial activities for the deceased child and communicating condolences to family survivors. Children need to express their sorrow and to participate in activities such as attending memorial activities, writing notes or drawing pictures for the bereaved family, and creating a memorial book, bulletin board, or memorial garden.

## Sudden and Traumatic Death

Many children and adolescents die from accidents, suicides, or homicides. Regardless of the cause, the death of a child or adolescent should never be ignored. Young people should have opportunities to discuss the death and to have their questions answered in a warm and open manner. Support and further assistance in dealing with the death should be provided for all students who feel the need.

When death is the result of suicide, young people need a lot of help in understanding why the suicide occurred. It is common for surviving friends, siblings, and children to feel considerable guilt about something they said or did to the deceased individual, and to feel responsible for the suicide. When this occurs, the young person needs adult support and professional counseling to come to terms with the death and to find relief from this sense of responsibility.

Family survivors of a suicide victim are inclined to feel shame about the death. Many hold religious and personal views in which a person who commits suicide is condemned. These are difficult feelings for family members and friends to work through and require extra support.

In the school setting, it is helpful to allow expression of emotions surrounding the suicide, especially through classroom discussions of the death and memorial activities. Depressed students, who might view the suicide as a path to follow, need special help.

Survivors of suicide victims need to talk and ventilate their feelings. Listening on the part of friends and school personnel is one of the most important types of support. Let them relate their feelings over and over if they desire. It is in the relating of their feelings that they begin the healing process. While listening, one should be careful not to place blame or rationalize reasons for the suicide. Affirm their right to feel the way that they do.

Avoid making comments such as these:

- ❖ It was God's will.

- ❖ You must forget her or him.

- ❖ He or she must have been insane.

- ❖ Don't cry.

- ❖ You have other friends.

- ❖ You have other children.

- ❖ I know how you feel.

- ❖ Time will make it easier.

Realize that there is no appropriate timetable for the grief process. Allow time for recovery, even if it takes months or years.

## When Tragedy Comes to School

This section provides an actual account of how a school coped with the tragic death of a student.* Their experience provides an example of all the different needs and issues schools must address in these types of situations.

### Coping with the Trauma of a Violent Death

A member of the junior class was murdered one weekend, following a party with friends. She was killed by her boyfriend, a classmate. Both students were well-known and well-liked in the school. As can be imagined, there was considerable anguish and confusion on the part of all who knew them. The student body was stunned, the small New England community shocked.

The loss of their classmate prompted a variety of emotions among the students. After initial shock and grief, our students experienced anger and varying levels of fear and depression. It was not unusual that at times these emotions commingled indiscriminately. The students needed to be guided through this difficult time so they could deal with their grief and the grieving period would be brought to some sort of acceptable closure.

During a sad time like this, students, staff members, community members, and the family of the deceased need assistance as they attempt to cope with their feelings while desperately trying to bring normalcy back into their lives. School officials must act sensitively, decisively, and with a plan that addresses the needs of all.

I hope you never have to deal with such a condition. However, if it does occur, perhaps by knowing our experience you may be better able to manage the situation. The following was our reaction and process.

### A Meeting with Classes

Each grade level was addressed on the next school day following the tragedy. The first class to meet was the class of the victim. The students were talked to softly and gently, told that their grief was natural and had a purpose. They were told that the grieving period and subsequent time would help to heal the hurt while preserving the memory of their classmate.

Many students were afraid after the tragic event. They envisioned themselves as experiencing the same tragedy. Many said that they were afraid to be alone, or that they were afraid of the dark. They were comforted and urged not to live their lives in fear. The mere statement gave considerable reassurance. Repeated with confidence and conviction, it had a calming effect.

---

* This section on coping with the trauma of a violent death is taken from J. P. Franson, "When Tragedy Comes to School: Coping with Student Death," *NASSP Bulletin*, October 1998, 88–91. It is reprinted here with permission.

Finally, students were warned to give no credence to rumor. Rumor, whether true or false, has a destabilizing impact on the entire school. One cannot stress this point often enough. Students must be given as much information as possible from credible sources. They should be urged to reject all statements that begin with, "I heard that . . .". In the absence of personal knowledge, they must assume nothing.

The main office, guidance office, and library were set up as in-school information centers. Students were urged to seek factual information there.

## A Place to Be Apart

Grieving students were allowed a place in the school where they could express their grief. They were often too upset to go to their classes, and needed a place where they could talk, cry, or simply sit and reflect. The library was closed for general use and made available to anyone who needed to be apart from classes or classmates.

## A Memorial Service

A memorial service conducted in the school gym had a considerable healing effect. Probably its most significant accomplishment was to bring closure to the period of public grieving, while accelerating the end of personal grieving.

The service was primarily for the students; however, since the parents of the victim did not have a memorial service open to the public, we were able to provide a medium by which friends of the family could participate and express their sentiments. The parents also attended the service, and they, too, were consoled.

The service was held after school and was primarily directed to the students. They had "reserved" seating by the podium. Other guests were given the remaining available seats and bleacher seats. More than 1,000 persons attended.

Journalists from all media were invited to the service, although cameras of all types were prohibited. Advance notice of this restriction was given the media where possible; others were informed of the restrictions at the entrance to the gym. This decision lent much to the dignity and solemnity of the service.

A clergyman known to many of the students delivered the eulogies and the prayers. As principal, I spoke, and at various times during the service, the choir sang.

At the conclusion of the service, there was no rush to leave. People stood around talking quietly. Students hugged each other, cried softly, or otherwise consoled one another. Townspeople came by to talk. They were pleased with the sensitive way in which the school managed events. It was an important part of the healing process. Great care should be taken not to miss this opportunity.

## Student Support Services In-House and Out-of-House

When students left the memorial service, they were given a paper that told them how they could find support during the next five days in school, and indefinitely out of school. This information was also posted in the halls and office area.

In school, a hotline and drop-in center were established by the guidance directors. The school was open 24 hours a day for the next five days (which included a long weekend).

The telephone numbers of area emergency services and mental health centers were made available. An area outpatient clinic was also available to provide immediate therapeutic services to those in need.

The hotline was active during the first couple of days of its availability. By the fourth and fifth days, there were only one or two calls. Seemingly, the students who used the outreach opportunities felt satisfied. Others may have found comfort simply in knowing that the help was available.

### Bereavement Counseling for Staff

It was important not to overlook the emotional needs of staff members during this time. Teachers often have deep personal ties to their students. We contacted a mental health clinic in a neighboring town and requested the services of their bereavement counselors. (The counselors donated their services.) The counselors came to school and talked to the staff members, explaining the stages of the grieving process and the symptoms that the staff members could expect to see in themselves and in the students. They gave suggestions on how to cope with the different situations. Further, they explained how just their coming together had a therapeutic effect that contributed to the healing process.

The knowledge and comfort that staff members gained in this session contributed greatly to their ability to calm themselves and their students.

### Staff and Administrative Presence

The first school day after the tragedy was the most difficult day of all. There was much congregating in the halls, cafeteria, gymnasium, and other places with general access. The professional staff members were visible and accessible to students at every opportunity. Questions were answered. Opinions and solace were given with love, caring, and sensitivity. Nothing would have been more devastating than a "business as usual" approach.

Class time was given up freely for the discussion of events. School rules regarding punctuality were relaxed. A caring and sheltering atmosphere pervaded the school building. The students responded with relief and affection. As mentioned earlier, the staff counseling contributed much toward the effectiveness of staff-student counseling.

### Civil Officials

The local police chief and an officer came to school to meet with interested students to explain the sequence of legal events that were to follow. They shared as much information as possible, and further explained the potential consequences for their other classmate.

At the courthouse where the trial was to be held, the district attorney met with a delegation of students to discuss the legal process in homicides. Both meetings provided authoritative information with which students could make personal judgments.

## The Media

The media provided one of the thorniest problems during the entire process. While some journalists behaved with sensitivity and in a professional manner, others could best be described as carnivores. The latter sought to sensationalize events and intruded on the grief of students with impunity and without apology.

Journalists have a vested interest in all news, but particularly in the spectacular. A middle ground must be found whereby the school can help them meet their professional responsibilities and yet protect individual privacy.

To this end, on school grounds, all interviews with journalists were done exclusively by school administrators and guidance counselors. Journalists and students were kept apart. Any student interviews initiated by journalists were conducted off school grounds. We did not do this until the second school day after the tragedy. In that short time, considerable student animosity developed toward the media.

One young-looking female reporter hid herself in the girls' room, eaves-dropped on conversations, and printed them in the evening paper out of context. In another incident, our students were photographed in their grief and ended up on the 6:00 news. It was not surprising, then, that the students requested that their privacy be protected. We supported their request wholeheartedly. From that point on, the members of the media behaved much more responsibly.

During the entire process, no student file information was released. There are statutes that prohibit release of private information; however, in the absence of such statutes, it is still a good idea to maintain confidentiality.

## Memorial Tributes

Different kinds of memorials were established on behalf of the deceased student. Members of the school and community sent contributions for a memorial scholarship. The company for whom the victim's father worked matched all contributions on a two-for-one basis. It has turned into our largest scholarship award with an endowment of approximately $20,000.

During the week following the girl's death, the school flag was flown at half mast.

Students planted a cherry tree and provided a memorial stone. A dedication ceremony was held for the junior class and all others who wished to participate. The school choir also participated.

A page in the class yearbook was dedicated to the student in memoriam. When the class graduated, the parents, in a private meeting with me, were presented a diploma granted in memoriam.

Strength is supposed to come from adversity. I would have to say that such was the case here. In addition, there was a certain coming together of the school and community as a result of heightened sensitivity by those who sought to comfort and those who sought to be comforted.

We are all changed by the past events and yet we are still the same. We shall never forget that year. But there is comfort in knowing that in this very difficult time, we helped.

## Cultural Perspectives on Death and Dying

Trends in culture, religion, and society have profound influence on our attitudes and customs concerning death and dying. These influences affect the decisions family members make regarding organ donation, autopsies, embalming or cremating the body, and funeral and/memorial services. Today, many diverse burial traditions are emerging as people seek ways of making services more personalized. If you were to ask a funeral director about his last 10 funerals, he would very likely report 10 unique services. Part of this trend has been a shift toward cremation. In 1963, only 4% of Americans were cremated; today, that number is almost 24% and expected to rise even more.

It is helpful for teachers to have some understanding of their students' perspectives on death and dying. This understanding will help educators feel more comfortable in attending funeral services and talking to grieving students and family members. Teachers can obtain this type of information by talking to clergy or members of the community with the same religious or cultural background as the students. It can also be helpful for teachers to talk with funeral directors for additional insight and understanding.

# Death Education

No matter how hard we try to deny death, we cannot escape its inevitability or universality. Death will come to each of us, to some in childhood or adolescence, to others in the middle adult years, but to most in their later years. We will have to face the possible deaths of parents and grandparents, other relatives, friends, those we work with, and perhaps our own students or children.

Education about life and death assists students and teachers in confronting one's own mortality and that of others. This awareness allows the development of the mature perspectives necessary for decision making about matters of life and death. Students will be able to find more depth and meaning in family relationships and friendships, to set goals and priorities, and to better understand the feelings of those who experience dying and bereavement.

Through death education, students acquire skills to help others deal with bereavement. In addition to gaining an understanding of bereavement and grief processes, students practice and acquire listening and communication skills to assist others through grief-work. These skills also help in coping with personal losses (see Box 9-1).

Yarber lists several possible areas of study in a death education unit or course:[8]

❖ Definitions, causes, and stages of death

❖ The meaning of death in American society

❖ Cross-cultural views and practices related to death

❖ The life cycle

❖ Funeral ceremonies and alternatives

❖ Bereavement, grief, and mourning

❖ Cremation

❖ Cryogenics

❖ Organ donations and transplants

❖ Suicide and self-destructive behavior

❖ Extending condolences to a relative or friend

❖ Religious viewpoints of death

❖ Legal and economic aspects of death

❖ Death portrayed in music and literature

❖ Understanding the dying relative or friend

❖ Preparing for death

❖ Euthanasia

Before a teacher initiates a death education unit, she or he must confront personal feelings about death and come to terms with these feelings. The teacher, of course, must also be knowledgeable about the subject matter. Rosenthal suggests that persons planning to teach death education ask themselves the following questions to assess their readiness:[9]

❖ Will I have enough knowledge to answer factual questions and have an understanding of what is happening in the subject area of death and dying?

❖ If I do not know the answers to questions, do I know the resources available to obtain the answers?

❖ Will I have time to preview all materials that I plan to use and evaluate the worth of these materials?

❖ Do these materials help to achieve my objectives?

❖ Will I be willing to plan and use alternative exercises for those students who do not want to participate in the experiences planned for the day?

❖ Will I be willing to go to all field trip sites before taking my class there?

❖ Will I go to the cemetery, funeral home, etc., so that I know what the students may expect to encounter?

❖ How will I feel when students ask me difficult questions?

❖ Am I willing to share my points of view?

❖ How will I feel if students seem quite upset when discussing death?

❖ Will I be able to help a student who expresses suicidal thoughts?

❖ Will I be able to help a student whose parent or sibling is dying?

❖ Am I able to talk about death without using euphemisms (e.g., "passed on," "gone away")?

❖ Am I able to listen and not try to "cheer up" a grieving person?

❖ Am I able to express the fact that I care?

Death education is controversial in some areas. Some feel uneasy having teachers discuss issues that touch the very core of peoples' personal beliefs. Others contend that teachers are not sufficiently trained to deal with the emotions that come from facing one's own mortality or that emerge from grieving survivors. Before beginning a death education unit, teachers should check to see if the topic is permitted in state, county, and school guidelines and should consult with the principal.

IN THE
CLASSROOM
*9–1*

## Teaching Loss as Part of Life

Here are some examples of teaching activities that deal with loss and seeing death as a part of life. The appropriate grade level for each activity is indicated.

### Falling Leaves

Collect leaves and make a display in the classroom of a variety of shapes, sizes, and colors. Liken them to the uniqueness of individual lives. Discuss the finite nature of life and the reassurance that our world goes on.   (P, K, I, J, H)

### Pets

Allow children to talk about the death of pets or of relatives. This gives you an opportunity to teach the acceptance of death as part of life.   (P, K, I, J)

*continued*

## Literature

Comment on death and loss as it occurs in the literature that you read in the classroom. Discuss how grieving characters act and help your students understand the need for grief-work. Reinforce that loss is universal, that it hurts, and that life goes on.   (I, J, H)

## In the News

Discuss violent deaths that are prominent in local or national news. Help students empathize with grieving families. Teach students safe ways to verbally or nonverbally express any anger they feel.   (I, J, H)

## Draw

Have students draw a picture entitled "Death." This is a good groundbreaking activity for the subject. It will also give you a quick preview of who has experience with death, who sees it as an abstract cartoon, and who may have fears concerning death. These pictures can then serve as a starting point for discussions on death.   (I, J, H)

## Obituary

Have students write their own obituaries. The purpose of this activity is to help them identify all the things they want to fill their lives with. It demonstrates the fact that there is a beginning and an end to each of their "stories." Provide your students with examples of actual obituaries from newspapers. Instruct students to select the age and cause of death and to enumerate on their accomplishments and activities.   (I, J, H)

## Two Years

Have students close their eyes, take a deep breath, and relax. Tell them: "Imagine yourself in your favorite place to be alone, someplace you like to go when you want to think something through. It is very comfortable, warm, and quiet there. You feel very calm and relaxed, and at peace. Your feelings are a little surprising, because you have been told you have only two years to live. You have already gone through denial, anger, bargaining, and have come to accept your circumstances. You have come to this special place to think about what it is you want to do with the time you have left. Take a few moments now and visualize what it is you want to do with the two years you have left." Give

*continued*

*continued*

students about five minutes to think this through. You may need to occasionally speak, helping them through this visualization. At the end of the visualization, instruct students to take a deep breath, let it out slowly, and to slowly come back to the present and open their eyes.

Discuss their visualizations and what they wanted to do with their limited time. This activity helps students identify their priorities in life. It can also help illustrate the point that everyone dies, but not everyone lives. (J, H)

### Role-play

Have students role-play the following situations: talking to a very ill grandparent, talking to a terminally ill friend, asking their healthy parent about their living will or funeral desires, talking to a grieving person, and talking to a person with suicidal thoughts.   (I, J, H)

### Panel Discussion

Invite representatives from different religions to discuss their beliefs about death and life after death. Have students prepare questions for panel members in advance.   (H)

### Roots

Have students fill out a family tree with their parents or guardians. In addition to becoming familiar with ancestors' names and dates and places of birth and death, suggest that students inquire about their ancestors' personalities and characteristics.   (I, J, H)

### Funeral

Have students plan and enact a funeral for an imaginary person or animal. (I, J, H)

### Other Customs

Have students research other cultures' perspectives of death and funeral customs. Have them also look for changes that have taken place in their own culture over the past two hundred years.   (I, J, H)

*continued*

### Mortuary

Have students visit a mortuary and report on itemized costs of funerals and other services.   (H)

### Living Will

After discussing the importance of organ donations and transplants, create a living will as a class.   (I, J, H)

### Hospice

Ask a representative from a local hospice to speak to your class about the needs of the terminally ill and about hospice services.   (I, J, H)

## Key Terms

grief-work   336
preparatory grief   340
denial   340
anger   340

bargaining   341
depression   341
acceptance   341

## Review Questions

1. How does our society hide death from the living?
2. What needs do children have concerning death?
3. How do preschoolers, middle-childhood-age children, and adolescents, respectively, view death?
4. How do adults typically deal with topics associated with death, especially when children are involved?
5. What is grief-work?
6. What are some of the responses a child or adolescent can have to the death of a parent?
7. What is recommended that a school do when a student's parent dies suddenly?
8. What behaviors in a bereaving child indicate the need for additional support or counseling?
9. Explain the particular needs and possible problems a child or adolescent might experience when a sibling dies.
10. Discuss the needs of children whose pets die.
11. Explain why dying children are often encouraged to attend school for as long as possible.

12. Explain the important role a classroom teacher can play in the life of a terminally ill child.

13. Explain how a teacher can help a terminally ill child continue to feel included as a member of the class.

14. How does open communication about death with terminally ill children help them cope with impending death?

15. What losses do dying children experience in their lives?

16. According to Dr. Elizabeth Kübler-Ross, what stages do dying individuals progress through during preparatory grief? Briefly describe each of these stages.

17. What needs do children have during preparatory grief? How can teachers and other school personnel assist children in their preparatory grief?

18. Discuss how a school should deal with a student's death, including information on meetings, informing students, dealing with rumors and grieving students, attending memorial services and having memorial tributes, providing counseling and support services, and dealing with the media when necessary.

19. In what ways can death education assist students and teachers?

20. In what ways can a teacher assess his or her readiness to teach death education?

21. What precautionary steps should a teacher take before initiating a death education unit in his or her classroom?

# References

1. Berg, D. W., and G. G. Daughterty (1984). "Teaching About Death." In J. L. Thomas, ed. *Death and Dying in the Classroom: Readings for Reference*. Phoenix: Oryx Press.

2. Wass, H., and J. M. Stillion (1988). "Death in the Lives of Children and Adolescents." In H. Wass, F. M. Berardo, and R. A. Neimeyer, eds. *Dying: Facing the Facts*. Washington, DC: Hemisphere.

3. Butler, A. R. (1984). "Scratchy Is Dead." In J. L. Thomas, ed. *Death and Dying in the Classroom: Readings for Reference*. Phoenix: Oryx Press.

4. Bertoia, J., and J. Allan (1988). "School Management of the Bereaved Child." *Elementary School Guidance and Counseling*, 23: 30–39.

5. Brenner, A. (1984) *Helping Children Cope with Stress*. Lexington, MA: Lexington Books.

6. Bryant, E. H. (1984). "Teacher in Crisis: A Classmate Is Dying." In J. L. Thomas, ed. *Death and Dying in the Classroom: Readings for Reference*. Phoenix: Oryx Press.

7. Keith, C. R., and D. Ellis (1984). "Reactions of Pupils and Teachers to Death in the Classroom." In J. L. Thomas, ed. *Death and Dying in the Classroom: Readings for Reference*. Phoenix: Oryx Press.

8. Yarber, W. L. (1984). "Death Education: A Living Issue." In J. L. Thomas, ed. *Death and Dying in the Classroom: Readings for Reference*. Phoenix: Oryx Press.

9. Rosenthal, N. R. (1986). "Death Education: Developing a Course of Study for Adolescents." In C. A. Corr and J. N. McNeil, eds. *Adolescence and Death*. New York: Springer.

# Index